Age through Ethnic Lenses

Age through Ethnic Lenses

Caring for the Elderly in a Multicultural Society

EDITED BY LAURA KATZ OLSON

ROWMAN & LITTLEFIELD PUBLISHERS, INC.
Lanham • Boulder • New York • Toronto • Oxford

ROWMAN & LITTLEFIELD PUBLISHERS, INC.

Published in the United States of America
by Rowman & Littlefield Publishers, Inc.
A wholly owned subsidary of The Rowman & Littlefield Publishing Group, Inc.
4501 Forbes Boulevard, Suite 200, Lanham, Maryland 20706
www.rowmanlittlefield.com

PO Box 317
Oxford
OX2 9RU, UK

British Library Cataloguing in Publication Information Available

Library of Congress Cataloging-in-Publication Data

Age through ethnic lenses : caring for the elderly in a multicultural society / [edited by]
Laura Katz Olson
     p. cm.
   Includes bibliographical references and index.
   ISBN 0-7425-0113-2 (alk. paper). — ISBN 0-7425-0114-0 (pbk. : alk. paper)
   1. Minority aged—Government policy—United States. 2. Minority aged—Long-term
care—United States. 3. Aged—Government policy—United States. 4. Aged—long-term
care—United States. I. Olson, Laura Katz, 1945–

HQ 1064.U5 A63327 2001
305.26'0973—dc21   2001019089

Printed in the United States of America

∞™ The paper used in this publication meets the minimum requirements of American National Standard for Information Sciences—Permanence of Paper for Printed Library Materials, ANSI/NISO Z39.48–1992.

For George, Alix, Mom, and Anne,
the very special people in my life

Contents

Foreword

Every book represents the time in which it is conceived and produced. This is certainly true of the present volume. A book focusing on care for the ethnic elderly written one hundred years ago surely would have had many fewer groups represented in its individual chapters. The inclusion of Vietnamese, Chinese, and Haitian elderly, for example, would not have been deemed necessary since these groups were not recognized as major components of American society in 1900, or even in 1950. What the editor and her colleagues offer here for us, therefore, is a book of the new millennium in which the United States has clearly become a mosaic of diverse cultures and a country with major immigrant inflows. As comprehensive as this volume is, even it cannot represent all of the groups that are now shaping American society. These range from the other major Latino populations, such as Cubans and Salvadorans, and other Asian groups, including Cambodians, Hmong, and Indians, to the growing but underexplored subpopulations of Arab Americans. Each of these groups has its own exciting history and potential contribution to make to our thinking. This early in the twenty-first century it is hard to predict how all aspects of American culture, including attitudes and care provided to older persons, will be affected by these new, diverse ethnic cultures.

A book written in 1900 also would not have risked any focus on specific issues facing gay and lesbian elderly or perhaps even questioned the appropriateness of the role of women as caregivers. The inclusion of the chapters in part VII hopefully is an indication of our increasing openness to issues of diversity stemming not only from ethnic background but also from gender and sexual orientation.

As many of the authors and the editor point out, traditional practices are always under pressure to change. Patterns of family relationships that exist in countries such as Korea are transforming in the United States under the stresses and influences of American patterns of social and economic mobility. Health conditions also are changing because of the adoption of American eating and living practices. The emergence of these new cultural forms will be a major area of research for social scientists in coming years.

The types of relationships among groups that have long been represented in American society, such as Italians, Greeks, and Jews, also are altering. An awareness of the complexity and evolution of ethnic customs is important for service providers and policymakers because of the increasing numbers and proportions of older persons in each of the groups discussed in this book. Without an understanding of the emergent patterns of these divergent cultures, all of our best-intentioned efforts to ensure that all older persons maintain or improve their quality of life and health may go for naught, or even create problems.

As the new millennium progresses volumes similar to this one will update the ongoing changes and needs of older people from a variety of cultural perspectives. It will be exciting to see how these needs shift and what groups are represented in American society. At this time, we can only be grateful to Laura Katz Olson and her colleagues for their effort to increase our consciousness of the current requirements of each of these groups and possible programs and policies to meet them.

—Donald E. Gelfand

1

Multiculturalism and Long-Term Care: The Aged and Their Caregivers

Laura Katz Olson

Since the 1990s, the politics and policies of aging and long-term care have emerged as one of the more important issues in American society. Older people are disproportionately greater consumers of health care, social services, and related benefits of public programs, garnering about 40 percent of the federal budget (Binstock, 1999). And the number of elderly is growing rapidly, reaching over 34 million, or 12.8 percent of the population. In another thirty years, they will comprise 20 percent of the total, mostly due to the aging of 76 million baby boomers and the entrance of 2 million new immigrants (Senate, 1998b).

The fastest-growing sector of American society is those people aged eighty-five and over, a group that has increased fivefold since 1950 and will grow from nearly 4 million today to 8 million by 2030. Prolonged life spans into the extreme age groups generate large numbers of frail individuals, many of whom experience debilitating illnesses, chronic conditions, and/or functional impairments. At least half of people over the age of eighty-five require some help in performing their daily activities (Abel, 1991). For the vast majority, the need for care is ongoing.

Currently, about 7.3 million older people require assistance with personal care, chores, and/or their financial arrangements; this is projected to nearly double to almost 14 million over the next twenty years (GAO, 1999). Nearly 80 percent of functionally impaired elders live in the community, whether alone, with spouses or adult children, or in community-based settings such as assisted living facilities, boarding homes, or continuing care retirement communities. The rest, 1.5 million individuals, reside in nursing homes or other institutions (AARP, 2000).

Costs for elder care have been mounting rapidly, especially for nursing homes. By 1995, the federal government spent over $51 billion annually on long-term care, with $30 billion funded through Medicaid alone; fully 90 percent of the latter went to institutional facilities (Wiener and Stevenson, 1998). Medicaid currently pays for about half of all nursing home expenses. Although the program finances some home and community services, it is mostly for postacute skilled medical care. Only a very limited amount (through waivers, scattered demonstration projects, and small pilot programs) pays for personal assistance, household maintenance, or other support for day-to-day living. Moreover, stringent eligibility requirements limit aid only to those who are impoverished. At-home services under Medicare, which is short-term and also focused on skilled medical care, amounted to about $22.7 billion in 1995, or only about 9 percent of its outlays (Senate, 1998b). Consequently, publicly funded aid to help frail older people remain in their own homes is not widely available and certainly is inadequate relative to need. Nearly 40 percent of formal long-term-care costs are paid for by the elderly themselves or by their families (Kingson, 1996).

The politics and policies of long-term care are not easily addressed. Despite the attention devoted to the subject in recent years, there has been limited concern for, and understanding of, the differences among the elderly population. The diversity of the nation continues to increase, and while many groups become "Americanized," they often retain some distinct characteristics and face unique social, political, economic, and cultural problems. Importantly, the degree of incapacitation, vulnerability, and powerlessness created by the chronic conditions of old age is largely dependent on the social, cultural, economic, and political context in which the elderly function.

Although policymakers, gerontologists, and practitioners alike often give short shrift to the specific elder-care needs of various racial, ethnic and socioreligious groups, they will be forced increasingly to confront these concerns as we advance through the twenty-first century. Minority populations already represent slightly over 16 percent of the sixty-five-and-over population (U.S. Census, 1998). In 1998, older blacks, including individuals of African heritage as well as those from the Caribbean, represented 8.4 percent of the elderly. Latinos (people from Mexico, Puerto Rico, Cuba, and Central America) and Asian and Pacific Islanders represented another 5.2 percent and 2.4 percent, respectively. The percentage of elderly American Indians and Alaskan Natives, though small, also has grown more rapidly than the rest of the older population overall.

Immigration has had a significant impact on the growth in the number of racial/ethnic elders over the last several decades. Since 1965 there has been an influx of Latinos and Asians, consisting of those receiving new visas, refugees, and illegal aliens (Gelfand and Barresi, 1987a). Most Koreans in the United States have arrived since the 1970s, and many soon invited their elderly parents to join them, often to help maintain their households. The Japanese and Chinese, too, rapidly increased their numbers, with the Chinese population of the United States doubling between 1980 and 1990, mostly because of immigration. In contrast to the Japanese, the majority of Chinese are foreign born, including over 83.5 percent of its elderly population. In 1975, largely because of the Vietnam War, over one hundred thousand Vietnamese emigrated here; since that time their numbers have grown 600 percent. Puerto Ricans, Cubans, and especially Mexicans also have significantly increased both their overall and elderly populations.

In addition to immigration, major changes in the racial and ethnic distribution are due to higher fertility rates among some groups. Blacks and Latinos alone currently represent nearly 16 percent of the under-eighteen population and 12.5 percent and 11 percent, respectively, of individuals age eighteen to sixty-five (U.S. Census, 1998). Thus, though the number of elderly among certain groups is increasing, some of them, including Mexican Americans and Mormons, also will remain younger than the general population for some time. Others, such as Puerto Ricans, Cubans, and American Indians and Alaskan Natives, are experiencing aging within their own groups.

Over the next thirty years, minority populations are projected to become even larger, reaching 25 percent of the elderly by 2030 (U.S. Census, 1998). The number of older Latinos is expected to grow by 238 percent; blacks, 134 percent; Asian Americans, 354 percent; and American Indians and Alaskan Natives, 159 percent, as compared to only 79 percent for the white, non-Latino elderly (Williams and Temkin-Greener, 1996). Moreover, large numbers of Americans are first- and second-generation immigrants from Europe, and some of these ethnic groups have particularly large and growing numbers of older people. Even those who are native born and mostly Americanized, such as the Irish, Poles, Italians, and Greeks, retain distinctive characteristics that affect aging and long-term care.

Women overall (including lesbians) also will make up an increasing percentage of the elderly, especially among the oldest old. Nearly 72 percent of the rapidly growing eighty-five-and-over population currently is female: 2.2 million women versus 850,000 men. It is expected that by 2010 one-fifth of all older women will be over the age of eighty-five (Steckenrider, 1998; Hooyman, 1997).

The Goal of This Book

This volume seeks to delineate the diversity of approaches to long-term care among the various racial, ethnic, socioreligious, and other groups in the United States. The intent is to accomplish six interrelated purposes: (1) to explain the nature and extent of the disparate problems and special needs of these groups in caring for the functionally impaired elderly; (2) to discuss the different cultural values, attitudes, and behaviors related to long-term care options for older people and their informal caregivers; (3) to evaluate the social, political, and economic context in which elder-care decisions are made; (4) to examine the shared values, issues, and goals among the frail elderly and their caregivers in American society and the common forces affecting them; (5) where appropriate, to assess the social, economic, political, and cultural issues for younger and middle-aged people in their role as formal service workers (e.g., nurse's aides); and (6) to provide suggestions for changes both in policymaking and in program implementation (e.g., offer strategies that respect diversity and are more responsive to persistent cultural differences).

The book consists of twenty-one chapters, each focusing on a specific sub-group of older people and their families. The selections, which represent a broad spectrum of our elderly, include Asians, Latinos, individuals of European and African origins, Native Americans, socioreligious groups, women, gay men and lesbians, and people living in rural areas.

Each chapter considers such issues as gender roles; dependency, individualism, and interdependency; the extent of any community support networks; economic situation and class; intragroup inequalities; religion and the role of religious insti-tutions; migration experiences and stresses; status within the larger society, in-cluding degrees of oppression, discrimination, and cultural stereotyping; filial and other caregiver obligations/burdens, intergenerational accommodations, struggles, and challenges, and types of family ties; beliefs, barriers, and practices related to government aid, social welfare, and paid care in general, including nursing homes; special health concerns, disabilities, functional status, and mortality rates; attitudes toward old age, death, and disability; and other cultural practices, values, and is-sues—both positive and negative—that affect aging and long-term care. Also in-cluded is key demographic information about each group, including its legal and/or undocumented immigrant status, its relative or changing role in American society, and its use of various long-term care alternatives.

The ultimate goal of this book is to present a comprehensive overview of the complex problems facing our nation in coping with a growing but diverse frail, aging population. Our portrait focuses on two of the three major participants in long-term care: older people and their informal, unpaid caregivers. The intention is to broaden our perspective on the issues of elder care and provide a guide for future public policy in this area. Political leaders and policy analysts must learn to recognize, understand, and respect differences among older people, workers, and informal caregivers while addressing common problems and objectives.

In this introduction, I will weave together some of the highlights of the vari-ous chapters and discuss major themes that have emerged.

Demographics

While many racial, ethnic, socioreligious and other subgroups in American soci-ety are scattered throughout the United States, some are concentrated in certain parts of the nation, imposing particular challenges—and costs—for certain states and localities. For example, most Mexican Americans reside in the Southwest, primarily in California and Texas; Puerto Ricans immigrate mostly to New York City, while Cubans prefer South Florida. Most Haitians also live in New York City, though a few retirees who have attained middle-class status are leaving for Florida.

Slightly over half of all African American older people live in the South and only 9 percent in the West (U.S. Census, 1997). The majority of Japanese Amer-icans are found in Hawaii and California. The Chinese live largely in major cities on the West and East Coasts, with elderly immigrants congregating in China-towns. The Amish are clustered in Pennsylvania, Ohio, and Indiana and the Mormons in Utah. About half of American Indians are concentrated in Oklahoma, California, Arizona, New Mexico, and Texas; one fourth of the elderly live on reservations.

Older ethnic and minority groups also are more urbanized than the overall population. Latinos, Asians, and African Americans, along with individuals of European heritage such as Greeks (concentrated in New York City) and Poles (concentrated in New York City and Chicago), are overwhelmingly urban.

Socioeconomic Status, Health, and Long-Term Care

Elderly minorities, as a group, experience higher poverty rates than other older people. Only 8.2 percent of non-Latino whites age sixty-five and over live below the official poverty level, compared to 26.4 percent of blacks, 21 percent of Latinos, 12.4 percent of Asian and Pacific Islanders, and 20 percent of American Indians and Alaskan Natives (U.S. Census, 1998). Among Latinos, Mexican Americans and Puerto Ricans have the lowest incomes, with approximately half of their elderly living near or below the poverty level. Of Asians, Vietnamese Americans tend to be the most economically deprived; more than one-fourth are in poverty.

Because of their inadequate incomes, these groups tend to face other problems, including lower life expectancies, poorer health, and a greater number of functional disabilities than the more advantaged sectors of society, including certain European-origin whites and Asian Americans (Markides and Mindel, 1987; Kane, Kane and Ladd, 1998). Gannon (1999) points out that "there is considerable evidence documenting a strong influence of socioeconomic status on health, disability and mortality," an association that increases with age. Latino and black elders are more vulnerable to certain diseases and disabilities and "are more likely to be 'less healthy' and experience limitations in activity due to poor health" (Villa, 1998). In fact, the prevalence of chronic diseases among blacks is twice that among whites. Mexican Americans also have high levels of chronic illness and disability, requiring more informal aid and for longer periods than some other groups. For example, the rate of end-stage renal disease among Mexican Americans is six times, and of non-insulin-dependent diabetes two times, that among non-Latino whites (Du Bois, Yavno and Stanford, chapter 6). American Indians and Alaskan Natives are ten times more likely to have diabetes than are whites (Polacca, chapter 10).

Research shows that we cannot easily separate issues of race and ethnicity from those of socioeconomic status (Cool, 1987). Markides and Mindel (1987) argue that many ethnic-related differences and inequalities among the elderly persist despite considerable assimilation, mostly because of their subjugation in American society. They note that most Mexican Americans, whether immigrants or born here, have lived in economic and cultural isolation from the American mainstream. Many cannot read or write and considerable numbers cannot speak English. Throughout their lives they worked at economically marginal jobs and rarely were given the opportunity for upward economic mobility. Like Blacks, they have suffered much discrimination, prejudice and stereotyping.

American Indians and Alaska Natives, too, have suffered high unemployment, low-wage jobs, limited education, and high levels of illiteracy.

Barriers to Long-Term Care

Coupled with higher morbidity rates among low-income ethnic and minority elderly is their greater need for long-term care. Yet those groups with the most functional and chronic impairments tend to use the fewest formal services, relying heavily on their families instead (Markides and Mindel, 1987; Hooyman and Gonyea, 1995). Inadequate resources and cultural and religious barriers, along with exclusionary and discriminatory practices, have limited their access to private and public sources of assistance. Many needed services are not located within ethnic communities, are difficult to reach without adequate transportation, and are not sensitive to particular food preferences, distinctive lifestyles, or the traditions and beliefs of the elders they are supposed to serve. American Chinatowns, for example, sorely lack adequate health care and social services (Wong, chapter 2). American Indians and Alaskan Natives, who face considerable obstacles, have even less access to public programs than some other ethnic/minority groups (Polacca, chapter 10).

Illiteracy and an inability to speak English pose significant problems since few programs provide bilingual staff or translators. In fact, a lack of English may prevent some groups, such as older Haitians, from seeking American citizenship, rendering them ineligible for any government programs (Laguerre, chapter 9).

Moreover, while ethnic and minority older people have long-term care needs similar to those of the dominant sectors of society, they may experience them differently. As Barresi (1987) puts it, cultural precepts can shape the life course and one's perception of it, including how old age and its vulnerabilities are viewed. For most people, old age inevitably entails frailty and reliance on others for assistance, conditions that are at variance with the American values of individualism and self-sufficiency. In addition, the specific meaning and significance of terms such as dependency, autonomy, and community depend on ethnicity, race, and other group identities. There also is significant cultural variation in ways of thinking about other issues related to old age, including notions about health, illness, medicine, death and dying, and physical prowess, which also can affect elder care.

Regardless of background, families are the primary providers of assistance to functionally disabled older people in the United States. However, for some racial and ethnic groups, because of barriers to paid care as well as cultural and/or religious mandates, adult children may have even greater responsibility for their parents than in other sectors of society. And, though most older people—even those with functional limitations—reside in their own homes, certain cultures expect or encourage frail elders to move in with their kin, rendering multigenerational households more common among them.

Divergent Attitudes and Values

Attitudes also vary toward social welfare, needs-determined public aid, and paid care itself. While many overburdened families turn to publicly supported services when they are available, some groups are reluctant to do so. These elderly place inordinate stress on their informal caregivers or even forgo help entirely (Harel, McKinney and Williams, 1987). Sometimes frail older people who are averse to paid help are more willing to receive aid from racial/ethnic/religious organizations in their community. However, as Harel, McKinney and Williams (1987) observe, the vast majority of these support networks cannot provide sufficient expertise, resources, or services for everyone, especially as needs continue to grow.

For groups that stress collectivism, interdependence, and close family ties, dependency of frail elderly parents is an expected and accepted phase of the life cycle. The lifelong socialization of Italians, which emphasizes family over individual interests, creates strong bonds within the extended family and a high status for older kin. These values are translated into an extensive support system for frail elders (Johnson, chapter 17).

Greek Americans, too, have a familistic/collectivist orientation; their sense of self is tied to the family. Both filial piety and respect for elders encourage a high level of obligation and support for older parents. They are more likely than some other groups to have multigenerational households, although older Greek Americans prefer to live independently if possible. A few Greek elders obtain help from the American Hellenic Educational Progressive Association, which provides limited senior housing, including a nursing home (Constantakos, chapter 18).

Among Asian Americans, dependency also is viewed in a more positive light than in the general American culture. They tend to have long traditions of interdependence, which is viewed as basic to the human condition, and filial piety tends to govern relationships between the generations. However, in the United States such relationships may become strained in multigenerational households.

The Japanese are subject to Confucian ethics, which includes obeying parents, upholding obligations to one's kin, and not bringing shame to the family. Respect for parents and ancestors is reinforced by Shintoism, which maintains that elderly parents become spirits at death and protect the family system. A significant number of single older women (generally foreign-born) live with their adult children. According to Japanese culture, elders must passively accept any assistance they receive and feel obliged to the caregiver unless they can reciprocate in some way, a particularly troublesome issue for frail Japanese American older women without resources of their own.

Japanese American elders tend to live on their own. While they would rather not use formal services, there is some indication that increasing numbers are willing to do so rather than impose on their children or jeopardize their close relationship by becoming dependent on them. Most Japanese communities provide some services, such as congregate meal programs and recreational activities, and a few, such as Little Tokyo, even have a nursing home or residential facilities (Shibusawa, Lubben and Kitano, chapter 3).

The Chinese, whose filial piety also has its roots in Confucianism, have a long tradition of interdependence and high status for the aged. According to their concept of loss of face, the family is viewed as more important than the individual, and any dishonor brought on oneself will shame all family members. Together, these values promote self-sacrifice, devotion, and care of elderly parents—according to prescribed roles based on gender, age, and birth order—without question or resentment. Though maintaining separate residences is becoming the norm, it can be a source of embarrassment both for the aged parents and their adult children (Wong, chapter 2).

According to the contemporary Vietnamese family code, all children are expected to care for their frail elders on a rotating basis. While most older Vietnamese Americans do not want to burden their children and would choose to live on their own, the reality is that most are forced by economic necessity into multigenerational households (Tran, Ngo and Sung, chapter 5).

Under traditional Korean custom, the main family relationship is between parents and their eldest son. As with other Asian families, Korean immigrants expect to live with them and be taken care of by their daughters-in-law. However, growing numbers of Korean immigrant elders, who live with their adult children when first coming to the United States, eventually move out, preferring their autonomy to the myriad difficulties they encounter in the homes of their Americanized families (Kim and Kim, chapter 4).

Some Asian American immigrants seem to resist any move to the suburbs with their adult children, preferring to live independently in ethnic enclaves, relying on government services. A large number of Korean elders, for instance, prefer to live in government-subsidized senior housing rather than depart from central cities with their adult children (Kim and Kim, chapter 4). Similarly, many Chinese immigrants choose to live alone in Chinatown rather than leave familiar surroundings (Wong, chapter 2).

Latinos tend to deemphasize individual problem solving, viewing the needs of the family as a whole as taking precedence over individual wants. *Familismo* is important to Mexican Americans and Puerto Ricans, both of whom have strong identifications with immediate family and extended kin. For example, interdependence between and among generations and communalism are basic to Puerto Rican culture, with a strong emphasis on filial responsibility; however, other relatives can be counted on in times of need, as can "fictive kin"—adopted or special friends—in their large, informal network. Latinos are more likely than non-Latino whites to live in multigenerational settings, though that may be due to financial need as much as to any cultural imperative (Sanchez, chapter 7).

Despite a serious underutilization of formal services by Mexican Americans, they are not particularly averse to using some paid care and will do so when structural barriers are reduced. Among Latinos, they have a particularly difficult time attaining legal residency or citizenship, rendering many of them ineligible for public aid. For Latinos generally, the informal family network tends to serve as a liaison between elders and service providers, facilitating their access to government assistance (Du Bois, Yavno and Stanford, chapter 6).

Older African Americans, who tend to have close, large extended families, often seek care across households, fostering a collectivist (two or more caregivers) approach to elder care. The aged, of whom a large percentage live in multigenerational households, are held in high esteem. In addition, the black church traditionally has served as a support system for African American elders and their families, including the provision of some health-based interventions and social programs. Because of high levels of spirituality among African American families, the church also contributes to their feelings of well-being. However, because of competing and growing needs among children, teens, and young single mothers, especially in urban areas, emphasis on, and help for, frail older people and their caregivers is limited (Dilworth-Anderson, chapter 8).

American Indians and Alaska Natives elders, who are still a highly respected sector of the community, also receive the vast majority of care from relatives. In fact, they are four times more likely than their white cohorts to live in multigenerational households, particularly on reservations. They tend to value cooperation and exchange and are guided by a need to maintain harmony and balance among the individual, other people, nature, and the spiritual world (Polacca, chapter 10).

Arab Americans stress mutual assistance, but they expand the concept of kin to include "aunts" and "uncles" who are not blood relatives. Their ethic of filial piety, which encompasses respect for, and duty toward, elders, is buttressed by religious law, chiefly through the Quran. A large percentage of Arab American older people, especially widows, live in multigenerational households, and they are particularly unwilling to accept paid care. However, elders receive some assistance through their religious and social organizations, including the Arab American Council and the Chaldean Council (Fakhouri, chapter 14).

The Amish stand in even starker contrast to the American concept of individualism: not only do they encourage reciprocal family assistance but the entire Amish community is responsible for helping each other, including elders. This concept of mutual aid is based both on religious belief and on historical tradition. The Amish view that illness related to aging is a natural part of life allows them to accept help easily. Though older parents live in a separate dwelling (the Grossdaadi Haus), generally on the family farm, for the Amish the true meaning of independence is a separation from the world, especially government (Zook, chapter 12).

In traditional Polish society, reciprocity governed family relationships; care of vulnerable parents was assumed to be normal and natural. If elders had to turn to government assistance, there would be a sense of shame for themselves and their families. Since many Polish American children do not feel an obligation to provide hands-on care for their older parents–or do so reluctantly–disabled elders often forgo help entirely rather than face the embarrassment of seeking it elsewhere (Berdes and Erdmans, chapter 15).

Some groups, such as the Irish, are reluctant to express or even acknowledge dependency needs. The culture emphasizes independence and self-reliance, which is important for self-esteem, thus encouraging older Irish Americans to make it on their own. When adult children do provide care, it can be particularly stressful for both parties. Moreover, because the Irish define good health as being able to perform physical labor, older Irish Americans fear disability and sickness more than some other groups. When they can no longer care for themselves, the Irish elderly often view formal assistance as a viable and attractive alternative to family care. The Irish also tend to be intricately tied to the Catholic Church and receive some help from their parishes (Fanning, chapter 16).

Mormons, too, stress self-reliance as fundamental to their church doctrine; members must be industrious, defer immediate gratification, and prepare to take care of themselves and their families on their own. Family ties and obligations are strengthened both by cultural/religious expectations and by low levels of geographic mobility. In addition, Mormon culture provides a particularly positive approach to health, with a focus on preventive care throughout the life cycle. The Word of Wisdom forbids the use of coffee, tea, alcohol, and tobacco and encourages health foods. Elders are advised to keep up their physical fitness and activity, including service to others, contributing to their high level of health and long life expectancy as well as fewer disabilities among their elderly and briefer periods of illness than other groups.

Mormons eschew any government aid, viewing it as undermining independence and the work ethic. Instead, they provide assistance for the needy, regardless of age, through an extensive church welfare program. However, help is available only after all personal and family resources are exhausted. Moreover, their community support system requires some work in exchange, even for older people, and supplies only temporary relief (Campbell, chapter 11).

Other racial/ethnic/socioreligious groups are less reluctant to secure paid services, especially among better-off families. Instead of hands-on family care, they prefer to focus on emotional bonds and let professionals take care of one's physical needs (Dwyer and Coward, 1992). American Jewish families, for example, tend to use more outside assistance than some other groups, possibly because of high levels of mobility among adult children and elders alike. Moreover, with their strong tradition of charity *(Zedakah)* and the commandment to "honor thy father and mother," a variety of Jewish agencies and federations—relying on some government funds—provide housing, services, community centers, and nursing homes for many (but not all) Jewish elders in need (Harel, chapter 13).

The rural elderly, who tend to be poorer and less educated than their urban counterparts and have more functional impairments, also have limited access to health and social services. They experience problems with transportation, a deficiency of services and service providers, and greater costs to deliver care. Moreover, their adult children tend to move away, leaving them with fewer kin to provide care for them (Scott, chapter 21).

While lesbian and gay elders are not an economically deprived group overall, they often suffer compromised health care, medical neglect, or fewer available social services because of homophobia and discrimination. Although gay men and lesbians have formed a large number of community groups to meet their health and service needs, these organizations tend to focus on younger people and their social, political, and health needs. More recently, groups such as Rainbow Gardens and Senior Action in a Gay Environment (SAGE) have been developing informal housing networks and retirement and assisted living complexes, along with information and referral services, transportation management, and other support for elders in some larger metropolitan areas, particularly for the middle class (Claes and Moore, chapter 19).

Institutional Care

Most Americans view nursing homes as a last resort; however, certain racial/ethnic/socioreligious groups, including African Americans, Latinos, and Native Americans, have particularly low levels of institutionalization. For many of them, placement in a nursing home is tantamount to abandonment. While these groups may have an aversion to these facilities and "choose" to provide care at home, we must be careful to differentiate between cultural imperatives and structural factors. As suggested earlier, discrimination as well as a paucity of facilities in specific communities, language problems, financial constraints, and other barriers may restrict access considerably.

Some groups increasingly are accepting nursing home placement when families have no other viable option, especially for elders experiencing dementia. More Arab and Jewish Americans, Asians, and European ethnic older people have been willing, albeit reluctantly, to move into a nursing home when they can no longer take care of themselves. Others, such as the Amish, eschew institutional care entirely.

While isolation and mistreatment of elderly residents are common in nursing homes, some sectors of society are particularly vulnerable. For example, groups with a large number of non-English-speaking aged, such as the Chinese, Haitians, and American Indians, may feel especially threatened and isolated. Some families live far from their institutionalized elders, limiting visits from relatives and friends substantially. Lesbian and gay elders, many of whom have remained in the closet, often feel alienated; others face physical and emotional abuse because of their sexual orientation.

Impact of "Americanization"

Many students of ethnicity point to the evolving nature of cultural values, attitudes, and practices as racial and immigrant groups encounter the dominant American society and its views. Gelfand and Barresi (1987a) call it the "emergent" nature of ethnicity. Traditional ethnic culture can become "Americanized," with results that sometimes bear little resemblance to the practices of either the home country or the United States. Parents and their adult children may increasingly diverge as the former hold on to some older traditions that are abandoned by their offspring. Further, given the nature of American society today, many adult children may be incapable of meeting ethnic expectations. As Markides and Mindel (1987: 120) conclude, "Change is a feature in present-day American life that constantly affects the interplay of traditional cultural values and patterns with the demands of modern life." For example, Greek filial obligation appears to be more conditional in recent decades, depending on situational factors such as whether children can afford to take care of their parents (Constantakos, chapter 18). Because of changes in women's roles in this country, including their increasing participation in the workplace, at-home care for elders is more difficult to provide for all groups.

Korean women's economic participation in the household has dramatically affected cultural mandates. Since most Korean American wives contribute equally to the family finances, it is difficult to maintain the patriarchal family structure or the primacy of parents over wives, thereby modifying many aspects of filial piety. For many of these working women, only limited time, energy, and resources are available for elder care (Kim and Kim, chapter 4).

High rates of intermarriage, affecting such groups as Japanese and Polish Americans, may seriously erode traditional expectations of care. However, despite a significant level of intermarriage among Italians, resulting in less traditional behavior patterns overall, parent–adult child ties and obligations appear to be relatively resistant to change (Johnson, chapter 17).

Immigration itself can cause a change in cultural values that depend on reciprocity. Many immigrants lose their income, assets, position, authority, and reputation when they leave their homeland, especially when they do so at older ages. For instance, in traditional culture, older Haitians are respected by their children and sought after for advice, wisdom, and folk medical knowledge. However, Haitian immigrant elders, who often are forced to leave everything behind, have little to offer their adult children in exchange for their care. Consequently, though they tend to live in multigenerational households in the United States, their children refuse to submit to their authority and control as they would have in Haiti (Laguerre, chapter 9). Moreover, groups with a high percentage of immigrants, such as the Chinese, face a greater risk of depression and other forms of mental illness because of the stresses of immigration and acculturation (Wong, chapter 2).

Other Stressful Experiences

Some elderly and their families face issues tied to their particular culture, religion, experiences, and/or outsider status. The problems of vulnerable Jewish elders who are Holocaust survivors, for instance, are compounded by their past traumas, particularly for those forced into nursing homes (Harel, chapter 13). Institutionalization also can be particularly stressful for American Indians and Alaska Natives who were forcibly placed into government educational facilities during their youth (Polacca, chapter 10). The internment of people with Japanese ancestry during World War II has had lingering effects on Japanese elders, including a mistrust of the U.S. government (Shibusawa, Lubben and Kitano, chapter 3). Extensive periods of revolution and war destroyed much of the traditional fabric of Vietnamese society and its family structure and forced many people, including elders, to leave the country, often without sufficient means (Tran, Ngo and Sung, chapter 5).

Lesbians, gay men, and bisexuals face homophobia, discrimination, and the devastating impact of AIDS, which can lead to earlier and longer caretaker roles, loneliness due to death of a significant other and numerous friends, and loss of one's own independence at an early age. They also have difficulties negotiating a long-term care system that denies same-sex partners the rights and privileges accorded to spouses (Claes and Moore, chapter 19).

Intragroup Differences

There also are significant differences within the groups themselves. Even among better-off sectors of society, foreign-born aged tend to have fewer financial resources than those born in this country. They often are not eligible for Social Security and become dependent on means-tested government aid such as Supplemental Security Income, food stamps, and public housing and/or on their adult children. Noncitizens receive no public assistance or social services.

Intragroup variations occur between current immigrants and those coming to this country in earlier periods. They tend to have different migration experiences, stresses, geographic locations, and socioeconomic status. Each of the several waves of Polish immigration, for example, involved people with different levels of education, status, and income (Berdes and Erdmans, chapter 15). Many Asian immigrants arriving recently in the United States are vulnerable and economically dependent. However, a large number of families who have lived here for several years have attained middle-class status.

Some groups, such as African Americans, can be divided along urban and rural lines as well (Dilworth-Anderson, chapter 8). American Jews are split between religiously affiliated and unaffiliated elders as well as by national origins. Jewish subgroups with the greatest need, such as unaffiliated Soviet immigrants, have the least access to services (Harel, chapter 13). Similarly, Arab Americans have emigrated from various Middle Eastern countries, each with different languages, religious affiliations, and other characteristics (Fakhouri, chapter 14).

Women, Race, and Ethnicity

Gender poses a particular challenge for analysts and policymakers of long-term care. Among other factors, older women tend to live to more advanced ages, have more chronic illnesses and disabilities, and experience greater poverty than older men. They disproportionately live alone or in nursing homes. However, age-related problems faced by women tend to be compounded by those associated with race, ethnicity, and socioreligious identity. For example, the material conditions of racism are experienced most dramatically by women of color throughout their life cycle. Latinas, too, encounter, more obstacles as they age and shoulder more elder-care burdens than those who are white (Katz Olson, chapter 20).

Compared both to men of similar backgrounds and to women from the dominant culture, older ethnic females, especially immigrants, suffer from greater poverty, illiteracy, lack of English, transportation problems, and other barriers to private and public assistance. They tend to be more isolated and lonely as well.

Although we must respect diversity and devise government programs that are more responsive to racial and cultural needs, we also should be aware that certain norms, behaviors, and policies affect the well-being of women and men in divergent ways. Though ethnicity can provide positive means for dealing with aging (Gelfand and Barresi, 1987a), in some cultures strict patriarchal structures seriously limit females' options and opportunities throughout their life cycle, including old age.

As suggested throughout this book, nearly all cultural mandates for filial piety and elder care translate into women's work, whether for wives, daughters, or daughters-in-law. With rising longevity, these females may have several generations and large numbers of kin to care for. They also tend to have only limited resources themselves. Many of them, out of necessity, now participate in the paid labor force, often in low-wage, mostly exhausting jobs that do not offer flexible hours. Therefore, even as we strive to keep cultural values intact, we must bear in mind that, for a large percentage of ethnic women and women of color, elder care entails particularly burdensome financial, physical, social, and psychological costs.

Moreover, there are serious workforce issues that inevitably, and shortly, will arise as growing numbers of vulnerable older people require paid assistance. Staff shortages are prevalent, especially in rural areas, and are expected to grow dramatically. Nursing home and in-home service jobs are emotionally and physically demanding, tend to be low paid, and offer few benefits. More and more, front-line employees—mostly women—are younger and middle-aged documented and undocumented immigrants, with cultural, economic, and social issues of their own.

Latinas, particularly Mexicans, tend to be overrepresented in these job categories, as are Haitians and other immigrants of color. These aides sometimes work two shifts, live in dire economic circumstances, and often have responsibilities for their own kin, whether children or elderly parents. Their caregiving labor is exploited not only by nursing homes and home health agencies but also by the better-off, mostly white families in American society. As Chang (2000) observes, "Perhaps the real issue is that privileged women of the First World, even self-avowed feminists, may be some of the primary consumers and beneficiaries of this trade."

Nursing home assistants and their mostly white clients also tend to target each other. Nursing assistants are subject to difficult patients who sometimes inflict racial slurs and physical violence on them. However, a large number of patients suffer from neglect, mistreatment, and a general disregard of their needs by the aides. Insufficient staffing, lax hiring practices, low wages, and rigid, harsh, and strenuous working conditions have contributed substantially to such abusive behavior (Katz Olson, chapter 20). As Foner (1994) notes, the racial and ethnic differences "feed into and intensify, rather than create, divisions between groups in nursing homes."

Among other changes, nursing homes, home care agencies, and political leaders must address the problems faced by overworked and underpaid staff along with those of residents. And they also have to provide for the diverse religious and cultural needs of both groups.

Conclusion and Policy Implications

Faced with rapidly growing expenditures on care for an expanding vulnerable and disabled population, policymakers and analysts have been experimenting with alternatives to institutional care and searching for more efficient, cost-effective ways of delivering services. The national government also has increasingly shifted responsibility—and expenses—to the states. Formal long-term services for older people now account for slightly over 11 percent of state budgets. Political leaders at all levels of government also are cutting funding drastically for publicly supported services overall, including those for the aged. Consequently, as the number of disadvantaged ethnic and racial elderly is increasing and their needs are growing, resources to care for them are declining.

The chapters in this volume show the likely negative impact of these changes on Americans of diverse ethnic and racial backgrounds. They suggest, for example, that any efforts to cut government costs for the aged will impose greater burdens on families. Despite different cultures and attitudes among groups, spouses and children continue to provide most of the care. Reduced public aid further limits any meaningful choices such individuals have when faced with ailing spouses and parents. At the same time, there appears to be a growing disinclination among elders of diverse backgrounds to live in multigenerational households. Indeed, the

Americanization of younger generations can produce different expectations—and clashes—between elderly immigrants and their adult children. In addition, the former tend to be reluctant to move to the suburbs with their children, preferring the familiarity of their ethnic neighborhoods.

It has long been recognized that frail elders, whether at home or in an institution, value "emotional work" at least as much as help with the physical aspects of their care (Foner, 1994). As this volume makes clear, one undervalued component of this affective role has been respect for the traditions and culture that often are an essential part of an older person's life. Culturally sensitive care contributes to the well-being of older people, enhancing both their self-respect and the quality of their lives. For nursing home residents, in particular, it provides a sense of continuity, allowing them to keep a piece of their identity intact (Gelfand and Barresi, 1987a). When we ignore their racial/ethnic/socioreligious backgrounds, we treat our vulnerable elders as objects.

Certain groups tend to be underrepresented in the limited government programs providing old-age assistance. Substantial barriers prevent many of these groups from obtaining whatever aid may be available. As suggested in this work, some racial/ethnic subgroups of elderly are particularly isolated and underserved because of concerns about their undocumented status, shame that their family is not providing care, unrealistic expectations from the larger community about the availability of family assistance, and language problems.

Virtually all of the authors in this volume conclude that, as a minimum, if we want to meet the needs of our minority/ethnic elders, services must be provided in specific languages (and sometimes several dialects), more low-cost housing and long-term services should be available in minority/ethnic communities, and staff should be trained in the culturally appropriate values and customs of the people they serve. Social workers and others also must engage in aggressive outreach, targeted to isolated elders who may lack information and be apprehensive about government programs generally.

Though retrenchment policies imply an unwillingness to fund any new, specialized services, the need for such assistance is obviously growing. Clearly, American society requires more, not less, social responsibility for dependent elders, including affordable housing alternatives and publicly funded services to help with personal care, day-to-day living, and household chores. Without such programs, minority and ethnic elders and their families will face increasing hardship and isolation along with decreased levels of care.

2

The Chinese Elderly:
Values and Issues in Receiving Adequate Care

Morrison G. Wong

"With their strong, traditional values about the sanctity of the family and the revered position of the elderly, the Chinese elderly do not have any problems." "Filial piety, a value instilled in the Chinese child since birth, virtually assures that the needs of the elderly Chinese parents will be taken care of during their golden years." These are just a few of the common conceptions regarding the Chinese and the Chinese elderly. How accurate are these statements when compared with the realities of the Chinese experience in the United States?

There are many misperceptions and much misinformation regarding the Chinese elderly. Explanations abound as to why this is the case. It has been argued that because of their high socioeconomic status, the Chinese in the United States do not suffer from, or else have overcome, the social and structural barriers that affect other racial or ethnic minorities. This view of them as a model minority may lead some to believe that the Chinese and Chinese elderly do not have any problems. There are those who place great emphasis on the differences in cultural values, arguing that belief in the traditional Confucian ethic and its emphasis on strong family responsibilities and obligations such as filial piety still permeate and guide the lives of the Chinese family in this country. Finally, these stereotypes and misconceptions may be perpetuated by the dearth of empirical research on elderly Chinese.

The paucity of literature may be due largely to two factors. First, the Chinese constitute only a small proportion of the total U.S. population. In 1990, there were 1.65 million Chinese residing here. Although this represents a 103 percent increase from 1980 (U.S. Census, 1988, 1993a), they make up less than half of 1 percent of the total U.S. population. The vast majority of these Chinese are foreign born. Barring any major immigration reform, this number is expected to continue to increase. Second, the Chinese population tends to be concentrated in major cities on the West and East Coasts. Hence, their particular situation and the problems the elderly Chinese face usually draw only local attention (if that) and very little national concern.

This chapter will shed some light on the elderly Chinese population in the United States. It will (1) discuss the role of immigration in the formation of the elderly Chinese population; (2) present selected characteristics of the Chinese elderly population; (3) look at traditional Chinese values as they relate to older people and the aging process; (4) analyze some of the barriers that prevent the Chinese elderly from receiving adequate care; and (5) make some recommendations for improving their situation.

Chinese Immigration to the United States

The history of the Chinese in the United States entails a discussion of American immigration laws and policies since these have considerably affected the social and demographic characteristics and adjustments of the Chinese in this country. The Chinese were the first Asian group to immigrate to the United States in significant numbers. Although there had been Chinese in this country as early as the 1780s, the large influx did not begin until 1850. The discovery of gold in California was a major impetus for this massive inflow. The Chinese initially were well received, though they were often viewed as objects of curiosity. Providing supplementary labor rather than competing with members of the dominant group, the Chinese elicited few or no objections to their presence. However, they eventually gravitated toward the gold fields to make their fortune. It is here that one notes the beginning of anti-Chinese sentiment. By 1852, antagonism against the Chinese was well established.

From 1851 to 1860, 61,397 Chinese immigrated to the United States, while another 64,301 arrived during the next decade. Almost all were adult males. The frenzy of anti-Chinese agitation in the 1870s coincided with the peak of Chinese immigration when 123,201 Chinese came here. Despite these high rates, many Chinese did not stay, and their total population never exceeded 106,000.

Up until 1882, Chinese immigration increased continually and dramatically. After several decades of anti-Chinese agitation, inspired by real or imagined competition with white workers along with racist propaganda (Sandmeyer, 1973; Saxton, 1971), Congress passed the Chinese Exclusion Act of 1882, the first immigration act to specifically prohibit a nationality group from entering the United States. This law barred both skilled and unskilled Chinese laborers for ten years. It also prohibited the naturalization of the Chinese. After its passage and the enactment of subsequent exclusionary acts, Chinese immigration declined precipitously until sometime in the 1920s. For the next six decades, the Chinese population not only failed to grow but actually declined (Wong and Hirschman, 1983).

In 1921, Congress enacted legislation denying to an alien-born woman her husband's citizenship. Such restrictive changes imposed tragic hardships on American-born Chinese males. Because of the unbalanced sex ratio and antimiscegenation laws in the United States, they had been forced to seek wives in China. As aliens ineligible for citizenship, the wives could not immigrate to the United States. Another barrier was the discriminatory features of the Immigration Act of 1924, which made it impossible for American citizens of Chinese ancestry to send for their wives and families (Chen, 1984: 44; Chinn, Lai and Choy, 1969: 24; Sung, 1971: 77–81).

Significant demographic changes in the Chinese population began in the 1920s and 1930s. The long population decline that was triggered by the passage of the Chinese Exclusion Act had ended, and a small upturn due to natural increases and ingenuity in evading immigration regulations had set in. Even more significant was that by 1940 native-born Chinese Americans for the first time outnumbered the alien segment of their community. Nearly 20,000 Chinese American babies were born over the next decade. For the first time in history, the most numerous five-year cohort of Chinese Americans was persons under five years of age (Kitano and Daniels, 1988: 37).

On December 13, 1943, President Roosevelt signed the Magnuson Act repealing the Chinese Exclusion Act of 1882 and making Chinese immigrants, many of whom had been living in the United States for decades, eligible for citizenship. A token quota of 105 persons per year was set for Chinese immigration. Although small, the quota did open the door to further immigration.

In 1952, the Immigration and Naturalization Act, also known as the McCarran-Walter Act, was passed, eliminating race as a bar to immigration and giving preferences to relatives (Chen, 1980: 211–13; Lee, 1956; Li, 1977). This act, which was more of a rationalization of existing immigration policy than a reform, continued the token quota of 105 Chinese immigrants per year (Wong and Hirschman, 1983).

In the mid-1950s, more than half of the Chinese American population was native-born, and this segment of the population, reinforced by stranded students from China, was becoming increasingly middle class. Its members increasingly disassociated themselves from the concerns of the American Chinatowns and strove for acculturation into American society (Lyman, 1974: 119–57).

The reforms of the 1965 Immigration Act had important consequences for the Chinese community in the United States as well as American society at large. Perhaps the most significant result was the dramatic increase in the number of Chinese immigrants to the United States (Wong and Hirschman, 1983). By 1980, the majority of the Chinese population in the United States was foreign born.

A second outcome was its influence on the family life of the Chinese in America. With its emphasis on family reunification, this act granted each country a quota of 20,000 immigrants annually. During the 1970s, approximately 22,000 Chinese immigrated to the United States each year. Unlike the pre-1965 immigrants who came over as individuals, most of the new Chinese immigrants came over as family groups—typically husband, wife, and unmarried children (Hong, 1976). A family-chain pattern of migration developed (Glenn, 1983; Li, 1977; Sung, 1977; Wong and Hirschman, 1983).

From 1980 to 1990, the Chinese population in the United States doubled from 812,000 to 1,645,000, maintaining its distinction as the largest Asian group in the United States. About 53 percent (444,962) of this increase was due to immigration. During the 1980s, approximately 44,500 Chinese immigrants entered the United States each year. More recently, between 1991 and 1997, the average annual rate increased to 56,472 people (U.S. Dept. of Justice, 1999). A significant impact of immigration policy is that currently about 70 percent of the Chinese population are first-generation immigrants, most arriving after 1965. Consequently, a vast majority of the elderly Chinese population is foreign-born.

Characteristics of the Chinese Elderly Population

What are the social and economic characteristics of the elderly Chinese in the United States? What is the nature of their Social Security benefits? What sort of residential patterns do they exhibit? How do they differ from the general population, and what are the implications of these differences?

Because of their small population size, data on the social and economic characteristics of the Chinese in the United States are hard to ascertain. The only current data file with a large enough sample of Chinese for empirical analysis is the 1990 U.S. census. Case studies, although dated and less generalizable, provide additional sources. The following observations regarding the social and economic characteristics of the Chinese population have been based on these resources.

Education

The Chinese as a whole are better educated than the general population (Wong, 1994). This is also true for the elderly Chinese male population: in 1980 proportionally more Chinese older men (18.5 percent) than those who are white (10.5 percent) had completed four or more years of college. However, only 6.8 percent of elderly Chinese females have achieved such educational attainments, slightly less than the rate for white females. Moreover, a greater proportion of aged Chinese males and females (about 15 percent and 35 percent, respectively) than whites (1.5 percent each) had no education (Yu, 1986).

Social Security Income

Miah and Kahler (1997) and O'Hare and Felt (1991) found that the elderly Chinese were much less likely to receive Social Security benefits than whites. Only 64 percent of the Chinese elderly received these pensions in 1989 as compared to 92 percent of non-Hispanic whites. In addition, the average Social Security benefit for the elderly Chinese ($6,291 per year) was less than that of the white population.

As noted, immigration has had major implications for the Chinese elderly population. Because nearly 83.5 percent of Chinese Americans sixty-five years and older in 1990 were foreign-born, they had minimal or no Social Security retirement benefits. Moreover, pension amounts varied considerably between the foreign-born and American Chinese elderly population: the latter were receiving about $1,200 more than the former (about $7,200 compared to $5,965).

Residence

Owing to the increase in immigration, the population of Chinatowns has grown throughout the United States. It was once postulated that the restrictive immigration policies that prohibited the Chinese from entering this country would result in the rapid disappearance of these places (Lee, 1956). However, within the past three decades, we have seen a resurgence in their vitality and functionality everywhere in the nation. Many Chinese immigrants, especially the elderly, are taking up residence in Chinatowns. During the 1960s and 1970s, the aged residents of central locations in Chinatowns increased by 45 percent, the districts just outside the core by 34 percent, and the extended areas by 17 percent (Carp and Kataoka, 1976). Such trends continued throughout the 1980s and 1990s.

The concentration of the Chinese elderly in Chinatowns has implications for their adjustment and acculturation. Because of their lack of facility with the English language, their strong ethnic identity, and their fear of the unfamiliar in the non-Chinese environment, many older Chinese immigrants prefer staying in Chinatown where they can speak and communicate with others in their own language, eat food that is much more agreeable to their palates, and consult with familiar herbalists or Chinese doctors in times of need. Such isolation hinders the acculturation process. Moreover, many of the elderly who immigrate to the United States would prefer to live in China. Ikels (1983a) found that their decision to migrate usually is based on the traditional value that children should take care of their older parents.

However, because of the differences in culture and the economic demands placed on the family in the United States, multigenerational households are atypical, and separate residences for elderly Chinese parents are rapidly becoming the norm (Ikels, 1983a; Chen, 1979; Cheung, 1989; Lum et al., 1980; Wong, 1998). Although many of the elderly remain in Chinatown where their social needs can be more easily met, their second- and third-generation American-born children have left the central cities for the suburbs. In essence, a modified extended family exists among the Chinese, where the children still remain in the general vicinity of the parents but in separate households. Some of these children may feel less obligated to take care of their elderly parents as tradition would dictate (Cheung et al., 1980), and others may wish to divorce themselves from the patriarchal influence of their parents in their own family decisions and practices (Chen, 1979; Cheung, 1989).

Table 2.1 Age Distribution for the Elderly Chinese Population in the United States by Nativity Status: 1990

	Total	Native-Born	Foreign-Born
Total	1,646,696	506,116	1,142,580
65–74 Years	86,889	14,934	71,965
75–84 Years	36,358	5,401	30,957
85+ Years	8,515	1,420	7,095
Total 65+ Years	131,772	21,755	110,017
Percent 65+ Years	8.0	4.3	9.6
Median Age	32.3	16.3	36.7
Female	827,164	245,539	581,615
65–74 Years	45,181	7,408	37,773
75–84 Years	20,146	2,824	17,322
85+ Years	5,255	856	4,399
Total 65+ Years	75,582	11,088	49,494
Percent 65+ Years	8.4	4.5	10.2
Female Median Age	32.9	16.4	37.1
Male Median Age	31.7	16.1	36.2

Source: U.S. Census, 1993b.

Age Distribution

In 1990, about 8 percent of the Chinese population were sixty-five years of age and over. The foreign-born Chinese population is much more likely to be elderly than its native-born counterpart and is older as well. For each age category, the proportion of foreign-born elderly Chinese was at least twice as large as the native-born. Similarly, the proportion of females was greater than that of males (see table 2.1).

Health Characteristics and Disability Status

The Chinese appear to be relatively healthier than white Americans, at least as measured by the death rate. In 1980, the age-adjusted death rate for the Chinese was 3.5 per 1,000 resident population compared to 5.6 for white Americans. The former also held an advantage in old age: for those aged sixty-five to seventy-four, the rates for Chinese and whites were 18.9 and 29.1, respectively, rising to 52.3 and 66.2 for those aged seventy-five to eighty-four. Interestingly, nativity status seems to make a greater difference than gender. The death rate among the foreign born is almost twice as high as that of U.S.-born Chinese. Among the Chinese population sixty-five to seventy-four years old, the death rate for the foreign-born is almost six times higher (Yu, 1986).

The Chinese elderly are much less likely to report that their health is good or excellent than their white counterparts. In a study of 138 San Francisco Chinatown

Table 2.2 Mobility or Self-Care Limitation of Chinese Elderly by Nativity: 1990

	Total	Native-Born	Foreign-Born
65–74 Years	86,314	14,796	71,518
Limitation	13,313	1,997	11,316
Percent	15.4	13.5	15.8
75+ Years	43,300	6,451	36,849
Limitation	13,346	1,861	11,485
Percent	30.8	28.8	31.2
Percent by Nativity		14.5	85.5

Source: U.S. Census, 1993b.

residents, Carp and Kataoka (1976) found that twice as many Chinese (30 percent) as white (15 percent) elderly identified health as their most serious problem. As expected, the younger age group of the Chinese American elderly had better health than the older ones (Chen, 1979). Moreover, elderly Chinese men tended to rate their physical health higher than their female counterparts (Mui, 1996).

Various gerontological studies suggest that the older one gets, the greater the likelihood of physical or mental impairments. Such is the case for the elderly Chinese in the United States. Table 2.2 shows that 15.4 percent of individuals aged sixty-five to seventy-four and 30 percent of those aged seventy-five and over have one or more mobility or self-care limitations. There does not appear to be a significant difference based on nativity status. However, given the overwhelming numbers who were born outside the United States, this group comprises the vast majority of the disabled older Chinese population. In addition, researchers have found a greater prevalence of dementia among Chinese elders than for the general population (Yano et al., 1984).

Many stresses are associated with immigration and acculturation. Poverty, low educational attainment, lack of language skills, poor physical health, high rates of family disruption, the splitting of households, and a lack of physical and emotional resources to cope with such anxiety-producing events are prevalent among ethnic elders, including older Chinese immigrants. They are more likely to develop mental health problems and are at a higher risk of depression than elderly white Americans (Mui, 1996; Ying, 1988). Unfortunately, the Chinese are less likely to be identified by service providers as suffering from these illnesses and are less likely to receive treatment for them (Carp and Kataoka, 1976; Mui, 1996).

Numerous researchers also have found evidence of high suicide rates among the Chinese elderly, greater than among older white Americans overall (Yu, 1986). The percentage for older Chinese women is even larger, ten times that of their white counterparts (Browne and Broderick, 1994; Liu and Yu, 1985). Further, in 1980, three times more elderly Chinese immigrants committed suicide than did those who were native born (Mui, 1996; Yu, 1986).

Traditional Values and the Aged

One of the major values that affects the lives of the Chinese is the strong emphasis on the family, on family togetherness, conformity, and the interdependence of family members. Implicit in the strong family value is adherence to specific roles, obligations, and responsibilities. These teachings have major implications for the adjustment of elderly Chinese to old age.

Filial Piety

Filial piety is not simply a casual or customary practice; it has deep historical roots in Confucianism (Moody, 1998; Okada, 1988; Wu, 1975). A highly cherished precept among the Chinese, it was a set of moral principles, taught at a very young age and reinforced throughout one's life, of mutual respect for those of equal status and reverence toward the dominant leader and one's elders. Duty, obligation, loyalty, respect, devotion to parents, importance of the family name, service, and self-sacrifice for the elders, all essential elements of filial piety, characterized Chinese family relations (Hsu, 1971b; Kung, 1962: 206; MacKinnon, Gien and Durst, 1996; Wong, 1998).

Hierarchy is important, and family members have prescribed roles and responsibilities according to gender, age, and birth order. For example, one prescription is that children must obey and care for their parents without question or resentment. Another is that the firstborn son has the greatest authority and responsibility for the care of elderly parents. It is considered culturally desirable for aging parents to live with a married adult child, preferably a married son (Hong and Ham, 1992). Today, however, all children are expected to display filial piety and to repay their parents for sacrifices they have made for them (Braun and Browne, 1998; Char et al., 1980; Elliot et al., 1996; Huang, 1991).

Within the larger American society, adult children are encouraged to leave their parents' home and establish an independent household. However, such an action is often very stressful for the elderly Chinese. It may engender great disappointment, shame, and loss of face. Older parents living alone tend to perceive themselves as failures for not doing their part in rearing their children with proper values and a sense of filial piety, and this may be perceived as a source of embarrassment among members of the Chinese community.

Respect for Authority

Respect for, and deference to, authority is a major tenet of the Confucian ethic. Thus, individuals are expected to comply with social authority, even to the point of sacrificing their own desires and ambitions (Ho, 1976). Such a value may produce miscommunications. Courtesy and dignity may become an issue when the Chinese person is saying yes but really means no, and vice versa. Yee and Weaver (1994) point out that positive head nodding may indicate to American physicians that the Chinese patients agree with and understand what is being said. However, in reality, Chinese patients may be simply deferring to authority, not wishing to contradict or embarrass the physician.

Elders are viewed as family decision makers and the keepers of family traditions and cultural wisdom. As a consequence, the elderly within Chinese culture are viewed with considerable respect because they represent a link to the past. They preserve Chinese customs and are proud of their cultural heritage, which has lasted more than five thousand years. Because of the prominent and venerated position of the elderly in Chinese culture, younger adults have been said to look forward to old age as a time when they can sit back and enjoy the fruits of their labor while family members honor them and seek their advice on important life issues (Cheung, 1989; Kalish and Moriwaki, 1973; MacKinnon, Gien and Durst, 1996; Ujimoto et al., 1993; Wu, 1975).

The Concept of Losing Face

The concept of losing face is central to many Chinese. Roughly translated, it denotes shame, shame brought by individuals to themselves and to their families. In fact, the family is viewed as more important than the individual. It is imperative that one not do anything to bring dishonor upon one's self or, indirectly, upon one's family or family name. Thus, personal indiscretions, mistakes, or even mental illness and disabilities may reflect badly on the entire family and cause shame or loss of face (Braun and Browne, 1998; Huang, 1991).

One way to counteract the loss of face is to enhance the family name. This can be accomplished by an outstanding achievement in some aspect of life, whether it is educational honors, occupational accomplishments, or awards (Ho, 1976; Wong, 1980, 1984a, 1990).

In this discussion, the values of filial piety and respect for those in authority and the aged and the concept of losing face have been looked upon as separate, independent, and unrelated ideas. But in traditional Chinese society they interact and intersect in many different and complex ways, promoting caring relations between children and older Chinese parents. Hence, unlike in American society, age is an important source of status for the Chinese (Chen, 1979; Cheung et al., 1980; Nagasawa, 1980; Cheung, 1989). Growing old is regarded as a blessing.

The Role of Traditional Values in the United States

How applicable are these traditional values to the lives of the elderly Chinese in the United States? Do they still hold a prominent place in this country? Does the concept of filial piety continue to play a major role for adult Chinese children? Can aging Chinese parents look forward to a life where they will be respected and revered by their children?

Various researchers have questioned the prominence of these traditional and ancient values in the lives of the Chinese in America (Browne and Broderick,

1994; Chen, 1979; Cheung, 1989; Lum et al., 1980). They argue that the concept of filial piety has lost its place within the Chinese American family. Adult children are not supporting their elderly parents either financially or emotionally.

The erosion of this value may be due to several factors. First is the absence of social and community pressures on adult children in American society to take responsibility for their aged parents (Chen 1979; Miah and Kahler, 1997). Individualism (as opposed to collectivism) and the nuclear family structure (as opposed to the extended family) have become the foci of younger people's lives. As a consequence, the role and authority of the elderly are less prominent.

Second, the American-born Chinese have become more acculturated to the beliefs, traditions, and customs of U.S. society, many of which are at odds with Chinese culture. As a consequence, it is becoming more common to hear foreign-born Chinese parents express disappointment and complain that "my son is just like an American" (Chen, 1979). In addition, the Chinese precepts and how they should be put into practice may be perceived differently by older Chinese immigrants and their more Americanized children (Cheung, 1989). Thus, the type of support from Chinese families for their elders may be changing (Chan, 1983; Kalish and Moriwaki, 1973; Kalish and Yuen, 1971; MacKinnon, Gien and Durst, 1996).

Third, because of the emphasis on the independence of family members within American society, the Chinese family in the United States is experiencing a weakening of its tradition of interdependence. Hence, the importance of the role of the father's position as the patriarch and the mother's position as the emotional center of the family, as well as the obligation to take care of them regardless of their worthiness, is greatly diminished. (Browne and Broderick, 1994; Chen, 1979; Miah and Kahler, 1997).

Fourth, the admixture of individualism, materialism, nuclear-family autonomy, and urbanization often creates pressures on the American-born children of Chinese immigrants to disregard and sometimes even to reject their elderly parents (Lum et al., 1980).

In conclusion, because of different experiences between the generations, shifting values within the Chinese community and within the family, and the rapid acculturation of the second- (and third-) generation Chinese into American society, many American-born Chinese may not place the same significance on caring for their elderly immigrant parents as the latter did for their own parents.

Barriers to Adequate Care for the Chinese Elderly

The elderly Chinese in the United States face many barriers to receiving adequate care. Although many of these obstacles are similar to those experienced by all elderly persons, others are unique to the elderly Chinese. Certain impediments, including their cultural values, financial hardship, distrust of government programs, language and literacy problems, difficulty in dealing with government and/or private agencies, lack of information about the American health and social service delivery systems, and a belief that services based on a Western model of wellness are irrelevant, may result in an underutilization of needed heath care and social services even if they are available (Browne and Broderick, 1994; Cox, 1991; Cuellar and Weeks, 1980; Dhoomer, 1991; Gelfand and Barresi, 1987b; Gould, 1988; Kamikawa, 1981; Sue and Sue, 1977; Tsai and Lopez, 1997; Wong, 1984b; Wu, 1975). For instance, a strong sense of family responsibility—that one's children should be taking care of them—may arouse feelings of shame or loss of face, preventing older individuals from seeking formal services. Some Chinese elderly persons may be afraid of racial discrimination or may believe that the staff is not culturally sensitive (Chen, 1979; Cheung, 1989; Fuji, 1976; Ikels, 1983b; Nagasawa, 1980; Wong, 1979). Let us investigate these issues more fully.

Language Barriers

The ability to communicate in English is a major contributing factor to the successful acculturation of the Chinese to American society. However, about 70 percent of the Chinese population are foreign-born. Many of these older people, especially those who arrived in the United States late in their lives, remain linguistically isolated. In 1990, about 46.5 percent of the overall Chinese elderly population faced such a situation; only 15.3 percent of the native-born American Chinese were linguistically isolated, compared with 52.6 percent of those born elsewhere (U.S. Census, 1993b). The inability to speak English constitutes a serious impediment to service delivery or provider–client communications.

About 50.5 percent of the total Chinese population state that they do not speak English "very well." What that actually means is uncertain, especially when it is noted that about 15 percent of the native-born Chinese give a similar response. In any case, almost 84 percent of the foreign-born elderly and about one-fourth of those born in the United States indicate that they have only limited facility with the language. Approximately 84 percent of the total Chinese population, and fully 90.6 percent of the elderly, tell us that they speak a language other than English (U.S. Census, 1993b). However, we can't be sure how fluent they are or whether they are bilingual.

For those in institutions (nursing homes, convalescent centers, senior citizens retirement centers, and the like), lack of facility with the English language may result in problems of adjustment, mistreatment, and inadequate care (Wong, 1984b). A related issue is the lack of bilingual aides who can address and attend to the particular needs of the Chinese elderly. As the number of foreign-born Chinese elderly immigrants increases over the years, we can expect this problem to grow.

Moreover, health care and social services in the community cannot be dispensed effectively without providers who are able to communicate with their patients as well as be culturally sensitive to their plight. Because of the lack of bilingual/bicultural staff, many elderly Chinese must rely on their adult children to translate their physical or mental maladies to the doctor. There are several problems with this. Yeo (1996–1997) notes that in cross-gender discussion of topics that are taboo, such as the breast or genitourinary organs, young family members may change, or not ask, a question considered inappropriate, even at the risk of their parents' receiving inadequate care. Moreover, placing the responsibility of translation on young family members can be especially traumatic. They may feel inadequate, awkward, or embarrassed if the discussion is seen as demeaning to the parent or if they are asked to give him or her grave news.

Western Legalese versus Chinese Tradition

Living wills, durable powers of attorney for health care, and informed consent are Western concepts that have no counterpart in Chinese society. Service providers or translators have a dual problem. First, they must attempt to explain these new and seemingly strange concepts and their implications to the immigrants. Second, they must try to overcome the reluctance among the elderly Chinese to discuss death and dying. It is believed by many Chinese that just talking about death can bring bad omens (Braun and Nichols, 1997).

American medical practice values individual autonomy. As a consequence, informed consent by the patient, as practiced in the United States, is inconsistent with Chinese traditional values in which the family may be expected to protect, and make decisions for, their elders. In fact, the American orientation conflicts with filial piety and family solidarity, values that are deeply embedded in Confucianism (Moody, 1998). For example, some Chinese families have a strong preference not to tell elders that they have a terminal disease such as cancer so as not to destroy their hope (Fung, 1994; Orona, Koenig and Davis, 1994; Yeo, 1996).

The reluctance to sign legal documents may reflect the cultural importance that the Chinese place on the honor of the spoken word and verbal agreements (Eleazer et al., 1996). Hence, written agreements may be viewed as an insult to their honor and an affront to their sense of responsibility and obligation. In addition, since many of the first-generation older Chinese immigrants are illiterate in English, they may hesitate to sign a document that they can neither read nor understand.

Chinese Concept of Disease and Difficulties with Western Medicine

Different cultures have different interpretations of, and explanations for, the causes of disease and even health itself. For example, Elliot et al. (1996) found that recent Chinese immigrants in California may interpret dementia symptoms as mental illness (which is shameful) resulting from a retribution for individual or family sins, an imbalance of yin and yang, improper alignment of the house (according to feng shui), or the possession of the body by an evil spirit. In a study of recent Chinese immigrants in Honolulu, Braun and Browne (1998) found that informants believed that obvious symptoms of dementia observed among older

Chinese were a natural part of old age and that they were caused by the elders' move to a new environment.

Balance is central to Chinese cosmology. The Chinese believe that physical and mental health result from a state of equilibrium among humans, society, and cosmic forces. In traditional Chinese medicine, health is achieved if one can balance the yin and yang energy forces. Yin (the female element) represents the passive principle or bodily forces described as darkness, cold, wet, and emptiness. Yang (the male element) is equated with the active principle, characterized by light, heat, warmth, dryness, and fullness. It is believed that eating certain foods can bring about the balance or imbalance between the yin and yang. For example, because of their age and physical conditions, elderly people are naturally predisposed to yin, or cold, energy forces. Therefore, they should avoid eating too many "cold foods," such as leafy green vegetables—an avoidance that, by Western standards, is not conducive to good health (Kuo and Kavanagh, 1994; Yee and Weaver, 1994). One must also maintain the unobstructed flow of *chi*, or vital energy, through the body to maintain health and prevent illness or injury (Lam, 1994; Yeo, 1996–1997).

When there is an imbalance of the chi traveling through the body, the attending "physician" (who may be a doctor with Western training, an acupuncturist, or an herbalist) may take an active role in restoring its flow or correcting the disequilibrium between yin and yang. The physician may apply acupuncture, acupressure, or moxibustion (the laying of hot coins on certain points on the body) or prescribe food and herbal medications with strong yin and yang qualities (Char et al., 1980; Lam, 1994; Yeo, 1996–1997).

Such therapeutic interventions are not used just by the Chinese in China. Investigators and practitioners have found that a significant number of Chinese in America employ a combination of Western and Chinese medical services (Braun and Browne, 1998; Char et al., 1980; Hessler et al., 1975; Liu, 1986). When my father had a stroke, he would see a physical therapist (Western medicine) as well as a Chinese herbalist and an acupuncturist (illegal at that time). Hessler et al. (1975) reported that Chinese patients in Boston sought both Western and Chinese health care (predominantly herbal medicine) and never used one type to the exclusion of the other.

Chinese elders who use Western medication, herbs, and homemade Chinese remedies are susceptible to drug interactions and toxic substances. For example, the contents of the Chinese treatments may interact with those in prescription or over-the-counter medication, creating serious side effects (Yee and Weaver, 1994).

Kraut (1990) notes that whether because of their lack of facility with English or unfamiliarity with Western medicine, some Chinese immigrants rarely seek the care of Western physicians. Many of the elders in Kraut's study expressed a sense of fatalism and were reluctant or unable to communicate with service providers. Because of their traditional values and their concept of the nature of the origins and nature of disease, they often mistrusted health care professionals and the motives of the health care system. These factors lead many immigrants to refuse to use any Western medicine, even when such facilities and resources are available (Liu, 1986; Moody, 1998). In a study of residents in Boston's Chinatown, Liu (1986) found that 61 percent of the sample did not have a private physician, relying instead on herbalists, acupuncturists, and pharmacies operating in the classic tradition of Chinese medicine. Lack of familiarity with, or lack of belief in, medical insurance further handicaps these immigrant families.

Stereotypes

One of the most accepted stereotypes regarding the Chinese elderly is that they do not have any problems with regard to long-term care. It is believed that because of their adherence to traditional values, the Chinese family will provide for their elderly parents, and without any outside help. However, as suggested earlier, owing to such factors as acculturation, changes in filial expectations, altered socioeconomic environments, and diverse lifestyles, the reality is that the elderly Chinese can by no means count on their children for all of their care.

Outdated views must be discarded so that policy may be implemented to deal with the real needs of the Chinese elderly (Kalish and Yuen, 1971; Kuo and Kavanagh, 1994; Lam, 1994; Lee, 1986; Liu, 1986; Mui, 1998). Their problems are beyond individual and family resources, and the family's efforts need to be complemented with community and government services and programs.

Conclusion and Policy Implications

Increase Transcultural Nursing/Social Work

Transcultural nursing and social work involves anticipating, recognizing, understanding, and accepting views of life and the world that may differ from one's own. As it applies to the Chinese, this involves such things as knowing about the family structure, authority and decision-making processes, cultural views regarding death and dying, and the use of herbs and other alternative medical therapies. Transcultural skills allow the integration of unique sociopsychological factors in nursing care and social welfare plans, interventions, and evaluations (Kuo and Kavanagh, 1994). Curricula in nursing programs and social services should include courses that encourage and promote a transcultural or multicultural approach (Richards, Browne and Broderick, 1994; Browne and Broderick, 1994). This is especially crucial in areas where there is a large concentration of Chinese.

Increase Bilingual/Bicultural Staff

Because many immigrant Chinese lack facility in English, they experience great difficulty in understanding or communicating when they seek services. Therefore, it is crucial to have bilingual staff available. Such staff should not be used solely as translators for non-Chinese professionals but should be engaged in the coordination and implementation of outreach services to ensure sensitivity to the values within the Chinese population (Salcido, Nakano and Jue, 1980; Browne and Broderick, 1994; Carp and Kataoka, 1976; Chen, 1979; Lum et al., 1980). The On Lok Senior Citizen Center in San Francisco (Suzuki, 1978; Dang, 1999), the Kin On Health Care Center in Seattle (Otsuka, 1999), and Project Open Door in New York (Harlan, 1998) can serve as models that take into consideration the values, family structure, language, religion, gender-role differences, and institutional structure of the Chinese community. It is also important to have nursing homes staffed by people who can understand Chinese ways and communicate with the elderly in their native dialects.

Encourage Both Western and Eastern Medical Therapies

It has been suggested that the Chinese elderly have a greater faith in traditional folk therapy than in Western medicine. However, many of them prefer a combination of medical therapies, utilizing Western medicine with traditional herbal prescriptions and acupuncture. This admixture tends to create a better psychological condition for improving their health (Miah and Kahler, 1997)

Consequently, medical curricula should include courses that encourage and promote a transcultural approach. Such a program could provide courses on acupuncture, acupressure, and Chinese herbal medicine and could also prove useful to others seeking alternative forms of medicine.

Locate Services in or near Chinatown

Older residents of Chinatown, in particular, have severe barriers to obtaining medical and other types of care. These reflect their extreme isolation, poverty, and inadequate information about the American delivery system as well as the lack of adequate medical, social, and health care facilities in their community.

Services, including senior citizen clubs, nutrition programs, and clinics, should be located in or near the Chinese community. Lum et al. (1980) and Salcido, Nakano and Jue (1980) point out that when medical, social, and health care agencies are located within the immediate neighborhood, utilization by the Chinese elderly is enhanced. Part of the reason for this is that most of the Chinese aged do not use public transportation; they prefer to use health and social services that are within walking distance from their residence. For example, Carp and Kataoka (1979) found that 70 percent of the elderly Chinese interviewed walked to the doctor and about 66 percent walked to get their medicine.

Increase Effective Outreach Services

Because of the assumption that the Chinese take care of their own, there has been very little outreach. The linguistic diversity of the Chinese population, including different dialects of Cantonese, Mandarin, and so on, makes such efforts even more problematic.

To ensure that the Chinese elderly have access to services, outreach should be incorporated into the service programs of public welfare agencies. Since the problems of the Chinese elderly are beyond the ability of the family system alone, they require public support through health and welfare programs.

To reach the Chinese elderly community, one's message must be heard and understood. Pamphlets, brochures, program information, eligibility requirements, and location of available community resources should be translated into the language of the Chinese elderly, including their different dialects. In areas with a large concentration of Chinese, usually some form of Chinese-language media is available. The use of Chinese-oriented television, radio, or newspapers has proven to be very effective in increasing their utilization of services and programs (Markides and Mindel, 1987).

In conclusion, the Chinese elderly face many barriers to adequate care, including their lack of facility with English, the conflict between Western legalese and Chinese tradition, the Chinese concepts of disease, and stereotypes that imply that the Chinese family can and will take care of their own. Implementation of these recommendations will lower some of these barriers, allowing us to provide more adequate care for the Chinese elderly.

3

Japanese American Elderly

Tazuko Shibusawa, James Lubben, and Harry H. L. Kitano

In traditional Japanese culture, the primary responsibility of caring for frail elders belongs to the family. This, in large part, is due to the influences of Confucian values, which emphasize filial piety. Japanese Americans have preserved many of the values of their country of origin, including the respect for elders (Kiefer, 1974; Kitano, 1976; Osako, 1979). In the late 1960s and early 1970s, as the *Issei,* or first generation of immigrants, began to age, Japanese American communities throughout the United States became involved in developing services for their elders. A number of these services were named *Keiro,* which means "respect and admiration for the elders." The majority of first-generation Japanese immigrants have now passed away, and currently, the senior generation consists of second-generation Japanese Americans known as *Nisei* and recent immigrants known as *Shin Issei,* which means new Issei. There are two groups of Nisei: those who grew up in the United States, and those known as *Kibei Nisei,* who were sent to Japan during childhood. The latter are less acculturated, prefer to speak Japanese, and share similarities with later-arriving immigrants from Japan (Shin Issei). The older Japanese American population today presents a spectrum of values and preferences regarding long-term care.

Historical Background

The main wave of Japanese immigration to the United States occurred between the late 1800s and the early 1920s (Kitano and Daniels, 1987). The Chinese Exclusion Act of 1882 had created a shortage of workers for Hawaiian plantations, and Japan was viewed as a source of cheap labor. After Hawaii was annexed by the United States in 1898, many Japanese moved to the West Coast, where they initially worked in agriculture and railroad maintenance (Kitano and Daniels, 1987). The first immigrants were exclusively single men. Many acquired a wife from Japan through an arranged marriage that often included an exchange of photographs, from whence the term "picture brides" is derived. Others made brief visits to Japan to marry and then returned to the United States with their new brides (Nishi, 1995).

Immigration from Japan took place during an era of intense anti-Asian sentiment. Japanese immigrants were not allowed to gain U.S. citizenship, and alien land laws prohibited them from owning land. In 1924, the enactment of the Immigration Exclusion Act banned all immigration from Japan. The doors for Japanese immigration did not reopen until the immigration act was revised shortly after World War II, largely to accommodate the war brides of American servicemen. A large majority (86 percent) of Japanese immigrants to the United States during the 1950s were women, and almost three-quarters of them were the wives of American citizens (Nishi, 1995).

Anti-Japanese sentiment on the West Coast culminated in the internment of all persons of Japanese ancestry during World War II. Close to 120,000 Japanese Americans in Arizona, California, Oregon, and Washington were classified as "enemy aliens" and were incarcerated in internment camps in remote areas of Arizona, Arkansas, California, Colorado, Idaho, Utah, and Wyoming. The internment, which lasted for four years, had devastating effects on Japanese Americans. Most lost their property, and families were torn between loyalties to Japan and the United States. The internment experience has cast its shadow on subsequent generations of Japanese Americans; there is a lingering distrust of the majority society and a perception that they are vulnerable to similar acts of racism and discrimination based upon racial/ethnic identity (Nagata, 1993; Yoo, 2000).

Demographic Characteristics

According to the 1990 census, there are close to 850,000 Japanese Americans (U.S. Census, 1993d), with the majority living in either Hawaii or California. Japanese Americans have the longest average life span among ethnic groups in the United States. According to a study based on the 1980 census, the average life expectancy at birth for Japanese males in Hawaii was 77.7, while the average life expectancy for white males in Hawaii was 74.2 (McCormick et al., 1996). Among Asian and Pacific Islander groups, Japanese Americans also have the highest proportion of U.S.-born elders (Tanjasiri, Wallace and Shibata, 1995; Lubben and Lee, 2000). According to the 1990 census, 63 percent of Japanese American elders are U.S. born, in contrast to 16 percent of Chinese American elders (Elo, 1997).

Overall, the median family income among Japanese Americans is $51,550, which indicates middle-class to upper-middle-class status. Close to 90 percent have a high school education (U.S. Census, 1993d), and over 35 percent have a bachelor's degree or higher (Lee, 1998). The poverty rate among Japanese Americans in 1989 was estimated to be somewhere between 3 percent and 7 percent, which is similar to that of the white population (Lee, 1998). Families tend to be very small, and the total fertility rate for Japanese American women is 1.1. The low birth rate is associated with high educational levels and high average incomes (Lee, 1998).

Health Status

As with other Asian American groups, population-based data on health statistics among Japanese Americans are relatively limited (Zane, Takeuchi and Young, 1994; Curb et. al., 1996). Much of the information about the health of elderly Japanese Americans is provided by cross-national studies that compare Japanese elders in Japan and the United States. The Ni-Hon-San studies, which were conducted among Japanese in Japan, Hawaii, and San Francisco, examined the relationships between genetic and environmental factors in the development of coronary heart disease, cerebral vascular disease, and different types of cancers (Reed et al., 1983). The results show, on one hand, that Japanese Americans have a much higher risk of cardiovascular disease than their cohorts in Japan. Change from a traditional Japanese lifestyle to a Western one that is more sedentary, along with a diet that is higher in animal fat, may be responsible for the increase. On the other hand, the mortality rate from cerebrovascular diseases is lower for Japanese Americans than their Japanese cohort. This may be attributed to a lower intake of salt in the Western diet. Both Japanese and Japanese Americans have relatively high death rates from cancer. Moreover, in comparison to other ethnic groups in the United States, Japanese Americans have a high incidence of stomach cancer.

The Ni-Hon-Sea study, another cross-national research effort, has been investigating the prevalence and incidence of dementia among elderly Japanese in Seattle, Honolulu, and Japan (Graves et al., 1999). Recent results from the Seattle population indicate a lower incidence of Alzheimer's disease among Japanese Americans who are less acculturated. Those who had traditional Japanese lifestyles and/or were exposed to the Japanese language as children have lower risks of experiencing cognitive decline.

Japanese American Families

The first-generation Issei immigrated to the United States during the Meiji era (1868–1919), a period in Japan when families were legally organized according to an extended family system known as the *ie*. The ie was based on a primogeniture system headed by a male figure, so the household succession was through eldest sons. Family relationships were highly structured in a hierarchical order, and interactions were determined by prescribed roles. Family rules also were reinforced by Confucian ethics of filial piety, which included obedience to, and respect for, one's parents, obligation and loyalty to the family, the duty to ensure the succession of the family line, and the obligation not to bring shame to the family (Johnson, 1993). In addition to Confucian ethics, respect for one's parents and ancestors was reinforced by Shintoism, the indigenous religion of Japan, which maintains that elderly parents become spirits upon their death and protect the ie (Kinoshita and Kiefer, 1992).

Despite acculturation, Japanese American families have retained many of the values and norms of their culture of origin. Differences in parenting have been observed between later-generation Japanese Americans and European Americans in the areas of child rearing, including developmental goals and educational expectations (Ching, et al., 1995; Kitano, 1976, 1988; Matsui, 1986), communication patterns (Johnson and Marsella, 1978), and filial obligation (Kiefer, 1974; Osako, 1979).

Living arrangements among Japanese American elders differ from those of their white cohorts. According to a study based on the 1990 census data, 37 percent of older unmarried Japanese American women lived with their adult children (Kamo and Zhou, 1994). This is quite high in comparison to the coresidence rate of their non-Hispanic white counterparts, which was 9.4 percent. Japanese elders who lived with their adult children tended to be foreign born, recent immigrants, and not as acculturated as those who resided alone (Kamo and Zhou, 1994). Among married elderly Japanese American females, 6.9 percent lived with their children, while only 2.2 percent of their white counterparts did. Although fewer Japanese American than white elders live on their own, larger numbers of elderly Japanese than other Asian elders live alone or only with their spouse (Himes, Hogan and Eggebeen, 1996; Lubben and Lee, 2000). Osako and Liu (1986) found that while half of the Japanese American elders in their study lived with their daughters, their preference was to live nearby but not to coreside.

Studies of first-generation immigrants (Issei) report that Japanese American elderly are able to relinquish authority in the family and become dependent on their children without losing self-esteem (Kiefer, 1974; Osako, 1979). Researchers contend that this is because Japanese American elderly receive more respect from their children than white elders and because dependency is viewed in a more positive light in Asian cultures.

In East Asian cultures, the interdependent nature of human relationships is accepted as a basic human condition, and, consequently, less emphasis is placed on autonomy and independence. In Japanese culture, relationships are understood in the context of *amae,* which is defined as a state where a person presumes on the indulgence of another for care and gratification (Doi, 1977). The prototype of amae is the parent–child relationship, especially the mother–infant relationship, where mothers indulge their children and are solicitous of their emotional and physical needs. Role reversal is expected when parents become frail, and the elderly are expected to receive active nurturing from their children. In such a cultural context, dependency is viewed as a normal part of the aging process (Kiefer, 1974).

According to Osako (1979), role reversals between first-generation parents and second-generation children took place long before the former started to age.

During World War II internment, most Issei did not speak English and had to yield their authority to their English-speaking Nisei children who were either adolescents or young adults at the time.

Studies of older Nisei, on the other hand, indicate that, unlike their Issei parents, they do not expect to become dependent on their children (Tomita, 1998). Yanagisako (1985) reports that the Nisei in her study, however, hoped that their children would be "Japanese enough" to take care of them in the future should the need arise.

The reluctance among Nisei to depend on their children may be the result of a number of factors. First, the Nisei have, to a large extent, embraced the Western values of independence and autonomy. Second, they have fewer expectations of their children than their Issei parents (Kitano, 1976). For example, the Issei expected their children to grow up with a sense of Japanese identity. Further, traditional expressions of filial piety are declining among later-generation Japanese Americans, and thus the Nisei cannot expect their children to care for them in old age in the same manner as earlier generations did (Ishii-Kuntz, 1997). According to Tomita (1998), the Nisei express few expectations of support from their children in old age, in part to avoid disappointment.

In many ways, the Nisei resemble their cohort in Japan, known as Showa *hitoketa*. This cohort was born between 1926 and 1935 during the single-digit years of the Showa era. (*Hitoketa* means single digit.) In their early years, the members of the Showa hitoketa generation were indoctrinated with Confucian values of caring for and respecting the aged. Once World War II ended, they were educated under the new democratic system, which was introduced by U.S. occupation forces. They are committed to caring for their frail parents but are ambivalent about being cared for by their own children. They hope that their children will be willing to care for them when they become frail; at the same time, they do not want to impose on their children. Nisei went through similar experiences. They were exposed to two cultures, that of their parents and that of the dominant society (Kurashige, 2000). Nisei who were adolescents or young adults during internment faced shame and humiliation with respect to their Japanese heritage as well as pressure to prove their loyalty to the United States by assimilating into the dominant society (Mass, 1991). Like the Showa hitoketa generation, the current cohort of Japanese American elders took care of their parents but do not expect their children to care for them. At the same time, the Nisei would prefer that their children take the initiative to care for them if they become frail.

Another factor that affects elder care among Japanese American families is the high rate of out-marriages. The rate of interracial marriages among Japanese Americans has been increasing over the years. According to the 1980 census records, the out-marriage rate for Japanese American women was over 40 percent, and over 20 percent for men (Lee and Yamanaka, 1990). According to the 1990 census, there were 40 percent more Japanese–white births than monoracial Japanese American births (1990 census as cited in Root, 1996). An increasing number of Japanese American elders will have children-in-law and grandchildren of diverse cultural backgrounds. Both Japanese American elders and their offspring will need to learn to negotiate among a diverse set of cultural expectations regarding elder care.

Japanese American Elders and Informal Care

Japanese Americans believe that the family is ultimately responsible for the care of frail elderly (Kitano, Shibusawa and Kitano, 1995). However, this does not mean that elders necessarily want their children to carry out actual caregiving duties. In fact, a number of factors cast doubt on the notion that Japanese American elders would be comfortable receiving personal care from their adult children. First, the social context in which adult children care for frail parents has changed. In traditional Japanese society, family relationships were governed by hierarchical structures that were supported by social norms of reciprocal obligations referred to as *on* (Fugita et al., 1991). Parents expected children to care for them when they were frail, in part because at a previous stage they had sacrificed on behalf of their offspring. Since *on* was the social norm, elderly parents felt that they had a right to be cared for. Oftentimes it was not the eldest son but his wife, the elderly parents' daughter-in-law, who provided the care for her parents-in-law. However, *on* norms of reciprocal obligations assured the daughter-in-law that in the future, if she became frail, her daughter-in-law would provide the necessary care for her. Thus, caring for elder parents was based on an elaborate set of intergenerational social obligations.

These expectations have greatly diminished both in Japan and in Japanese American communities. Social norms no longer demand that offspring care for their frail parents, and receiving care from family members has been made more complex and problematic. When people receive assistance in Japanese culture, they are expected to accept the care passively without voicing complaints or asserting their desires. To complain or assert their own wishes would be a betrayal or a sign of lack of appreciation toward the caregiver. Those receiving care are expected to *enryo*, which means hold back or restrain one's wishes. In traditional Japanese parent–child relationships, elders supposedly did not have to *enryo* toward their children because of the norms of filial obligation.

In Japanese culture, there is an implicit understanding that a person who receives care is indebted and, therefore, obligated to the caregiver unless he or she can reciprocate the favors. Most elders cannot reciprocate the care that they receive. In addition, the Japanese, who are sensitized to consider the burden on the care provider when they receive help, tend to feel that they must accept the assistance passively lest they offend the provider. Thus, dependence comes with a cost: one must passively accept the help and not assert oneself or negotiate for the kind of aid desired. Therefore, some elders prefer not to receive help.

The following example is illustrative of this situation:

Mrs. F, an eighty-nine-year-old Japanese American woman who is disabled, tries hard to maintain her autonomy. She walks two blocks around her apartment with her walker every day to maintain her muscle strength. She also tries to cook for herself every night, even though it is difficult for her to stand in the kitchen for an extended period. She grates vegetables, which is a physically taxing activity, and her arms hurt afterwards. Instead of acknowledging her efforts in a positive light, she views her wishes to maintain independence as a shortcoming. She says, "I am spoiled. I don't like to have people do things for me, even though I can't do things on my own." Mrs. F describes her determination to remain independent as "being spoiled," because she is unable to surrender her autonomy and become dependent on others. Mrs. F feels that it is a shortcoming on her part that she is not able to take on a passive help-recipient role.

Mrs. F's negative evaluation of her wishes to maintain independence is related to the fact that she feels that she is at fault for not being able to accept the reality of her dependent state. Traditional Japanese coping strategies are based on the values of accepting things as they are, believing in the value of silence, and practicing self-denial. The ability to accept things as they are is seen as an inner resource or strength of character. This capacity to endure hardships and difficult situations is known as *gaman*, the ability to "suppress complaints, conceal discomfort, and demonstrate a tolerance for adverse circumstances" (Johnson, 1993: 89). Suppressing the desire for autonomy and not imposing on the goodwill of others are viewed as positive traits among Japanese elders.

Attitudes toward Formal Care

Japanese Americans prefer to try to resolve problems on their own before seeking assistance from others. Usually, it is not until the situation has worsened that help is sought from the outside (Sakauye, 1989). Personal and family problems are kept within the family. This is because, traditionally, preserving family honor took priority over individual needs. As with other Asian American groups, Japanese Americans in general are reluctant to seek mental health services. This has been attributed to culturally fostered shame and stigma associated with mental illness (Kitano, 1976). Japanese, along with other Asian Americans, have higher rates of using psychiatric emergency services than other ethnic groups because they are reluctant to seek mental health treatment until there is a full-blown crisis (Sakauye, 1989).

The reluctance among Japanese Americans to acknowledge psychological disorders inhibits elders who are depressed or who have early stages of dementia from receiving appropriate and preventive interventions (Fugita et al., 1991). Suicide among Japanese Americans sixty-five years of age and older is almost twice as high as among younger Japanese American populations (Kitano, Shibusawa and Kitano, 1997). Suicide rates among Japanese Americans sixty-five and older are almost equal to those of white elderly (Baker, 1994). However, among Japanese elders over seventy-five years of age, the rate of completed suicides is higher than that of their white counterparts. Among Japanese American women ages seventy-five to eighty-four, it is 2.5 times higher than for white women. Among Japanese men age eighty-five and over, the suicide rate is almost three times greater than that for white men (Baker, 1994). These high rates of suicide among the oldest Japanese Americans are suggestive of the ancient practice of *obasute* in which self-imposed death was considered honorable when resources in rural villages were inadequate to sustain the whole population (Takamura, 1991).

Attitudes and preferences toward formal geriatric care vary among the current cohort of Japanese Americans (Adams, 1981). Japanese elders, like other ethnic elders, have traditionally been reluctant to use formal services because of language barriers, fear of prejudicial treatment, and inadequate financial resources (Sakauye, 1989). Lack of culturally appropriate services, such as bilingual staff, ethnic food, understanding of special holidays and customs, as well as lack of affordable quality services, has also led to underutilization of formal institutions (Sakauye, 1989).

Research on service preference among healthy Japanese American elders indicates that they would choose nursing homes over family care if they are permanently disabled by dementia. In the case of a hip fracture, they would choose paid in-home and family care over nursing homes. In general, Nisei who were acculturated and not married were more likely to be open to using nursing homes (McCormick et al., 1996). A study of Japanese Canadians found that elders would rather pay for formal services than burden family members (Matsuoka, 1999).

According to the 1990 census, the rate of institutionalization among Japanese American elderly is 1.6 percent (Himes, Hogan and Eggebeen, 1996). This is lower than the overall prevalence of nursing home use among U.S. elders, which is 5 percent. Institutionalization rates, however, are higher in geographical areas where Japanese facilities are available. For example, in the Seattle area, where there is a Japanese nursing home, the institutionalization rate is 5 percent (McCormick et al., 1996).

While an increasing number of Japanese American elders are willing to receive formal, paid care, some older persons, especially those who speak only Japanese, are reluctant to seek assistance from non-Japanese service workers (Shibusawa, Ishikawa and Mui, 1999). This reluctance is particularly evident with in-home care. Language barriers, and a discomfort with having a non-Japanese person in their homes, inhibit these older persons from obtaining in-home help. There is a shortage of Japanese-speaking home care workers because recent immigrants from Japan tend to have high levels of education and do not seek such low-paying positions. Consequently, some elders continue to struggle on their own without utilizing social services.

Japanese American Elderly and Community Support

The ethnic community has always played an important role in the lives of Japanese Americans. Historically, hostility and housing segregation led Issei to form their own communities and turn to each other for support (Brooks, 2000). Before World War II, the majority of urban Japanese Americans lived in ethnic enclaves, which offered physical and emotional protection from racial prejudice (Broom and Kitsuse, 1973). Religious institutions, including Buddhist and Christian churches, have always played a significant role in the Japanese American community, as have organizations such as the *kenjin-kai,* which are associations for people who came from the same prefecture in Japan (O'Brien and Fugita, 1991).

Most local Japanese American communities provide services such as congregate meal programs and recreational activities for their senior members. Some places, such as those in Los Angeles, San Francisco, San Jose, and Seattle, have skilled nursing and/or residential facilities. These services were developed by the communities in response to the lack of culturally appropriate programs in mainstream society.

One of the oldest Japanese American communities, Little Tokyo, is located in a business district in Los Angeles. The only residential facilities in Little Tokyo are a senior citizens' housing complex and a low-income housing complex. Although Little Tokyo is adjacent to a high-crime area, Japanese American elders, especially those who are Japanese-speaking, reside there because of its convenience. The elderly can walk to stores, banks, doctors' offices, social service programs, cultural organizations, and churches or Buddhist temples without having to depend on their children for transportation. Living in Little Tokyo is especially convenient for Japanese-speaking elderly since they can conduct all their personal business in Japanese. Most of the elderly in Little Tokyo plan to move to a Japanese American retirement home or nursing home if they can no longer live on their own.

Social workers in Little Tokyo engage in active community outreach because very few elders seek help even when they need assistance. Every spring, the kitchens in the senior citizen apartments are fumigated with insecticide, and residents are required to move things out of that area. This is a difficult task for elders with physical disabilities. The social workers seek out residents who need home care services and secure in-home services for them. Most elders do not know of the existence of in-home care services, nor do they know if they are entitled to receive them.

Non-English-speaking elderly and those who prefer to receive ethnic services are at risk for isolation when they do not live in Japanese communities. Nonethnic localities cannot provide the types of social and cultural support that are available in concentrated ethnic areas such as Little Tokyo. It is not only the content of services that facilitates autonomy and well-being among frail elders but also the way in which the services are delivered. For example, social workers in Little Tokyo are able to reach out to elders because their agencies are an integral part of the community network. There is close collaboration among churches, apartment managers, storekeepers, and service organizations, all of which are a part of the elderly person's daily network. One of the problems facing many Japanese American elderly today, however, is the shortage of facilities in ethnic communities. For example, there is a four-year waiting list for the senior housing facility in Little Tokyo.

Moreover, caregivers who do not speak English are at risk for burnout, depression, and especially social isolation. Such spouses tend to become more homebound than adult children who provide assistance to their parents. A number of social service agencies in Japanese American communities offer support groups and have volunteers who visit homebound caregivers. Funding for these services, however, is limited, and the lack of financial resources often restricts the expansion of these programs.

Community-Based Care

Elderly Japanese Americans, especially those who are Japanese-speaking, prefer to live in ethnic enclaves because it enables them to remain independent. Census figures indicate that older Japanese American women in ethnically concentrated areas are less likely to live with their adult children (Kamo and Zhou, 1994). Socially isolated elders also benefit from living in concentrated ethnic communities. One study found that isolated Japanese American men in Hawaii enjoyed better health than those living in less homogeneous communities (Reed et al., 1983).

English-speaking Nisei tend to live in suburbs and not in ethnic enclaves such as Little Tokyo, which tend to be located in inner cities. Regardless of where they live, connections to ethnic communities remain important for Japanese Americans, especially for older Nisei (O'Brien and Fugita, 1991). The reasons for this phenomenon are enormously complex; they constitute a topic that cannot be addressed adequately in this chapter. Still, we can point to these individuals' shared history of being an oppressed and marginalized group as one of the key factors. Another cause is related to culture. Although acculturated Nisei were born and raised in the United States, researchers have observed that they have a different style of interacting than their white counterparts. According to Miyamoto (1986–1987), certain traits, such as being less spontaneous in their communications, make them feel more comfortable interacting among themselves. Ethnic-specific services, therefore, continue to be important for older Japanese Americans. Most Japanese American geriatric facilities, as mentioned before, have long waiting lists.

As seen in the example of Little Tokyo, broad community support is necessary to enable frail elders to remain independent as long as possible. This does not negate the significance of families among Japanese American elders. Family ties are indeed important. Elders avoid becoming dependent on their children because it may jeopardize their close relationship (Osako, 1979).

Some researchers have suggested that Asian American elderly are a neglected minority group (Lee, 1987). More attention is required to address the needs of all ethnic groups of elderly, including Japanese Americans. An appropriate model for

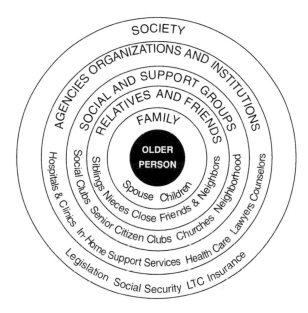

Fig. 3.1 Community care for aging societies. *Source:* Damon-Rodriguez and Lubben, 2000.

community assistance that is attentive to the role of kinship care in ethnic communities is presented in figure 3.1.

According to Damron-Rodriguez and Lubben (2000), care must first be directed to the elderly themselves and then extended to families and other members of the older person's social networks. For example, unrecognized dementia, especially in mild cases, is common among Japanese American men in Hawaii (Ross et al., 1997). Educational programs for families on early signs of the illness could prevent potentially treatable dementias.

Conclusion and Policy Implications

An overarching goal of community care for aging populations must be the preservation of their optimal functioning, dignity, and quality of life. It is also important to consider the families of the frail elderly, in part because they are the primary caregivers. Increased social investments that enhance an older individual's self-care capacity, as well as the ability of the family to provide aid, are likely to be both cost effective and preferred by older people (Damron-Rodriguez and Lubben, 2000; Stuck et al., 2000). In particular, ethnically sensitive programming improves the capability of elders to take care of themselves when appropriate and, if necessary, gain access to formal services on their own.

As seen in the case of Little Tokyo, agencies can be effective only when they are an integral part of the overall community. Formal services must not only be culturally appropriate, they also must be delivered in a culturally appropriate manner. When agencies are rooted in ethnic communities, seeking formal help becomes less of an onerous task for ethnic elders. Community-based ethnic agencies face constant pressure to secure funding and donations from the private sector. Care for frail elders must begin by helping ethnic communities strengthen their support systems for older persons and their families, which, in turn, will enable elders to enjoy as much independent living as possible. Increasingly, Japanese Americans will need to work together with other ethnic groups to build an integrated system of community-based care that facilitates the expression of new forms of filial piety in American society.

4

Intimacy at a Distance, Korean American Style: Invited Korean Elderly and Their Married Children

Shin Kim and Kwang Chung Kim

Immigration to the United States from Korea began at the dawn of the twentieth century, in 1903. Nevertheless, the great majority of the current Korean Americans are the post-1965 immigrants and their native- or foreign-born children from South Korea. (Korea was divided into North and South Korea at the conclusion of World War II. From that point on, North Korea has had no diplomatic ties with the United States.) There are two categories of Korean elderly currently living in the United States. The first is those who immigrated to the United States at the invitation of their adult children who were already settled here. Most of these immigrants were elderly at the time of their arrival in the United States. Min (1998) refers to them as the "invited elderly." The other group of Korean elderly is those who immigrated as adults with their own family and who recently reached the age of retirement—the "immigrated elderly," according to Min (1998).

These two types of elderly are quite different. The invited elderly generally have lost a considerable part of their preimmigration socioeconomic resources and status because of their migration. No matter how long they have been in the United States, they are not Americanized. Most of them have only a limited record of employment in this country, if any (Kim, Hurh and Kim, 1993). Therefore, these invited elderly are dependent on their children and the U.S. government for their living. In contrast, the immigrated elderly are expected to be financially independent owing to their long history of work in the United States. Their English proficiency and familiarity with the American system further help their retirement situation. Certainly, they tend to be better off financially and psychologically than the invited elderly (Min, 1998).

A great majority of the current Korean elderly in the United States most probably are the invited elderly, particularly those who are seventy years of age or older. According to the 1990 U.S. census, 35,200 of about 800,000 Korean Americans (4.4 percent) were age sixty-five or over (Yoo and Sung, 1997). Given the relatively short history of Korean immigration to the United States (a little over two decades at the time of the 1990 census), almost all of these older Koreans are presumed to be the invited elderly, although existing data do not provide this level of specificity.

Furthermore, the number of invited elderly is not likely to have increased substantially since the 1990 census. There are two reasons for this. First, there has been a drastic reduction in Korean immigration overall. Second, two 1996 laws—the Personal Responsibility and Work Opportunity Reconciliation Act (PL 104-193) and the Illegal Immigration Reform and Immigrant Responsibility Act (PL 104-208)—made inviting one's elderly parents quite difficult for adult immigrants. Nonetheless, the invited elderly still constitute a great majority of the current Korean American older population. This chapter is thus concerned only with the life experiences of the invited elderly and their relationship with their adult immigrant children.

The Immigration Context and Relevant Questions

Even though the number of Korean Americans is estimated to have reached between 1.3 million and 2 million by the year 2000, the heyday of Korean immigration was in the 1970s and 1980s. During the peak periods, over 34,000 Koreans came here every year. Beginning in 1989, immigration from Korea started to decline sharply, and by the second half of the 1990s it had fallen to less than half that of the peak periods (U.S. Dept. of Justice, 1970–1999). This trend has not shown any sign of reversal despite the recent Korean economic crisis. Unless North Korea unexpectedly opens its door to emigration, the number of new immigrants from Korea is likely to continue to decrease, albeit at a slower rate than previously. This decline has had an important consequence on the composition of the community: the so-called old-timers—those who have been in the United States for more than ten years—constitute the majority of the current Korean immigrant population, including the elderly.

When the invited elderly arrive in the United States, most of them initially live with the family of the adult children who officially invited them. Some live with other married children if the latter need help with child care or a business operation. A small number live with their unmarried children or other relatives. As their length of residence in the United States extends, though, only a small proportion of elderly parents remain with their married children's family; a large majority eventually move out to establish their own home (Kauh, 1997). The 1980 census shows that 75 percent of Korean elderly lived with their children; by the 1990 census, this proportion decreased to 57 percent (Yoo and Sung, 1997). Consequently, we expect that fewer than 50 percent of the invited elderly will be residing with their children's family in the 2000 census. In short, most of the invited Korean elderly now maintain a residence independent of their adult children.

Owing to a huge concentration of Korean immigrants in large metropolitan areas, this phenomenon is likely to be observed more readily in those regions (Yoo and Sung, 1997). Whether they currently live alone or with a spouse, invited Korean elderly parents living independently manage their own daily existence. Surprisingly, when their health no longer permits them to take care of themselves, they are more likely to move into a nursing home than back in with their children. Thus, it appears that most invited Korean elderly not only live independently of their adult children but also prefer such autonomy (Koh and Bell, 1987; Kim, Hurh and Kim, 1991). This leads to the first question, Why do the invited elderly parents prefer an independent residence?

Moreover, elderly parents with an independent residence are generally found to be more satisfied with their current life than those who stay with their children (Koh and Bell, 1987). This observation runs counter to the traditional expectation of filial piety (Kim, Kim and Hurh, 1991). Since the invited elderly are assumed to cling to this traditional expectation, they should be happier when they live with their married children. Considering the fact that these older people are not familiar with the American system, the higher life satisfaction of the independently living elderly is perplexing. In our view, this can be explained by looking at the actual situation in their children's homes. Thus, the second question is, What aspects of the experience of invited elderly parents who live with their married children push them to prefer independent living?

As the invited elderly parents move into their own places, their relationship with their married children is likely go through some transformations. Thus, the third topic explores the question, What is the relationship between the independently living elderly parents and their married children?

This chapter seeks to address these three questions on the basis of previous studies and our 1998 Chicago survey. In addition, we offer some policy suggestions to assist the Korean invited elderly and perhaps other Asian older people who live on their own.

Let us first place these issues in their proper context. Korean immigrants came from a society where most elderly parents still prefer to maintain traditional living arrangements, that is, to reside with their married sons. This is particularly true when the elderly parents do not possess sufficient resources of their own. Although they are currently residing in America, where multigenerational households are the exception, the invited Korean elderly parents are not Americanized. Also, they have lost a considerable portion of their resources through immigration. Typically, then, they do expect their married sons to practice the cultural norm of filial piety and take them into their homes.

This expectation was obvious during interviews we conducted in 1998. A great majority of the invited elderly parents living alone reported that they received more help from their daughters than from their sons. Nevertheless, almost all of them boasted of their sons' assistance and not that of their daughters. One implication we drew from these interviews was that no matter what they professed publicly, these Korean older people held onto the traditional expectation of filial piety. Indeed, there is a deep-down longing to live with one of their married sons. Thus, the invited Korean elderly parents' observed preference for an independent life of self-care is not necessarily an outcome of their transformed cultural norms.

Why Do Invited Elderly Parents Prefer Independent Living?

Mrs. K, eighty-one, lives with her husband in one of the senior citizens' apartment complexes on Sheridan Road in Chicago, where a good number of elderly Koreans reside. The couple immigrated to America in 1983 and lived with their eldest son's family for two years before moving into their current apartment. Her husband's health has been deteriorating over the last several years, and he is temporarily in a nursing home. These days she spends most of her time visiting her husband; in order to do so she must take several buses. "I have to make transfer twice [to get to the nursing home]. It takes more than an hour one way," she sighs. She also misses attending the only Korean adult day care center in town because of the long commute.

She is agitated, nonetheless, by the idea of moving in temporarily with her eldest son, who lives nearby. She emphatically expresses her desire to remain in her own place, despite the inconvenience. At the same time, she is clearly worried that she is giving an incorrect impression of her son. "He is a very good son," she says. "It is just darn too uncomfortable to live with children's family. Since we have this place of our own, why do I want to go back to such a life, even temporarily?"

The traditional family arrangement in Korea is a patrilineal and patrilocal extended family system. The root cause of the invited elderly parents' preference for independent living is the disappearance of this structure among Korean immigrants in America. In a patrilocal family system, married sons and their family are expected either to reside with their parents or live under their strong authority. Both sons and their wives are expected to take care of the parents faithfully (Choi, 1970). Worthiness of wives is often measured in terms of their ability and willingness to attend to their parents-in-law (Hsu, 1971b). In return, married sons keep the right to inherit their parents' wealth. Kin is viewed as a corporate body, with all male siblings maintaining the kinship group. Although this traditional patrilineal and patrilocal family system has been weakened considerably in recent years, it provides the basic framework for, and still exerts a powerful influence in, regulating family and kinship relations in Korea (Kim and Rhee, 1997).

In contrast, the prevalent family type among current Korean immigrants in the United States is quite divergent from the patrilineal and patrilocal extended family. Most Korean immigrants are exposed to a highly industrialized American economy (Kim and Hurh, 1991). As Goode (1963) contends, in such an economy, employment and occupational mobility depend largely on the ability and performance of individual workers. In this situation, family members have independent sources of income, and the head of the extended family has little control over his children's money or careers. Thus, the traditional extended family system weakens, and the conjugal family system emerges. By conjugal family, Goode

(1963) means the nuclear family with an independent residence (a neolocality), a bilateral kinship system (a nearly equal importance between the husband's and wife's kin lines), a narrow range of contact with affinal and blood relatives, and individual freedom of mate selection. Today, Korean immigrant families in the United States are rapidly developing a conjugal family system, with pretty much all of these traits (Kim and Hurh, 1991).

One may argue that the patrilineal family system is fast disappearing in Korea as well. Yet, two crucial elements differentiate the current family system in Korea from that of Korean immigrants. First, most of the invited Korean elderly parents in the United States possess very few resources of their own. They are unfamiliar with the American system and speak limited English. In most cases, their funds have been depleted by the time they arrive in America. In short, their loss of resources due to immigration basically renders them unable to sustain a patrilineal family.

Second, both husbands and wives are employed in almost all Korean immigrant families. (In Korea, married women still face formidable social obstacles if they want to work, and only the husband's breadwinner role is emphasized.) Quite often, wives contribute to the family income as much as husbands. As a result, a patrilineal family system, with an almost exclusive emphasis on male kin lines, is difficult to maintain. These two factors have expedited significantly the demise of the patrilineal and patrilocal family system among Korean immigrants in America.

The emergence of the conjugal family among Korean immigrants has, in turn, modified the basic idea of filial piety. In a traditional patrilineal family, the primary relationship in a family is that between parents and their married sons. If necessary, the sons are expected to sacrifice their marital relations for the sake of this primary one. In contrast, in a conjugal family, the relationship between a married couple is dominant; sons now are expected to forgo their relationship with their own parents, if necessary, in order to protect their marriage.

As mentioned, a high proportion of Korean immigrant wives are employed and make a substantial contribution to the family income. Such a financial contribution inevitably enhances the status and power of wives who do not want their husband's parents to interfere in their life. They are less inclined to sacrifice their marital relationship and family needs for the care of elderly parents-in-law. And resource-depleted invited elderly parents are not able to enforce traditional filial obligations. Thus, the primary family relationship has shifted to a couple-centered one, which, in turn, gradually has led to a new style of family and kinship relations (Kim and Hurh, 1991).

Filial piety traditionally obliges children to support only the sons' parents. As the emerging conjugal family strengthens the bilateral kinship system, making the distinction between male and female lines of kinship contact less sharp, it has become impractical to expect Korean immigrant wives to take care of their husbands' parents exclusively. Married children are now supposed to assist either the husband's or the wife's parents when help is needed (Kim, Kim and Hurh, 1991).

It is not yet a fait accompli among Korean immigrant families, but this new attitude is firmly entrenched.

Another component of traditional filial piety is the primogeniture system. Under this institution, the eldest son receives a greater portion of the inheritance from parents and shoulders the major responsibility for their care. The immigration process considerably disturbs this system of primogeniture. In the United States, the eldest son is not necessarily the one most capable of taking care of elderly parents. Thus, all married children are expected to share this responsibility, regardless of gender or birth order (Kim, Kim and Hurh, 1991). These circumstances lead to an interesting side question: which married child actually assists the parents more actively?

When elderly parents of Korean immigrants arrive in the United States, they are thrust into a family system different from that in Korea. It certainly is a far cry from the one to which they were accustomed. Thus, it is not difficult to imagine the distress they must experience living with their married children. Therefore, many of them prefer to live by themselves. Obviously, the availability of government subsidies greatly enhances their ability to move out. In short, an independent living arrangement is sought by the invited elderly as a relief from stressful conditions that originated from a changed Korean family system in the United States. As more elderly parents establish their own residence, "moving out" may even acquire an aura of fashionability and hence solidify the trend.

Experiences in Establishing Separate Residences

The Elderly Parents' Experience

When parents arrive in the United States, they are generally aware that their children's family system has changed drastically and that filial piety and related intergenerational relationships have been modified. Today, invited elderly parents often state that they do not want to be a burden to their children and that they would like to see their married children keep their family life free of parental interference. Deep in their heart, however, they still cling to the traditional expectation of filial piety, a natural inclination given their own lifelong socialization. In fact, as married young adults, they most likely took care of their parents as traditionally expected (Kim, Kim and Hurh, 1991).

From the perspective of the elderly parents, then, life in their children's homes is often filled with disappointment and grief. As they stay longer, they gradually realize that their adult children and their spouses are struggling much harder than they had imagined to settle their family in the United States, severely limiting the time, ability, and resources available to tend to them. Since the focus of the children has shifted to the needs of the nuclear family, elderly parents have become secondary in their lives (Kim, Kim and Hurh, 1991).

Consequently, elderly parents often feel that they are neglected, slighted, or even humiliated in their children's homes. Some even feel that their physical needs are not met adequately. Quite a few of them suspect that they are neither respected nor consulted on important family matters; their suggestions or advice, even when requested, is considered an interference (Kim, Kim and Hurh, 1991). In short, the invited elderly parents eventually become marginalized in their married children's home. It is true that many of them help with the housework or management of their children's small business. Still, the social condition of the invited Korean elderly parents creates a serious gap between "the expected role of respected elderly and the reality of degrading housekeeping" (Kang and Kang, 1981) or other menial tasks. In addition, many of these older parents experience isolation, since most children live in the suburbs.

Could the invited elderly parents' psychological experience of marginality differ depending on whether they are staying with a daughter's or a son's family? This is most likely the case, given their adherence to the traditional cultural norm of filial piety. Our 1998 interview data provide some information on this issue. First, more elderly parents who came to the United States at the invitation of an eldest son actually lived with them than those invited by an eldest daughter (76 percent and 65 percent, respectively). Second, before moving out, parents who lived with the eldest son had stayed with the family for much longer than those who lived with the eldest daughter (eighty-four months compared to forty-seven months). Third, when asked to describe the emotional experience of living with their children, parents residing with a son (particularly with an eldest son) used expressions like "It was the right thing to do" or "I had a right to do that." On the other hand, for those living with a daughter's family, typical responses include, "It was comfortable but uneasy" or "I felt a little bit guilty or was ashamed." Obviously, living with a son is culturally sanctioned as far as the elderly parents are concerned. Still, our interviews indicate that, overall, the invited elderly parents feel a sense of not belonging to their married children's family.

From the elderly parents' perspective, moving out of their children's home is the only possible relief, if they have the means to establish an independent residence. It certainly also helps to minimize the conflict between them and their children's family by protecting each generation's autonomy and privacy. Unlike American older people, however, the preference of Korean elderly parents for living alone clearly contradicts their traditional beliefs and the lifestyle they experienced in Korea and expected to continue in the United States (Kim, Kim and Hurh, 1991). It is ironic that because elders adhere to the traditional expectation of filial piety, they cannot tolerate the traditional living arrangements as they actually exist in the United States and prefer an independent residence.

Married Children's Experience

On the whole, married Korean Americans are generally in a position that makes it difficult to help their elderly parents. First, as immigrants, they tend to have jobs that require extensive time and involvement. For example, more than half of adult Korean immigrants work in a small business either as owners or employees. Quite often they operate the business for twelve hours a day, six or seven days a week. One can easily imagine their fatigue at the end of the day (Kim and Hurh, 1991). Second, the extremely long hours of work by both husband and wife in most Korean immigrant families severely restrict the time and energy left over for the care of their children, let alone elderly parents.

Their daily life is occupied with the three major adult roles: marital, parental, and work (Kim, Hurh and Kim, 1993). Many Korean immigrant families feel sandwiched between their children and elderly parents. Moreover, they are too busy and sometimes too young to comprehend their parents' stressful life conditions in America, the problems accompanying aging, and their hardships resulting from a limited ability to adapt to new ways. Whether overburdened with their own chores or not cognizant of their parents' life situation, adult children often seem to their elderly parents to be unconcerned. This appearance of insensitivity is sustained by the fact that the parents are usually in no position to help out in daily activities, such as transportation and grocery shopping. In short, whether intended or not, elderly parents may feel neglected, and this situation is likely to lead to a sense of guilt and shame in their children. In addition, elderly parents sometimes create friction between spouses and among siblings (Kim, Hurh and Kim, 1993).

In spite of these difficulties, most Korean immigrant married children maintain a strong sense of obligation to care for their elderly parents (Kim and Hurh, 1991). A great majority of Korean married female immigrants believe that the wives should take care of their parents-in-law as well as their own parents. Husbands also recognize a responsibility to attend to their parents-in-law, if necessary. However, most Korean immigrants no longer believe that the relationship between elderly parents and their married sons should be paramount (Kim and Hurh, 1991).

With these divergent expectations, the daily life of the invited elderly parents and married children under the same roof can easily become dangerously stressful. Therefore, the establishment of an independent residence for elderly parents becomes a sensible remedy. It does not mean, however, that the married children accept their parents' independent living lightly. Being a product of traditional Korean culture, they often feel some guilt and shame when their parents move out. It is our observation that as the size of the elderly population living alone has increased in recent years, along with the availability of social services, children's apprehension over this situation has lessened significantly.

The Relationship between Independently Living Elderly Parents and Married Children

In the analysis of Korean immigrants' intergenerational relationships, it is important to look at the geographic location of both elderly parents and their children.

This issue may be viewed from the perspective of either party. When it is examined from the perspective of elders who currently live in the United States, adult children can be classified into three types, depending on where they reside: (1) in the same metropolitan area as their parents; (2) elsewhere in the United States; or (3) in Korea or some other country besides the United States. Those who live in Korea are usually too far away to provide any meaningful assistance to their parents. All they can do is occasionally call them and send gifts or money. Although it is somewhat easier for children who live in the United States but at a distance, their ability to help is also highly limited. Therefore, a substantial portion of instrumental and expressive care provided to elderly parents comes mainly from children who currently live in the same metropolitan area as their parents.

The invited elderly parents rarely own a house. In fact, almost all of them with independent living arrangements currently reside in government-subsidized senior citizen housing facilities in the downtown areas of major cities. These older people tend to receive Supplementary Security Income (SSI), of which they pay a fraction for rent. In addition, a great majority use food stamps and have their medical bills paid by Medicaid. With such a heavy dependence on government for their daily living, it is not surprising to find most Korean elderly extremely grateful to the U.S. government. Fully aware that they themselves paid no taxes in the United States, they are impressed with the reliable monthly delivery of government checks. Many of them declare that the United States government is their true filial son, even more so than their own children. Furthermore, the life satisfaction of these elders is relatively high (Koh and Bell, 1987; Min, 1998). Still, only a small proportion of them manage to survive solely on government support. Assistance from their married children comes in the form of cash, groceries, or other household items. Many adult children do not send money to their parents on a regular basis but rather on special occasions like birthdays or holidays (Min, 1998).

Today most of the elderly parents have some Korean friends in the same housing complex. These friends provide good daily companionship, sharing everyday experiences and conversation with each other. A high proportion attend Korean ethnic church regularly as well, some going with their children. Many others use a church bus service when available (Kauh, 1997). Some members of the congregation are also their close friends. An ethnic church provides them a spiritual meaning of life as well as ethnic foods and companionship (Min, 1998).

Despite these extrafamilial networks, the independent-living elderly parents nonetheless depend considerably on their children for daily management of living. Such support goes beyond socioemotional and psychological comforts. In order to understand the intergenerational relationship accompanying an older person's independent living, in 1998 we interviewed 103 Korean elderly living in government-subsidized senior apartments in Chicago.

Most of the respondents (94 percent) are currently in their seventies or eighties. The two age groups differ in terms of their health conditions: the majority of those in their seventies report generally good health or some minor physical problems, while most of those age eighty or older indicate some serious health problems.

Most of the respondents (84.5 percent) came here in the 1970s and 1980s. Since they have been living in the United States for more than ten years, they are viewed as the so-called old-timers. Seventy-four respondents (71 percent) are U.S. citizens, and almost all of them have been naturalized since 1994.

Their current age and the timing of their immigration suggest that the majority of them arrived when they were too old to be employable—in their late fifties or sixties. Close to two-thirds of the respondents (62 percent) currently live alone, and the rest (38 percent) reside with their spouses. A great majority of the former are widowed mothers; elderly fathers rarely live alone. SSI was about $496 for a single older person and $775 for a couple in 1998. For almost all of the respondents, along with food stamps, SSI is the major source of income. Though meager, it allows them to enjoy economic independence. With occasional financial and in-kind support from their children, they manage their own daily living. As indicated earlier, the great majority of respondents (86 percent) prefer living on their own.

Two-thirds (65 percent) have four or more children, with a total of 451 for the sample as a whole. Virtually all of their children are currently married, and only a few of them have remained single, either being divorced or widowed. Half of them (111 sons and 110 daughters) live in the Chicago metropolitan area. Each elderly parent has one to three children—with an average of two—in that location. Certainly, the presence of their children in the Chicago metropolitan area is the major reason why the elderly respondents in this study have settled there. Twenty percent of their children (55 sons and 44 daughters) live elsewhere in the United States. About 30 percent of their children (68 sons and 66 daughters) currently reside in Korea. Very few live in countries other than Korea or the United States.

Virtually all of the elderly respondents (94 percent) immigrated at the invitation of their married children. Nearly half of the invited respondents (46 percent) indicate that it was their eldest daughter who extended the offer. Others report that their eldest son (22.3 percent) or other daughters (24.5 percent) invited them to the United States. In only a few cases did other sons (7.5 percent) issue the invitation. When the respondents arrived here, they usually stayed with the sponsoring child's family. In a few cases, they lived with noninviting children who needed child care or other help. The length of their stay with the inviting children's family was affected by both gender and birth order: two-thirds of those invited by the eldest daughter stayed with the sponsoring family for an average of 47.6 months; three-fourths invited by the eldest son stayed for 84.5 months; half of those invited by other daughters stayed for 38.8 months; and half of those invited by other sons stayed for 53.5 months.

These findings demonstrate the delicate state of current expectations of filial piety among Korean immigrants. Married daughters, especially the eldest ones, are significantly more likely to invite their parents to the United States than married sons. After arriving, however, a greater proportion of those invited by sons than by daughters live with the sponsoring family. In fact, these elders stay at their son's homes for a longer period of time. In brief, the findings suggest the emergence of the conjugal family and its accompanying changes in relations among Korean immigrant families. At the same time, owing to the lingering effect of the traditional expectation of filial piety, elderly parents feel most comfortable staying with their sons, particularly those who are the eldest. The length of stay with the eldest daughter is shorter than that with any of the sons. As traditionally expected, many parents still believe that their married daughters belong to the family of their sons-in-law (Kauh, 1997). Quite a few who had lived with their daughter's family after immigrating expressed such an uneasiness.

> Meet Mrs. L., seventy-seven: "I came to Chicago in 1972. My eldest daughter invited me to America because she had a baby son and needed me to take care of him while she went to their store. Yes, I lived with her for five years. But you know, I felt uncomfortable living with my daughter's family. The hardest part was seeing my son-in-law every day. No, no; he, of course, didn't say anything for me to feel that way. It was me who felt I did not belong there pretty much every day for five years. It might seem odd because I was really needed there. No matter, that was how I felt inside."

Most of the studies on the intergenerational relationship between elderly parents and their adult children report that Koreans keep in close contact with each other (Kauh, 1997; Kim, Hurh and Kim, 1993; Koh and Bell, 1987; Yoo and Sung, 1997). In our 1998 interviews, the respondents were asked about the frequency of telephone calls and visits from their children. The data show that they exchange information and opinions as well as provide support and comfort to each other through phone calls.

Our findings by gender and birth order as well as geographic location of children contain both the obvious and the unexpected. Three-fourths of the eldest daughters in the United States call their elderly parents once or more a week, whether they live in the Chicago area or elsewhere in the nation. Approximately two-thirds of the eldest sons, other daughters, and other sons who live in the Chicago area also report calling their parents once a week or more. Those who live elsewhere in the United States phone slightly less frequently than their counterparts in the Chicago area. About 80 percent of the children currently living in Korea call the respondents only few times a year or less. Children living in Korea are not in a position to maintain any meaningful communication with their elderly parents in the United States, creating considerable social and emotional distances between them.

Visits by adult children and their families, however brief, bring joy to the elders. When they meet face-to-face, the interaction is more real for them because of verbal and nonverbal cues. Their understanding of each other becomes deeper and more meaningful, and their children's support is more personal and effective. Many elderly parents eagerly look forward to their children's visits, often preparing presents such as Korean candy for their grandchildren.

Slightly less than half of all children living in the Chicago metropolitan area

(41 percent of eldest daughters, 45 percent of eldest sons, 47 percent of other daughters, and 38 percent of other sons) are found to visit their parents once or more a week. Most of these children (88 percent of eldest daughters, 78 percent of eldest sons, 80 percent of other daughters, and 84 percent of other sons) see their parents at least once a month. In contrast, most of the children who live elsewhere in the United States see their elderly parents only a few times a year (59 percent of eldest daughters, 80 percent of eldest sons, 71 percent of other daughters, and 70 percent of other sons). The majority of children who live in Korea manage to see their elderly parents even less frequently than once a year.

The respondents were also asked to indicate which child has been the most helpful in their daily living on the whole. Thirty percent of those who responded to this question note that they have more than one child who provides considerable assistance. Nevertheless, the eldest daughter is the most frequently mentioned, being identified as the most helpful by nearly a quarter of the respondents. Eldest sons were named next (13 percent), followed by other daughters (12 percent) and other sons (8 percent). Nearly 15 percent of the respondents indicate that they do not have any helpful children. Interestingly, the data suggest that sons aid their elderly parents when they face financial difficulties while daughters offer other types of support. Eldest daughters are found to keep closer and warmer ties with their elderly parents than any other children, including the eldest sons.

In summary, the Korean invited elderly parents who maintain an independent living arrangement are not necessarily isolated from their children. The latter keep close ties with their parents by telephone calls and visits. Obviously, the closest and most frequent contacts can occur when the child(ren) and elderly parents are living in the same metropolitan area. Those living at a distance, particularly in other countries, are limited in their ability to retain close contacts.

Second, invited Korean elderly parents depend substantially on the U.S. government for their daily living. Financial support from children is available, but it is secondary or minor and infrequent. As a result, adult children feel less economic stress in helping their parents (Kauh, 1997). In fact, a great majority of Korean adult children today would be financially hard-pressed to fully support their parents in a separate residence. Moreover, living with a child's family may create frictions in the latter's marital relations. The tension is likely to spill over to other siblings as well. In this sense, old-age social welfare programs are key to the well-being of both the parents and the children.

Third, the degree to which married children take care of their parents' needs depends primarily on two factors. As already reviewed, the first is the location of their current residence. The major instrumental and expressive supports can be provided mainly by children who live nearby. Even among those who live in the same metropolitan area as their parents, our study shows that the degree of their contact is related both to gender and to birth order. Unlike the traditional pattern of filial behavior, it is now married daughters who most actively support their parents. In addition, for both sons and daughters, birth order is an important factor in explaining the frequency of children's contact with their parents. Eldest children have the most contact, with daughters being far more active than sons in supporting their parents.

Another study, however, reports different results. Kauh (1997) concludes that sons are generally more active than daughters; among them, the eldest provide the most care for their parents. In fact, this study contends that elderly parents tend to live independently of their children when they have only daughters in America and to live together with their sons. Thus, the core of the traditional expectation of filial piety appears to remain intact. This finding is curiously at odds with our observations as well as some other studies (e.g., Yoo and Sung, 1997: Kim, 2000).

On the whole, most studies suggest the importance of gender and birth order in explaining the extent of children's support of their parents in the United States, revealing the Korean version of "intimacy at a distance." That is, invited Korean elderly parents and their married children maintain separate living arrangements, just as Americans do. Unlike Americans, though, immigrant Korean married children maintain a sense of filial obligation. This is a norm sanctioned by their culture. At the same time, there is clear evidence of change in the expectation and practice of filial piety, especially in terms of gender and birth order. In short, the Korean American version of intimacy at a distance reveals an adaptation to a changed environment.

Conclusion and Policy Implications

Currently the invited elderly constitute the majority of Korean older people in the United States, though their numbers have been declining since the 1990s. They are a specific group who immigrated here at their children's request. A great majority of them came in the 1970s and 1980s; few have arrived from Korea in recent years. In contrast to those immigrant older people who have a considerable employment history in America and therefore are self-reliant, the invited elderly are almost entirely dependent on the U.S. government and/or their adult children for support.

Most invited Korean elderly parents live separately from their married children, an arrangement that may seem odd given their cultural background and lack of resources. This chapter has attempted to explain why these older people seem to prefer living on their own and how they are able to do so. SSI and other government programs clearly facilitate their ability to move out of their children's homes. The primary stimulus, however, is the pursuit of the middle-class dream of suburban home ownership among young Korean immigrant families, which makes it necessary for both husbands and wives to work for long hours. Quite often, married children invite their parents to help with child care so that wives can remain employed. The elderly parents inevitably experience a cultural shock when actually living with their children's family.

The extent of uneasiness likely depends on the degree to which the elderly parents adhere to the traditional expectation of filial piety. They tend to stay at their eldest sons' homes significantly longer than at those of their eldest daughters, even though it is more often the daughter who invited them here. Thus, it appears that parents feel less discomfort living with their son's family than with their daughter's. Nonetheless, parents eventually feel marginalized at their children's homes, prompting them to move out. Once separate homes are established, elders and their married children maintain a close contact that exhibits both Korean and American cultural traits, or what we have dubbed the Korean American version of intimacy at a distance. One adaptation has been in the sharing of filial obligation among all children, regardless of gender or birth order.

The practice of intimacy at a distance is only possible if public programs are available. Today, there is a widely accepted myth about Korean and other Asian immigrants; they are viewed as model minorities who, because they are highly committed to the traditional expectation of filial piety, are able to solve their family problems without government supports. As shown here, however, this does not reflect the current reality of Korean immigrant family and kinship relations. The myth nonetheless has led the U.S. government to cut back on aid. We must realize that the elderly cannot manage their daily living without government supports.

In this regard, the 1996 Personal Responsibility and Work Opportunity Reconciliation Act (PL 104-193), which severely limits the nonnaturalized elderly's access to public programs, is myopic at best. Not only must the invited elderly wait at least five years to apply for U.S. citizenship but also the process of naturalization is arduous for them. Moreover, the requirement under the Illegal Immigration Reform and Immigrant Responsibility Act (PL 104-208) that sponsoring adult children must support their nonnaturalized parents does not take into account the reality of their lives. These laws are detrimental to the well-being of both the elderly and their adult children, and as such must be repealed.

Furthermore, government supports must be formulated with a consideration of the unique needs of these elderly. For example, there is a long waiting list in many senior citizen housing complexes in the Chicago area; Korean elderly need a lot more of these facilities than are currently available. Also, since Korean and other Asian invited elderly are not Americanized, such housing must be staffed by bilingual social workers and offer ethnic programs. Finally, Korean elderly and their children require a greater availability of ethnic social services, including adult day care centers.

5

Caring for Elderly Vietnamese Americans

Thanh Van Tran, Dung Ngo, and Tricia H. Sung

This chapter addresses issues involving the care of older Vietnamese Americans. When people grow old in a foreign society, they are compelled to modify their conception of the aging process in order to adhere to the cultural expectations of their host society. Immigrants and refugees are uprooted from their traditional society and social networks. For many, growing old in a foreign society requires a socialization that is often totally different from the one that they had acquired during their youth.

The goal of this chapter is to provide a preliminary analysis of the issues and problems concerning how to care for elderly Vietnamese Americans in their host society. These issues are examined through focus group meetings and in-depth interviews with a number of Vietnamese elderly, children, and community leaders. The chapter begins with a brief overview of the roles of the elderly in traditional Vietnamese society. The overview is followed by a description of the history of immigration and resettlement of the Vietnamese American community, the economic status of the Vietnamese community in America, and the means of caring for the Vietnamese-American elderly.

Aging and the Status of Old Age in Traditional Vietnamese Society

Unlike many Western societies in which the aging process has been subjected to scientific research and analyses, the Vietnamese have simply accepted aging as a fact of life without challenging why and how human beings grow old and die. Instead of questioning the aging process, they have celebrated longevity and prepared for their death when they can. In traditional Vietnamese culture, old age had been considered a leisured period of one's life. Because of the relatively short life expectancy of the general population in Vietnam, the oldest person in a village was considered elderly even when that person was fifty years old or younger. In ancient times, Vietnamese people got married at a young age (sixteen for men and thirteen for women), became grandparents in their mid-thirties, and became great-grandparents in their forties. Thus, the process of aging is considered more a function of changing social status than a specific chronological marker.

Traditional conceptualizations of aging in Vietnamese society are discussed to provide a background for better understanding the present perceptions of aging among Vietnamese Americans. It is important to distinguish clearly between the traditional Vietnamese community and culture within Vietnam and the Vietnamese American community and culture in the United States. Vietnamese Americans brought with them traditional values; however, these values have either been abolished, modified, or replaced by new cultural values as Vietnamese immigrants have acculturated into their host society.

As in many traditional societies (Keith, 1982), old age is respected and valued in traditional Vietnamese society (Toan, 1965). The older a person is, the higher his social status. For example, in the traditional village festival, the most important ceremony (Dai Te) was performed by men who were the elders or people with the highest education in the village (Le, 1992) Old people were respected because of their experience, skills, knowledge, and wisdom. They were also respected because of their longevity. Although elderly men and women are equally respected, the issue of social status is considered more important for men than for women.

During the greeting season, such as the Vietnamese lunar new year, people wish each other longevity. The formal words (Mung Tuoi) for the New Year greeting in Vietnamese literally means "congratulations for living one more year of age." In the wedding ceremony, people also wish the new couple longevity. Vietnamese children are taught to respect their elders so that they too can expect to live a long life (Kinh lao dac tho). Respect for old age has been shown in many ways. As Trung Vu Le (1992) reported, in the village of Lieu Doi, in the former North Vietnam, every year on the seventh day of the New Year celebrations villagers build a temporary thatched tent called the longevity tent where the elderly congregate. The people in the village came to wish happy New Year and to pay respect to the village elders. In many villages, it was a tradition to celebrate a longevity day. On that day, villagers organized a procession to honor the elderly in the village. The elderly were escorted around the community, and villagers offered their congratulations and wishes to the elderly. Villagers took turns bringing food and gifts to the communal hall to celebrate the longevity day (Cuu and Toan, 1967; Nhat, 1968; Toan, 1965; Dao, 1961).

These celebrations in honor of aging were more common among the wealthy and those of higher social classes than among ordinary people. Not all of the elderly who were interviewed in this study reported that they observed longevity day or the celebration of old age for their parents. It also should be noted that many traditional ceremonies were abjured by Vietnamese Catholics because they were taught by Catholic missionaries that such ceremonies are "superstitions."

Caring for the Elderly in Traditional Vietnamese Society

The traditional civil code required that children take care of their elderly parents. Those who mistreated their elderly parents were punished by caning, with a maximum of eighty lashes. However, the punishment was enforced only when elderly parents filed a formal complaint against their children (Dao, 1961). It is unusual for abused or neglected parents to bring their children to court, because of the fear of losing face among their neighbors and relatives.

A study of an ancient North Vietnamese village found a formal written village code of social conduct that specifically required villagers to assist the elderly. The village law stated that "anyone who met an elderly person on a street carrying heavy things must assist that elderly person. Those who ignored such an elderly [person] were subject to punishment" (Phan, 1992: 90). Contemporary Vietnamese family codes require that all children share equal responsibility for the care of their parents when they are unable to take care of themselves. Likewise, grandchildren are responsible for their grandparents' economic well-being if they do not have sufficient sources of support (T. G. Nguyen, 1993).

Age and Social Clubs in Traditional Villages

In many traditional villages, there are social clubs for people of different ages (Phan, 1992). For example, there is a club for children who herd water buffaloes (Hoi Muc Dong), a club for the elderly (Hoi Lao), and a club for older women and older widows (Hoi Chu Ba). Every social club has its own rules and regulations. The clubs serve the dual role of enforcing social control and offering social support to their members. Quang Ngoc Nguyen (1993) studied a number of traditional villages in North Vietnam and noted that in the Da Nguu village, men aged fifty or older belonged to the village elderly club, which was responsible for revising the village's religious and social ceremonies and providing support to members of families whose elderly members had died.

Vietnamese American Elderly Clubs

The contemporary elderly club in Vietnam as well as similar clubs overseas still provide social support to members in comparable situations. In the United States, these elderly clubs typically exist in areas where there are large concentrations of Vietnamese Americans. Members of the club get together at least a few times a year. Most gatherings celebrate major social, cultural, or religious events within the Vietnamese community.

The Vietnamese elderly club in Boston annually celebrates the Vietnamese lunar new year, or the Tet. Club members gather at a local senior center or the Vietnamese social service center. Members come to congratulate each other on their longevity and to thank their ancestors. The ceremony often begins with the burning of incense in front of a national ancestral altar. Thereafter, an elderly person reads a brief speech reviewing the club's activities and offering congratulations and good wishes to all members. The person selected to give the speech is often the most highly educated. Typically, elderly men were selected to give the formal speech at the Tet ceremony. However, recent changes in gender relations and roles among elderly Vietnamese Americans have led to opportunities for elderly women to fulfill the honored role of speaker.

The Changing Status of the Vietnamese Elderly

Before being exposed to Western civilization, Vietnamese society and culture were considered static. People were born, grew up, got married, had children, worked, grew old, and died according to a set of well-defined traditions and customs. During the twentieth century, French, Americans, Communists, and the Soviet Union exerted major influences on Vietnamese culture. As a result, many elderly Vietnamese gradually lost power and status because they did not adapt quickly to the rapidly changing world. The introduction of Roman Catholicism dramatically changed many traditional values and customs. This is illustrated in Vietnamese Catholic villages where the buildings were designed so that the church stands in the center of the village. The power and respect traditionally accorded to village elders were transferred to the priest and other clergy members.

One of the most significant factors that has changed the status of the elderly is the long period of revolution and war in Vietnam. For more than a hundred years, the Vietnamese have been at war constantly with the French and with themselves. The colonial domination of the French and the civil war involving the Americans practically destroyed the traditional fabric of Vietnamese society and family. Young men and women left their villages to look for work in French-owned mines, factories, and rubber, coffee, and tea plantations, leaving behind their elderly parents. Young men who once provided economic support to their elderly parents were killed or had to leave their parents because of the war. The division of the country in 1954 also destroyed several northern villages because many people decided to flee to the south to avoid Communism. One elderly woman noted that almost all of the families in her village fled to the south, and only a few families decided to stay. Forced migration no doubt also changed the roles and status of the elderly.

Research on migration has found that young people are more likely to make faster and more successful adjustments than older people. Although migration within a country is somewhat less traumatic than emigration, it still uproots a person from his or her familiar social network and support system. The elderly interviewed in this study revealed that it is very difficult for an older person to make friends and build a new support system in a foreign environment. For many, true friendship requires time and shared memories or histories. People who did not grow up together or who do not share the same memories of historical events may not have ties that bind them together.

Life in a Vietnamese village is somewhat isolated from the outside world. Each village has its own history and culture. In many cases, people who lived in the same village were trained for a specific trade or craft. Therefore, a person leaving his village to go to another one often would experience marked difficulties in adjusting to the new life as well as facing potential ostracism by members of the new village.

Like older people in other societies, the Vietnamese elderly have experienced a gradual loss of status due to technological advancements. Modernity has brought changes in all aspects of life. For example, with modern transportation, people are able to move from place to place in a relatively short period of time. Many of them are willing and can afford to move away from their place of birth to find economic opportunities or personal fulfillment elsewhere. New knowledge and skills are needed to survive in a technological environment. The ability to use a computer and navigate the Internet is now a necessary skill. The traditional power associated with the elderly has weakened, and in some cases disappeared, because they lack the capabilities needed in this rapidly changing, technology-based world.

Immigration and Aging among Vietnamese Americans

Even though migration from one village to another within Vietnam often proved devastating for many elderly because it uprooted them from their familiar environment and support systems, at least they were still surrounded by people who spoke the same language and shared the same national identity and culture. Emigration to another country is beyond the imagination of most young and old Vietnamese. Historically, the Vietnamese people have emigrated to countries such as Cambodia, France, Laos, and Thailand. However, in 1975 a large group of Vietnamese involuntarily emigrated to several Western countries. More than one hundred thousand Vietnamese emigrated to the United States. Since then, the Vietnamese population in this country has increased more than six hundred times.

During the French colonial period, some Vietnamese emigrated to France or its territories. However, the political upheaval of 1975 spurred the largest exodus of Vietnamese to foreign countries in the nation's four thousand years of history. A large number of Vietnamese people emigrated to the United States because of America's involvement in Vietnam.

Economic and Social Status of Elderly Vietnamese Americans

Among Asian American populations, the Vietnamese are one of the poorest groups. More than 25 percent of the Vietnamese population live below the poverty level compared with the national average of 13 percent. The national average per capita income was $14,143 compared to $9,032 among the Vietnamese (U.S. Census, 1993a). The majority of elderly Vietnamese Americans are poor because of their short length of residence in the United States. The Old Age Insurance (OAI) component of the Social Security Act mandates that a worker contribute to the system for at least ten years or forty quarters in order to qualify for benefits (Angel and Angel, 1997). Only immigrants who arrived from the mid- to late 1970s in their forties and early fifties could meet these eligibility requirements, and many of them have a private pension set aside as well. Immigrants who arrived in their late fifties often were unemployed. Even if they were able to find a job, they tended to earn little more than minimum wage, and/or they did not meet the required years of employment for Social Security benefits.

Many elderly Vietnamese who were employed continuously for eighteen years could not acquire adequate wealth to retire comfortably. Like other lower-socioeconomic-status elderly, the Vietnamese have limited sources of income and wealth.

> Mr. Hai Nguyen arrived in the United States at the end of the Vietnam War in 1975. After spending a few months in a refugee camp, his family was sponsored by an American family in Grand Rapids, Michigan. He resettled his family there and found a job in a warehouse of a paper company. He was forty-seven years old when he was initially employed, and he worked for the same company for eighteen years until his retirement at sixty-five years old. Mr. Hai Nguyen is one of the few elderly Vietnamese Americans who had been employed long enough to qualify for Social Security and to earn a private pension. His income, including both Social Security and private retirement benefits, is approximately $1,200 a month.
>
> Since his retirement, his wife left him, and he is now living with his daughter. He does not have to spend his income on housing, food, and clothing because his daughter helps him financially. If he had no children to live with, he would have to spend a major percentage of his income for housing and basic necessities. Compared to many of his Vietnamese American peers, he is a wealthy retiree. He is also relatively healthy and can do almost everything by himself except that he needs transportation and language translation assistance for his medical and social services.
>
> At this time his major health problem is poor vision. Although he can still function independently, caring for him is sometimes stressful for his daughter's family. She and her husband take turns providing transportation and translation when visiting eye doctors and going to church. Both his daughter and her husband are highly educated, and therefore they can provide for his needs. The family has begun to prepare for the time when he will no longer be able to perform his activities of daily living independently. It will be impossible for his daughter to give up her job to take care of him. At the same time, she is raising her own children.

Many elderly Vietnamese Americans are not as fortunate as Mr. Hai Nguyen. They do not have Social Security benefits or children who can afford to fulfill the traditional responsibility of providing both economic and social support. Many elderly Vietnamese Americans are aware that they are a burden on their children even though such caregiving is a traditional value. Given the choice, they would not want to depend on their children.

Socially, many elderly Vietnamese Americans are isolated. For those who live in neighborhoods that have no other Vietnamese families, social isolation is a fact of life. These elderly often are locked in their homes twenty-four hours a day without any meaningful social activities. Some take care of their grandchildren or do housework. Others are completely idle. The paucity of newspapers and television and radio programs in Vietnamese widens the gap between the elderly at home and the outside English-speaking world. Lack of transportation and language barriers are the two greatest issues facing many elderly Vietnamese Americans today.

Issues of Long-Term Care for Elderly Vietnamese Americans

Caring for the elderly is becoming an increasingly urgent issue within the Vietnamese American family and community, but because the elderly Vietnamese constitute approximately 2.3 percent of the total Vietnamese American population, most Vietnamese Americans do not pay attention to this issue. Many Vietnamese adults are more concerned about their present needs than their long-term needs. The typical Vietnamese adult is more worried about how to pay for housing and household bills than preparing for retirement through 401(k)s or IRAs.

This systemic lack of interest in the future often reflects a psychological need to focus on the present in order to survive, which could be attributed to the long-term effects of war. The majority of the Vietnamese arrived in the United States from a war-torn environment where people were only concerned about their day-to-day survival. Few people had any sense of control over their future. This learned helplessness profoundly affects the way they plan and prepare for their future. For the most part, Vietnamese Americans feel they have more control over their ability to satisfy their short-term needs than the long-term needs of a distant and uncertain future. This psychological phenomenon has influenced the attitudes of many elderly Vietnamese Americans toward their own old age as well as the overall aging process.

Health, welfare, and social service systems in the United States are, for the most part, still too complicated for many elderly Vietnamese Americans and their families. The inability of many Vietnamese to understand or navigate the medical and social service systems prevents many elderly Vietnamese persons from using services available in their communities. In addition, the majority of Vietnamese Americans do not have an adequate command of the English language. More than 92 percent of Vietnamese Americans speak Vietnamese at home, and 65 percent of them do not speak English well (U.S. Census, 1993a).

Unless local health, welfare, and social service organizations employ bilingual and culturally sensitive Vietnamese outreach workers to assist the elderly population, many elderly Vietnamese Americans will continue to be left out of the system. For example, of forty possible social and medical services that may be needed by disabled individuals and their families, all require that elderly Vietnamese individuals understand the English language in order to fully participate in or use these services (Binstock, 1998). The real challenge for elderly Vietnamese Americans and their families is to be able to access and use available health and social services that could markedly improve their quality of life.

Like the majority of elderly Americans (Binstock, 1998), elderly Vietnamese Americans do not like to live in nursing homes. However, there is a myth within the Vietnamese American community that all elderly individuals in the United States will eventually end up living in nursing homes. Many are frightened of the possibility that their children will abandon them in nursing homes where they will be completely socially, emotionally, and linguistically isolated. Elderly Vietnamese Americans who participated in some of the authors' focus groups and in-depth interviews have expressed a desire to live independently, but they also realize the economic, linguistic, and social realities requiring them to live with their children. Given the choice, most elderly Vietnamese individuals would prefer to live independently.

There is a cultural dilemma among many Vietnamese families concerning who is responsible for the care of their elderly parents. Many children still believe that it is their responsibility, and this is embedded in their cultural values. At the same time, they also face the reality that they are unable to devote all of their time, energy, and resources to this role. The struggle between traditional cultural values and the current breakdown of the extended family and traditional social networks has left many Vietnamese families with elderly parents in turmoil. Within the traditional Vietnamese extended family, brothers and sisters take turns caring for their elderly parents. Siblings share the responsibility of caregiving so that no single child is the parents' sole caregiver. An elderly parent who experiences a personal conflict with one child can easily move to live with another child; this helps to defuse many familial conflicts.

In addition to the disintegration of the extended family system, acculturation and assimilation pose new challenges for caring for elderly Vietnamese Americans. Many of them have sons or daughters married to non-Vietnamese-speaking individuals. Cultural and language differences between elderly parents and their sons- or daughters-in-law are very real and often threaten the continuation of the family caregiving system within the first generation of Vietnamese American families, as the following case example shows.

> Mrs. Pham is a sixty-nine-year-old widow who is still mentally and physically active. Unlike the majority of elderly Vietnamese American women, she is able to drive and has functional use of English. She has three daughters and two sons. They are all married and live in different parts of the United States. Two of her daughters married white American men. Her oldest son is divorced, and the youngest son is married to a white American woman. She cannot live with her non-Vietnamese sons- and daughter-in-law because of cultural conflicts and problems with commu-

nication. Nor can she live with her divorced son, because divorce is disgraceful to many elderly Vietnamese individuals.

The only daughter she can live with is the one who married a Vietnamese man. Nevertheless, there are many familial problems attributed to her interference in her daughter's family matters. For example, she and her daughter have different views on how to raise children, and this disagreement has created many conflicts within the family. On several occasions, she has threatened to move back to Vietnam or to move out to live by herself. This situation has been a constant source of emotional and physical stress for her daughter's entire family.

Intergenerational conflicts often affect the quality of long-term care for elderly Vietnamese Americans. During the course of the focus groups and in-depth interviews, some elderly expressed their reluctance to ask their children for help because of poor communication within the family. On average, an elderly Vietnamese American is more likely to live with a child than reside alone or with nonrelatives. Therefore long-term care is no doubt a family matter and responsibility for adult Vietnamese children. For the first generation of Vietnamese Americans, taking care of their parents' long-term care often involves offering linguistic services, transportation, and day care. These three areas directly affect the physicial and emotional care that the elderly parent receives.

Vietnamese American women still play the dominant role in caring for their elderly parents. A typical Vietnamese caregiver is middle-aged, has children, and works outside of her home in order to provide for the family's needs. Therefore, caring for an elderly parent, especially a frail one, is physically and emotionally stressful. Familial relationships and responsibilities are continuously being tested. A female caregiver said in a focus group that "I have to take care of my mother, who had a stroke, and it's almost impossible for a person to do everything for her, especially taking her to the bathroom and cleaning her. I just couldn't do it all by myself."

In some situations, Vietnamese men have to care for their parents when there are no women in the family or when their wives refuse to perform certain chores. A well-educated man in his late fifties talks about his caregiving experiences:

> I have to do things that my wife refuses to do for my frail mother, such as bathing and changing her. My wife does not mind cooking, washing, and looking after her, but she just won't provide assistance when my mother needs to defecate or unirate. I can't force her to do things she does not like. At the end, it is my mother. I suspect she would do these things for her own mother.

Most caregivers agree that government services such as translation, transportation, home care, and day care for their parents would be a tremendous help. Most elderly Vietnamese do not speak English and cannot drive or use public transportation. Having someone available to provide transportation and translation is essential for the well-being of both the elderly and their adult children. For the most part, all health and social services agencies require that the elderly Vietnamese speak English and have transportation to gain access to available services.

The following is a case example of a daughter struggling to care for her elderly parent.

> Mrs. and Mr. Nguyen work full time to support their family. They have a ten-year-old son and a six-year-old daughter. Mrs. Lan Nguyen works from 6:00 a.m. to 2:00 p.m. Her husband works between 5:00 p.m. and 1:00 a.m. By working different shifts, they can ensure that someone will always be available to take care of the children.
>
> This system worked fairly well until Mrs. Lan Nguyen's seventy-year-old father arrived from Vietnam to live with them. Mrs. Lan Nguyen was extremely happy to finally be able to bring her elderly father to live with her in the United States. She had felt extremely guilty about leaving him behind for several years. However, problems soon developed when her father needed health care and began to feel socially isolated. It was impossible for Mrs. Lan Nguyen to take time off from work to bring him for medical or dental appointments.
>
> Even when she is able to take her father to see a doctor, he refuses to discuss his health problems in front of her, despite his inability to communicate with the doctor in English. During the weekend, there are not many places that she can bring him for recreation or entertainment. Her family life is chaotic and difficult because of her elderly father's needs.

Mrs. Lan Nguyen's situation is similar to the stories of many Vietnamese middle-aged children who are taking care of their elderly parents. Unlike many elderly Americans born in the United States, most elderly Vietnamese Americans neither own a home nor have enough (or any) savings to live independently from their children.

Data collected from focus groups suggest that elderly Vietnamese Americans do not want to live in nursing homes or any kind of assisted living facilities. There is the general belief that only the elderly who are abandoned by their children and relatives end up in nursing homes. Elderly people are afraid of nursing homes and assisted living facilities because they do not want to live in unfamiliar settings with strangers who do not speak the same language, eat the same food, or share the same cultural understanding. They are afraid of becoming completely isolated. An elderly Vietnamese woman who visited a frail friend in a nursing home said, "She does not have any children or relatives. I visit her and bring her Vietnamese food. There [is] no Vietnamese food in the nursing home and my friend really missed the food she used to eat."

Home-based health and social services are preferred by both the elderly Vietnamese and their caregivers. They also would like these services to be provided by well-trained Vietnamese persons. Overall, there is an urgent need for skilled

Vietnamese and Vietnamese-speaking professionals to provide all types of assistance to the elderly in the Vietnamese American communities.

Conclusion and Policy Implications

In this chapter we have examined the issues of aging and long-term care within the Vietnamese American family and community. When people migrate to a new culture and society, they must acculturate to their host society to survive. Through this process of acculturation, individuals are compelled to assimilate aspects of their new culture while attempting to retain at least some of the customs and values of their homeland. It will take several generations for the Vietnamese American population to transform their experiences into a unique cultural identity within the host society. Each generation of Vietnamese Americans will grow old in a slightly different manner, and each will have different long-term care needs.

For the first generation of elderly Vietnamese Americans, our focus group data point to some critical issues that deserve attention from politicians, professionals, and Vietnamese community leaders:

1. Health and social service providers should establish culturally appropriate outreach programs to elderly Vietnamese Americans who are isolated from the general community because of language barriers and the lack of transportation.
2. Information about existing health and social services for the elderly should be made available to prospective Vietnamese caregivers in Vietnamese and English.
3. Home care for frail elderly should be culturally appropriate and meet the needs of both the elderly and their caregivers within the Vietnamese family context.
4. Prevention of elder abuse within the Vietnamese family should be a priority among health care and social service providers.
5. Community senior centers should reach out to elderly Vietnamese Americans by hiring Vietnamese-speaking staff and providing culturally appropriate services (e.g., recreation and food) as well as language skill training (e.g., conversational English or using the Internet in English)
6. Different options in long-term-care facilities, including nursing homes and assisted living facilities, should be designed to meet the cultural needs of Vietnamese American elders and their families (e.g., assisted living and group homes run by Vietnamese professionals).
7. Health and social service organizations should recruit and train Vietnamese persons to work with elderly Vietnamese.
8. Educational outreach programs in Vietnamese American communities should be implemented to encourage young and middle-aged Vietnamese

Americans to address critical aging issues as well as plan for their own long-term care.

9. Church- or temple-based caregiver-support groups should be promoted in Vietnamese communities. Not only do organized religious institutions have the infrastructure necessary to form social support groups but elderly Vietnamese Americans also tend to participate in them.

6

Care Options for Older Mexican Americans: Issues Affecting Health and Long-Term Care Service Needs

Barbara C. Du Bois, Carol H. Yavno, and E. Percil Stanford

The older Mexican American population is increasing in size faster than other Latino groups and is growing more rapidly than other age cohorts within the Mexican American population. The rates of growth are exceeding those in the United States overall, making Latinos the second largest ethnic group after Caucasians (Suarez and Ramirez, 1998; Villa et al., 1993). Older Mexican Americans have higher levels of disability, substantially greater need for long-term care services, and a pattern of underutilization of available services. They will remain underserved, with substantial care burdens placed on families, unless effective and culturally appropriate innovations are implemented in the formal as well as the informal long-term care service sector.

This chapter will focus on how Mexican Americans' long-term care preferences, access to services, and options for care are influenced by their culture, socioeconomic conditions, and family supports as well as structural barriers within existing health and long-term care systems. It also will develop programmatic and policy recommendations, with potential applications for practitioners in the acute care and long-term care service fields, those in the helping professions, government representatives, and policy advisers. Implications for the private and public service sectors will be discussed in the context of current cost-containment efforts.

This work will highlight the delivery and management of care systems for functionally impaired elderly. It will examine current literature regarding socioeconomic and demographic changes under way in the Latino community and their impacts on older Mexican Americans; levels of need and the nature of the problems faced by older Mexican Americans; and long-term care delivery issues and care options for an increasingly older group of at-risk elderly. This chapter will provide recommendations for enhancing the effectiveness of the long-term care delivery system for the Mexican American community, including an analysis of the kinds of services they and their caregivers are most likely to use.

Throughout the discussion, "Latino" is used instead of "Hispanic" to describe Mexican Americans. Not only is it more culturally appropriate for those who consider themselves Latin, but growing numbers of Mexican Americans, Cuban Americans, and Puerto Ricans identify themselves as such.

The field of Latino ethnogeriatrics began in the early 1970s in response to increasing demographic changes in the Latino groups nationally (Villa et al., 1993). Researchers identified serious age-related issues for the Cuban American, Puerto Rican, and Mexican communities. Between 1970 and 1980 the number of older Latinos increased 61 percent. Throughout the United States there was a growing visibility of older Latinos who resided mostly in Latino communities within large metropolitan areas. At the same time, Mexican American and Puerto Rican families became more mobile, with many Mexican American families traveling from coast to coast. Researchers began focusing on who would provide care to an increasingly older non-English-speaking group, what kinds of services they would need, and what medical insurance systems would be available. Other concerns included issues related to health and life satisfaction; the availability of family support; migration and isolation of immigrants; acculturation; the impact of these factors on retirement; and health and human services (Cuellar, Harris and Jasso, 1980; Weeks and Cuellar, 1983).

Latino elders represent a diverse group of nationalities that include Mexican Americans (both American-born and Mexico-born), Puerto Ricans, Cubans, Indians from southern Mexico and Central American countries, and other Latinos from the Caribbean and Central and South America. Currently, there is an expanding literature on older Mexican Americans; however, the literature base is uneven. Moreover, knowledge of Mexican Americans is more extensive than for the other Latino subgroups, with the least on Salvadorans and Indian immigrants.

Most Latinos are Mexican Americans located in the southwestern states of Arizona, California, Colorado, New Mexico, and Texas, with roughly three-quarters divided between California and Texas. Approximately 10 percent of Latinos are Cubans located in Florida and Puerto Ricans in New York. As a group, Latino adults are concentrated in cities, with approximately 90 percent located in urban areas. One out of every five adults has completed less than five years of schooling (Villa et al., 1993). They suffer from high unemployment rates, substantial poverty (approximately 30 percent of families live below the poverty level, in contrast to 15 percent of the overall U.S. population), and lack of adequate housing. They spend more of their disposable income on health care, do not have adequate health insurance coverage, and in many cases have no insurance whatsoever (Pousada, 1995). Fully one-third do not have such coverage, compared to 11 percent of the U.S. population. Although many qualify for medical benefits through public assistance programs, a large number of Latinos are considered the "working poor." They commonly are in occupations that provide few benefits. Although their wages are low, they do not qualify for public assistance; yet, they cannot afford private insurance.

Because of financial constraints, these families commonly postpone medical treatment until it is absolutely necessary; emergency room services often become their source of primary care. In fact, utilization rates of emergency rooms for Latinos are twice as high as for non-Latino whites (White-Means, Thornton and Yeo, 1989). The majority of medical care is received through large public hospitals with rotating staffs. Thus, for many Latino families, medical care is sporadic, discontinuous, and lacking in preventive services (Pousada, 1995).

Sociodemographic and Economic Factors

Sociodemographic and economic circumstances have a significant impact on the health of Mexicans in general and older Mexicans in particular. Most Mexican Americans today are of mestizo origin (mixed heritage of Spanish and Indian). More recently, in-migration of Indians from southern Mexico and Central American countries has increased Indian representation in the United States.

Nationally, the fastest-growing cohort in the United States is that of older Latinos (Villa et al., 1993; Williams, 1991). According to census data, the number of Latino adults over age sixty-five is estimated to increase from 906,000 in 1987 to 5.6 million in less than fifty years; older Mexican Americans are expected to account for the largest expansion (Villa et al., 1993). Of the 22 million Latinos presently in the United States, 61 percent or 13.4 million are of Mexican origin (Suarez and Ramirez, 1998). By 2010, the Latino population will increase to 41 million or 13 percent of the total U.S. population (Suarez and Ramirez, 1998).

Mexican Americans are the youngest of all Latino groups. Their median age is twenty-five, compared to twenty-seven for other Latinos (Suarez and Ramirez, 1998). Those over age sixty-five represent 5 percent of the total Mexican population as compared to 20 percent for Cubans, indicating even further the particularly young age structure of the Mexican American community in the United States.

Mexicans also have higher mortality rates at all ages than other Latino groups (Villa et al., 1993). Older Mexican American females outlive and outnumber older males but have higher mortality rates than non-Latino white females (Villa et al., 1993). Becker et al. (1990) argue that the leading causes of death among older Mexican Americans, a particularly vulnerable group, are "ill-defined conditions," probably related to their poor access to, and utilization of, health services, as well as lifelong poverty and poor nutrition.

Legal residency has immense importance for Mexican Americans (Villa et al., 1993). Puerto Ricans have citizenship by virtue of Puerto Rico's territorial status while most Cubans become legal residents upon reaching U.S. soil. However, Mexicans do not easily become legal residents, and many older Mexican Americans have not pursued citizenship papers. For individuals coming to live with their American relatives, lack of legal residency renders it difficult for them to find employment during their younger adult years and disqualifies them from public assistance and Medicaid throughout their lives (Villa et al., 1993). Many do not even receive pension income from the Social Security system.

Latinos tend to have less education than other demographic groups, with approximately half of those age twenty-five or older attaining a high school diploma. Mexican Americans are the least educated; only 46 percent have graduated from high school (Suarez and Ramirez, 1998).

Poverty rates are approximately four times as high among Latinos in general as they are for non-Latino whites. Cubans have the highest median income, $31,000 in 1992, followed by Mexican Americans ($24,000) and Puerto Ricans ($20,000) (Villa et al., 1993). However, since Mexican families tend to be larger than those of other Latino subgroups, their per capita income is the lowest.

The number of males to females aged sixty-five to seventy-four is approximately equal in the Mexican American and Puerto Rican sectors, while there are 91 males for every 100 females in other Latino subgroups. This ratio changes, however, to 70 males for every 100 females in all Latino groups after the age of seventy-five (Villa et al., 1993).

Burr and Mutchler (1992) examined the 1980 census data on unmarried Latino females age fifty-five and older, including their living arrangements. Mexican Americans had the largest number of children (4.1) of the Latino subgroups (3.8 for Puerto Ricans, 2.1 for Cuban Americans, and 3.1 for "other Latinos") and a higher number than non-Latino whites (who averaged 2.2). Thus, they had the greatest availability of kin with whom they could live. Overall, Latino elders are more likely than non-Latino whites to live with an adult child in a multigenerational family setting.

Cultural Practices, Social Norms, and Acculturation

Spanish is the preferred language for approximately 86 percent of older Mexican Americans (Villa et al., 1993). Older patients may be unable to answer questions in English during clinical encounters, resulting in misdiagnoses and other problems. Those who are not acculturated to American life are less likely to have health insurance or a regular physician or to seek medical specialists (Mitchell et al., 1990). Folk medicine continues to be practiced by the elderly, but its relative frequency is not known. *Curanderos,* or healers, as well as other forms of folk medicine, are commonly utilized as part of their overall practice of maintaining health and well-being (Villa et al., 1993).

Any discussion of Mexican Americans must include their levels of assimilation and acculturation. Mexican acculturation to American society is a complex process that encompasses the length of U.S. residence, the presence of cultural institutions and social norms and the degree to which Mexican Americans embrace them, language use and preference, level of education and income, the number of family members present, place of birth, age, and gender. Moreover, over the years a number of acculturation scales have been developed for use among Mexican Americans that today commonly include the cultural values of (1) *familismo—*

strong identification with family and extended relatives; (2) *respeto*—the respect that accrues to family members on the basis of age, sex, and social position; (3) *simpatía*—the quality of being pleasant and nice in social interaction to preserve honor; and (4) *fatalismo*—the belief that an individual has little control over things. The broad trends established from this acculturation research will be discussed below (Hazuda, Haffner and Stern, 1988; Marin and Marin, 1991).

Needs and Problems of Older Mexican Americans

The American health care system is faced with a rapidly growing geriatric population of Latinos (Institute for the Future, 2000). A 500 percent population increase of those over the age of sixty-five is projected by 2030 (U.S. Senate, 1989). Mexican Americans make up the fastest-growing segment of the older population relative to other Latino groups and have the lowest rate of health care coverage and the highest rates of poverty and unmet social and economic needs.

Problems associated with aging and the need for care among Mexican Americans are focused primarily in three broadly defined categories of need: special needs in the areas of health and functional status; financial and cultural barriers; and institutional barriers.

Special Needs in the Areas of Health and Functional Status

The less acculturated and those having low socioeconomic status are at particular risk for chronic diseases (Hamman et al., 1989). The primary morbidity conditions common among the older Mexican American population are non-insulin-dependent diabetes mellitus, a condition that is approximately twice as frequent as in non-Latino whites; hypertension and cardiovascular disease, which is less prevalent in non-Latino whites and Asians but somewhat more frequent in African Americans; and growing rates of certain types of cancer, specifically, that of the liver, pancreas, stomach, and cervix (Suarez and Ramirez, 1998; Villa et al., 1993). Mexican Americans also experience high rates of comorbidity conditions that predispose them for cardiovascular disease, including obesity, non-insulin-dependent diabetes, and hypertension (Stern et al., 1984; Villa et al., 1993). In the Hispanic Health and Nutrition Examination Survey (HHANES) data, which include self-reported and laboratory analyses, the prevalence of diabetes increases with age to approximately 33 percent among Mexican Americans aged sixty-five to seventy-four. The incidence of self-reported diabetes is much lower, indicating that Mexican Americans underreport their risks substantially (Perez-Stable et al., 1989). Hypertension and diabetes place Mexican Americans at greater risk for stroke than the older non-Latino white population (Villa et al., 1993).

Clearly, the comorbidity conditions associated with diabetes have a major impact on the health status of older Mexican Americans. Risks associated with uncontrolled diabetes are increased levels of hyperglycemia, retinopathy, clinical proteinuria, and end-stage renal disease (Perez-Stable et al., 1989). The incidence of end-stage renal disease is six times higher for Mexican Americans than for non-Latino whites (Pugh et al., 1988).

Depression is a serious mental health condition among elderly Mexican Americans, particularly at the oldest ages (Morton et al., 1989), lower income levels (Krause and Goldenhar, 1992), and lesser acculturation, as measured by an inability to speak English (Kemp, Staples and Lopez-Aqueres, 1987). It is also more prevalent among those who experience other debilitating medical conditions (Kemp, Staples and Lopez-Aqueres, 1987). But research indicates that Mexican Americans who prefer to speak Spanish have lower rates of affective disorders (Krause and Goldenhar, 1992), as do those born in the United States. The preference for using Spanish in a bilingual environment may in fact offer stress-buffering effects and reinforce Mexican cultural identity, thereby reducing the rate of mental illness. Those who speak only Spanish and whose depression rates are higher tend to be more recent immigrants. Immigrant women tend to have a higher risk of depression than men (Black, Markides and Miller, 1998). In general, taking into account sociodemographic risk factors and the presence of chronic comorbidities among older Mexican Americans, it is apparent that this group experiences high psychological distress (Black, Markides and Miller, 1998).

To determine the level of functional capacity in older persons, commonly used assessment methods include self-reports and observational ratings of activities of daily living (ADLs) (e.g., walking or ambulation, feeding oneself, dressing oneself, toileting, transferring) and instrumental activities of daily living (IADLs) (e.g., writing checks, running errands, cleaning house, preparing food, driving) (Kane and Kane, 1981). Other indicators of functional status and levels of disability may include health service criteria, such as bed disability days and geriatric assessment screens, that measure physiological performance (e.g., upper-versus lower-body mobility and strength).

The National Health Interview Survey (NHIS) functional status indicators show a higher level of impairment among Latinos generally when contrasted with non-Latino whites (Villa et al., 1993). All Latinos had higher levels of disability than non-Latino whites in restricted activities and bed disability days per year, more activity limitations, and a greater need for help with one or more ADLs. For restricted activity days per year, the Latino average was 46.5 versus 38.7 for non-Latino whites; the Mexican elderly had the highest rate—52.8 days per year (Villa et al., 1993). Bed disability days per year is higher among Latino elderly (20.7 days per year versus 12.9 for non-Latino whites), and again even greater for Mexican American elderly (26.1 days).

A national survey of elderly Latinos indicates that IADL levels are highest among those who are poor and uneducated, problems that increase with age (Tran and Williams, 1998). These data confirm the double-jeopardy hypothesis of many gerontological studies showing that indigent older minorities have the greatest risk of poor health and functional impairments.

A study of disability impairments in Mexican Americans indicated that lower-body difficulties were particularly high in older people (Markides et al., 1996). Older Mexican Americans develop disabilities earlier in life, with lower-body problems occurring most frequently. The inquiry, which included 3,040 older Mexican Americans in the Southwest, found the following functional limitations: inability to walk half a mile (29 percent), walk up and down stairs (25 percent), bathe (11.7 percent), walk across a small room (10 percent), dress (9.5 percent), transfer from bed to chair (8.8 percent), and groom (7.5 percent) or feed (5.4 percent) themselves.

Significantly, research among retirees in Los Angeles showed that 64 percent of the Mexican American men had to leave their jobs because of disability or poor health, as compared to 24 percent of the non-Latino whites. The higher prevalence of disability appears to occur among those in manual labor occupations that are more physically debilitating (Clark et al., 1997).

Do Mexican Americans really have higher rates of ADL disability, as some of these studies suggest? Some research has suggested that Latinos tend to overreport ADL limitations, which may account for a small part of their higher disability rates (Hamman et al., 1999; Markides et al., 1996). In a study among older people in rural Colorado, self-reports of ADL limitations were compared with standardized observational data of timed walking, rising from a chair, and stooping to pick up a small object. Difficulties for Latinos were found to be no greater than those for non-Latino whites, regardless of age. However, the results indicated that actual disabilities among Mexican American females were significantly greater than those for non-Latino whites, especially at the oldest ages (Hamman et al., 1999). Since the study was conducted only among community-based elders, their higher rate of disability may indicate that more functionally impaired Latino females remain at home than non-Latino whites. Indeed, the available data suggest that only the most severely disabled Latinos are institutionalized. Wallace and Lew-Ting (1992) provide evidence that older Mexican Americans have lower rates of nursing home utilization than both African Americans and non-Latino whites. In fact, they have lower rates of institutionalization than other Latino groups.

The Commonwealth Fund surveyed over 2,000 Latino elderly and found that 54 percent reported their health as fair or poor, compared to 35 percent of non-Latino elderly (Villa et al., 1993). However, the cultural notions of health may play a greater role than objective measures in how people perceive their health status. This may partly explain the higher rates of reported disability among older Mexicans and their poorer health status in general.

Financial and Cultural Barriers

Multiple studies on health status across the life span indicate that mechanisms for susceptibility to various diseases in middle and later life are quite complex. Latino subgroups experience widely varying medical problems, and in some sectors they are not markedly different from those of non-Latino whites. This is called the Hispanic epidemiological paradox (Kington and Smith, 1997; Markides et al., 1996). Where there are large differences in health and functional status, the generally accepted explanation is that it is because of socioeconomic inequalities (Kington and Smith, 1997). There is substantial evidence that low socioeconomic status contributes to risk factors for various chronic diseases and conditions.

Poverty. Forty-seven percent of older Mexican Americans live below or near the poverty level (Parra and Espino, 1992); these elders tend to be female, recent immigrants, and illiterate in English and to have the least education (Suarez and Ramirez, 1998; Villa et al., 1993).

The 1990 census data indicate that the median income for older Latinos living alone or with nonrelatives was $7,060 versus $10,798 for non-Latino white elderly. Older single Latino females had a median income of $5,543 in 1989 as compared to $8,486 for their male counterparts. Moreover, in 1998, only 77 percent of elderly Latinos received Social Security benefits versus 93 percent of non-Latino whites (Villa et al., 1993). Thus, more Latino elders (44 percent) depend on Supplemental Security Income (SSI) than other groups (Villa et al., 1993).

Labor Force Participation. Labor force participation among older Latinos is 11.4 percent, a rate that is similar to older non-Latino whites and African Americans. However, unemployment is higher for older Latinos than for the other groups (Cubillos 1987; Villa et al., 1993). As with Puerto Ricans, older Mexican Americans are more likely to have occupational histories of low-paying manual labor and service sector positions (Villa et al., 1993). Their lifetime employment patterns result in insufficient Social Security and private pensions upon retirement.

Health Insurance. Among older Mexican Americans, the single most important factor that negatively affects their access to health services, resulting in untreated or undiagnosed chronic conditions, is the absence of health insurance (Angel and Angel, 1996; Solis et al., 1990). Older Mexican Americans have the highest proportion of uninsured people—approximately 33 to 40 percent (Ruiz, 1993). Their lack of private or government health insurance (Medicare or Medicaid), coupled with limited finances, generally prevents them from seeking medical care or other health-related services. Out-of-pocket expenses for prescription drugs, emergency room care, hospitalization, and outpatient clinic visits also operate as deterrents for elder Mexican Americans (Parra and Espino, 1992). Younger Latinos overall, but especially Mexican Americans, have low levels of health care coverage, including public programs. Factors accounting for their lack of medical benefits are low levels of education; high rates of unemployment and underemployment; jobs that do not offer health benefits; and residency in states that have highly restrictive Medicaid eligibility requirements. Moreover, large numbers of Mexican Americans are not covered under the Social Security system and therefore lack Medicare benefits as well (Angel and Angel, 1996).

Cultural Barriers. Molina, Zambrana and Aguirre-Molina (1994) describe two primary domains of culture that are relevant for a discussion of health and service use by older Mexican Americans: (1) psychosocial aspects that include beliefs, behaviors, and social values, which are expressed through normative practices; and (2) objective measures of sociodemographic characteristics such as education and income.

The cultural construction of disease, and especially those conditions pertaining to aging and disability, should enable us to gain greater insight into how older Mexican Americans evaluate the meaning of disease and seek health services. Research on opinions regarding the causes and treatments of common diseases and how they are related to health behaviors was conducted on a cross-ethnic sample of noninstitutionalized African Americans, Latinos, and non-Latino white American men and women age seventy-five and older in Galveston County, Texas (Goodwin, Black and Satish, 1999). Close to 60 percent of both Mexican Americans and non-Latino whites considered arthritis a part of normal aging, followed by sleep problems (43 percent and 46 percent respectively) and heart disease (41 percent and 46 percent). A lower percentage of African Americans viewed these conditions as a part of normal aging. When asked to rank the reasons for heart disease, overwork and stress were identified by 16 percent of older Mexican Americans, as compared to 34 percent of African Americans.

Critically, more Mexican Americans (26 percent) thought nothing could be done to make heart disease better once a person was diagnosed. They even ranked potential cures for arthritis and sleep problems slightly lower than that for heart disease. Of the three groups, Mexican Americans had the greatest prevalence of fatalistic and nihilistic attitudes. The authors suggest that these views may contribute to inadequate health care use and may limit health-improvement activities.

Traditional cultural practices and the use of folk healers (curanderos), herbs, teas, and religious rituals also contribute to lower utilization of medical services by older Mexican Americans (Andersen et al., 1981). Additionally, the kin network seems to discourage doctor visits, even when the older person is ill (Hoppe and Heller, 1975). In one study, it was found that families sometimes rejected costly treatment for elders while encouraging prenatal care for pregnant women. This tends to support the notion that familism, or familismo, can work to encourage some types of access but may also discourage others (Queseda and Heller, 1977).

In terms of language ability, Schur and Albers (1996) found that monolingual Spanish speakers were more likely to be older, less educated, in poor health, uninsured, and in poverty. They were less likely than English speakers to have a usual source of care, to have seen a physician in the last year, and to have had blood pressure screening. An added risk for these older adults is that families and friends serving as translators may be ill prepared to explain complex medical conditions and drug regimens to older family members (Pousada, 1995). Thus, the importance of compliance with health care recommendations may not be appropriately conveyed. Furthermore, elders may shy away from any treatment for depression or other mental illness because they don't want family members to know the extent of their problem (Villa et al., 1993).

In examining ethnicity differences between African American and Mexican American elderly and preferences for Medicare hospice benefits, Gordon (1995) also found that lack of familiarity with the health care system and language barriers were more prevalent among older Mexican Americans and were serious deterrents to both their access to and use of these services. However, although language ability is important, higher socioeconomic status is the more critical factor for health care coverage and therefore access to a regular doctor and medical services overall (Angel and Angel, 1996; Solis et al., 1990).

Institutional Barriers

As suggested earlier, there are a number of obstacles to accessing and utilizing health care services and community-based long-term care for older Mexican Americans, including acculturation issues, Spanish monolingualism, poverty, lack of insurance, unemployment, geographic distance from services, transportation, cost of services, having someone to accompany the individual to appointments, and Medicare/Medicaid eligibility requirements (Wallace and Lew-Ting, 1992; Wallace, Campbell and Lew-Ting, 1994; Wallace, Levy-Storms and Ferguson, 1995). In fact, Mexican Americans are the most likely of the three Latino groups to be affected by these problems (Gordon, 1995). They are more likely to be monolingual, poor, and the least acculturated as well as to have little or no insurance and no regular place for receiving health care (Villa et al., 1993). However, lack of insurance coverage is clearly one of the more important factors in explaining their underutilization of services (Markides et al., 1996).

Researchers have examined the use of formal in-home services (visiting nurses, home health aides, and/or homemaker services), employing data from the 1988 Commonwealth Fund Commission's national survey of 2,299 Latinos age sixty-five and older. Wallace, Campbell and Lew-Ting (1994) found that the existence of a strong family network improved the ability of older Latinos to access community-based services. Moreover, lack of Medicaid coverage was a substantial barrier to service utilization, even for those people living in poverty. The authors conclude that a universal, publicly funded long-term care system is the only way to adequately meet the needs of older Latinos and other poorly served groups.

The paucity of Spanish-speaking health and long-term care professionals also poses a significant barrier to access and utilization of services by older Mexican Americans (Pousada, 1995; Villa et al., 1993). Given the substantial demographic increases in older Mexican Americans in the future, this situation will only worsen. Significant efforts need to be directed toward recruiting and training larger numbers of Latino or Mexican American providers. Of those students graduating from American medical schools, only 2 percent are Puerto Rican, 1.7 percent Mexican American, and 1.7 percent other Latinos. These figures, which show a substantial underrepresentation of the Latino community, have not changed substantially since 1985 (Pousada, 1995).

Latinos encounter many social and economic barriers in the American university system, including having few role models or mentors. High costs for college and graduate and medical schools prevent many qualified people from training for professional careers. Consequently, Mexican Americans occupy few high-level positions in the health and long-term care fields.

Pousada (1995) recommends that professionals in the health care field be trained in culturally appropriate values and methods. Sotomayor and Randolph (1988) suggested that formal systems are underutilized partly owing to the cultural insensitivities of such providers. Valle (1998) maintains that they must seek to understand the culture of Latino family caregivers. Research on African American, Mexican American, and non-Latino white families who have relatives in intensive care shows the benefits of culturally appropriate care for both patients and their kin.

Moreover, Latinos are overrepresented in low-paying jobs with few educational or other requirements, such as nurse's aides. In one study of ethnic groups in San Diego County conducted across thirty-three facilities (including convalescent hospitals, rehabilitation facilities, nursing homes, health care facilities and several continuing care settings), it was found that Mexican Americans alone accounted for fully one-third of the nursing assistants (Saghri, 2000). Moreover, they had high turnover rates, mostly because of their low pay, occupational stress, and high patient-to-worker ratios.

Older Mexican Americans and Their Informal Caregivers

The Latino kinship network is an important source of assistance for older people. For example, in contrast to quasi-formal support (civic and religious groups) and formal support (government and private programs), the informal support system of older Latinos is primary to posthospitalization recoveries (Wallace, Levy-Storms and Ferguson, 1995). One study revealed that fully 77 percent of Latino respondents with chronic functional impairments were helped by a spouse or adult child, with only 14 percent taking care of themselves (Commonwealth Fund Commission, 1989). This is in contrast to the 60 percent of the general elderly population that relied on their families for posthospitalization support; nearly one-third of these individuals had no help. Moreover, family members of older Latinos, especially those with whom the elderly person lives, are more likely than other groups to mediate between their elders and formal service providers (Wallace, Levy-Storms and Ferguson, 1995).

Although family and friends continue to be the primary source of personal assistance for older Mexican Americans, does this system provide sufficient and/or effective care to functionally impaired elders and to those suffering from serious chronic conditions? For instance, such aid may involve taking care of a diabetic family member who is obese, has visual impairments and difficulty controlling blood sugar, and is at risk for vascular disease and other end-stage renal conditions. Caregiver duties may include technical skills such as home blood-glucose monitoring, injections, weight control, and wound and foot care (Aranda and Knight, 1997). These are serious problems for Mexican Americans, who suffer from particularly high levels of chronic illnesses and disabilities early in life and thus require greater amounts of informal aid—and for longer periods—than do other groups (Wallace and Lew-Ting, 1992). The data suggest that Mexican Americans cannot provide adequate levels of in-home assistance even though they are not utilizing adequate formal sources of care to any great extent.

In some research among aged Mexican Americans, elders indicate their preference for direct family care (Gordon, 1995; Newton, 1980). However, other studies show that they do not view adult children as having an obligation to provide assistance (Crouch, 1972; Newton, 1980). For example, one inquiry in San Diego and Los Angeles found that a majority of older Mexican Americans did not want to be a burden on their families (Newton, 1980; Valle and Mendoza, 1978). It would appear that these conflicting views are related to levels of acculturation: the less-acculturated older adult is more likely to be Spanish monolingual, adhere to traditional notions of health and disease, and rely on the family for care. More-acculturated Mexican American elderly may, in fact, be exhibiting values that more closely approximate the larger, non-Latino white American culture.

Data from the 1988 Longitudinal Study on Aging and the Commonwealth Fund Survey of elderly Hispanics suggest that Latino families are not averse to using some levels of formal care and that, in fact, they elect to do so when structural barriers are reduced. In recent years, federal and state policy initiatives to control costs take advantage of Mexican American families by expecting them to provide even more in-home care. If public resources are withheld from Latino elderly on the basis that their informal support system provides sufficient aid, these policies actually penalize the caregiving efforts of Mexican American families. Moreover, since Mexican American elderly and their caregivers are more impoverished than most other groups, they cannot afford to purchase formal services to meet their growing needs (Greene and Monahan, 1984).

Conclusion and Policy Implications

Some program and policy recommendations that have the potential for addressing the areas of unmet need for older Mexican Americans are outlined below. They are based on model demonstrations and research results from interventions and community research programs.

Insurance and Improved Access to Community Long-Term Care Services

The Health Insurance Counseling and Advocacy Program (HICAP), funded through the Administration on Aging, could conduct specific education and outreach efforts in the Mexican American community to improve its knowledge of, and access to, health insurance. HICAP could work collaboratively with the Medicare and Medicaid systems to reduce the number of uninsured.

Innovative projects that utilize community health care workers as educators and translators as well as for outreach efforts have been effective in helping Latinos access and utilize community-based services. The California Health Care Foundation has funded a San Diego–based project to test and evaluate the role of Latino and Filipino community health advocates in reducing the access difficulties experienced by older adults in gaining entry to a Medicaid managed care health plan. Preliminary focus group results indicate strong support from physicians, nurses, medical case managers, home health agencies, community clinics, and administrators from long-term care facilities. There also are high approval ratings for the community health advocate role across culturally diverse groups. Everyone involved has emphasized the importance of integrating this role into normal health care infrastructure operations and other service delivery systems (Du Bois and Stanford, 2000). Demonstration projects should test the community health advocate role in different care settings to determine its feasibility.

As suggested earlier, the Mexican American family commonly provides the majority of informal care for frail elders. However, workplace realities are affecting family life today, and women may not be as readily available to serve as full-time caregivers. Consequently, the formal community long-term care sector needs to be developed as an adjunct to the informal system, and it must include more culturally appropriate programs.

State and county efforts are under way to consolidate the current fragmentary system of community-based long-term care into more coherent delivery systems at the local level. Given the pervasive underutilization of services by Mexican Americans, representatives from this group need to participate in long-term care efforts as planning partners.

Health Care, Prevention, and Health Promotion

The increasing development of Medicare and Medicaid managed care plans should target specific risk factors and physical impairments in at-risk older patients earlier in their development, including those for diabetes and cardiovascular diseases prevalent in Mexican Americans. For example, geriatric screening for these conditions could enhance early detection and treatment. Demonstration programs could test the value of various alternative services and programs as well as their cost effectiveness. Since many Mexican Americans use community clinics to meet their primary care needs, these facilities must be included in any demonstration projects.

Community service and medical case management programs could develop computer database systems linking medical and social systems. This would assist providers in assessing whether the community long-term care service plans are implemented following the patient's release from postacute care.

Greater emphasis should be placed on primary, secondary, and tertiary prevention programs available to older Mexican Americans and their families. The focus should be on improving knowledge of risk factors and morbidity conditions, and providing access to periodic screening (e.g., blood glucose levels) and rehabilitation services. Health promotion services should be enhanced in the areas of nutrition and diet, exercise programs, and injury prevention. Outreach activities must include use of the Spanish mass media (radio, Spanish cable television, and newspapers).

We should also expand the use of community volunteers through the Retired Senior Volunteer Program (RSVP), funded under the Older Americans Act. In particular, we must develop a Spanish RSVP program for Mexican Americans and include older volunteers as adjuncts to all aspects of family and community programs, as well as put together a volunteer reassurance program to link isolated Mexican Americans with a network of social contacts from the community.

Recruiting and Training Professionals for Careers in Health Care

Health careers opportunity programs (HCOP) are available at many universities in the United States for recruiting and training disadvantaged students for careers in the health and social service fields. There are approximately sixty training programs nationwide that receive their funding under the Department of Health and Human Services. These efforts recruit students through outreach and retention programs directed at precollege students. HCOP programs are making inroads in the professional development of Mexican American students; however, it is unlikely that they are sufficient to meet current or future needs.

The Texas Medical Center Collaborative Preceptor Program has developed curricula and training for hospital-based nurse preceptors to address cultural differences between staff and patients, resolve potential conflicts in their value systems, and identify methods of facilitating cultural understanding among providers (Williams and Rogers, 1993).

Cultural competency training refers to "the capacity of health professionals or of health service delivery systems to understand and plan for the health needs of a specific cultural subgroup" (Castro, Cota and Santos, 1998). Included in this training should be the promotion of cultural openness, competence, and awareness when designing programs and delivering services. Such efforts would be fruitful for all community-based agencies and institutional facilities serving Mexican Americans.

Forecasts for the Future

Access issues, as well as problems with the uninsured and those on Medicaid, will continue unabated unless significant changes are made. In fact, in light of ongoing efforts at cost containment at the federal and state levels, care for disabled older Mexican Americans most likely will worsen. For example, those on Medicaid increasingly will have more limited choices and tighter controls on services. Given the growing number of frail older Mexicans in the United States, their relatively low income, and their higher disability rates, if we are to meet their needs, we must begin to test, develop, and evaluate culturally appropriate community long-term care options for them and their families.

7

Puerto Rican Elderly

Carmen Delia Sánchez

In Puerto Rico as well as in the United States the sixty-five-and-over sector has been growing more rapidly than the rest of the population. The elderly population currently is the fastest-growing segment of Puerto Rican society. From 1899 through 1990, the number of people sixty-five and over increased from 19,000 to 342,059, at an annual rate of 3.2 percent. This growth has risen measurably since the 1950s as a result of a seriously reduced birth rate, decreased mortality rates in general, the massive emigration of young adults (ages twenty to thirty-four) to the United States during the 1950s and 1960s, and the return migration of older Puerto Ricans to the island. The Commonwealth of Puerto Rico, which had a total population of 3,522,037 in 1990, experienced significant shifts within age sectors during the prior three decades (Commonwealth of Puerto Rico, 1994). While the proportion of individuals aged fifteen years and younger was drastically reduced, from 43 percent in 1960 to 28 percent in 1990, those aged sixty-five and over increased from 5.2 percent to 9.7 percent during that time period. For every aged adult in 1960 there were three in 1990.

Census data for 1990 also show notable differences within the older sector itself: the seventy-five-plus group (the old-old) exhibits the greatest increase, 4.3 percent, as compared to 2.2 percent for those sixty-five to seventy-four (the young-old). The numbers of the very oldest age group are continuing to rise.

Projections for the year 2000 indicate that the percentage of elderly will increase to 14.4 percent, rising by 2020 to as much as 17 percent of Puerto Rico's total population. These forecasts are based on older Puerto Ricans' returning to the island, the aging of the baby-boom generation, continued emigration of young adults, crime rates that tend to affect younger rather than older age groups, a decreasing birth rate, and increased access to more advanced and specialized medical treatment.

Today, the possibility that a person born in Puerto Rico will reach old age is a concrete reality: 76 of every 100 persons born in 1996 are expected to attain the age of sixty-five. In fact, women's future longevity is predicted to reach eighty-five years, versus seventy-six years for males. Currently, life expectancy is seventy-nine years for women and seventy-four for men. Females represent the majority of the aged population in Puerto Rico, 54.2 percent, and this situation is expected to continue unless an extraordinary decline in male mortality risks occurs. At the oldest age group, eighty-five and over, there are only 70.8 men for every 100 women (U.S. Census, 1990a).

Close to 7 percent of the older population in Puerto Rico have never been married. Fifty percent are legally married or living with a partner, though there is a considerably higher proportion of married men than women. According to 1990 census data, 70 percent of men age sixty-five and over are married compared to only 4 percent of aged women. Significantly, nearly a third of the sixty-five-and-over population are widows; there are four widows for each widower. It is more common for men to remarry, particularly in old age. Culturally, men are encouraged to seek a new partner, while women are expected to live on memories and guard the remembrances of the spouse.

The sixty-five-and-over group has the least formal education in Puerto Rico. In 1990, approximately 48 percent of the aged population on the island had less than five years of schooling, and only 5 percent had a bachelor's degree or more (Centro de Investigaciones Demográficas, 1998). As age increases among this sector of the population, the proportion of persons with limited formal education is even higher. Moreover, older women evidence higher rates of illiteracy than older men. The low level of formal education should be taken into consideration when planning services for this sector of the population.

Socioeconomic Conditions

Puerto Rican elderly face a range of health and social problems, and formal medical and social services have not adequately met their needs. According to the 1990 census data, nearly one-third (31.8 percent) of those sixty-five and older have some limitations in their mobility and/or ability to care for themselves. This means that 107,247 elderly confront such problems and therefore have a high risk of dependency. Although there is little systematically obtained information concerning mental illness among the Puerto Rican elderly, the Puerto Rican Alzheimer Association estimates that approximately 25,000 persons are suffering from this disorder.

Socioeconomic barriers encountered by the Puerto Rican elderly may make them more dependent than some other groups. The social and health-care needs of this population cannot be fully understood without reference to their income, housing, and employment situation. Research on the Puerto Rican elderly on the island consistently demonstrates that most of them are quite poor; since they cannot afford formal services, or even their own residence, they are particularly dependent on their relatives (Sánchez-Ayendez, 1986; Sánchez, 1989). In 1990, fully 56 percent of the population sixty years of age and older lived below the poverty level, with an annual average income of $5,477 (U.S. Census, 1990a). Since Supplementary Security Income (SSI) does not exist in Puerto Rico, their income comes mainly from Social Security; for many, this is their only source of income. One out of every four older people lives on public assistance alone. Moreover, only 7.5 percent of Puerto Rican elders are in the labor force (Rodríguez, 1999), a percentage that has steadily declined as the economy has changed from predominantly agricultural to industrial.

According to the 1990 census data for Puerto Rico, 77.4 percent of persons sixty-five years of age and older were living in family households; many of these were multigenerational settings. Twenty-one percent, or 88,288, most of them women, were living alone or sharing a house with nonrelatives, and only 1.3 percent were institutionalized (U.S. Census, 1990a). As age increases, the proportion of elderly living in nursing homes grows larger. For example, institutionalization increased from 0.7 percent for the sixty-to-sixty-four age cohort to 5.1 percent for those eighty-five years of age and over (U.S. Census, 1990a). However, regardless of age, institutionalization is somewhat lower for Puerto Rican elderly than for older people in American society overall. Nursing homes or other long-term care facilities continue to be the last choice for elderly Puerto Ricans and their families. In fact, for the most part, families will go to extraordinary lengths before an institution is even considered.

The accessibility of a family support system appears to be the primary factor in reducing the probability of institutionalization for the chronically ill person on the island; this is the same pattern as in the United States (Brody, 1990). In addition, a substantial amount of care is provided by friends and neighbors. This accounts for the large number of persons who may need long-term care services yet are able to remain in the community.

The Puerto Rican Family and Elder Care

Parallel to the growth of the aging population, major demographic shifts affecting the family have occurred in Puerto Rico as well as in American society overall. The rapid socioeconomic changes that Puerto Rican society has undergone in the last three decades of the twentieth century have altered familial and community patterns of interaction. However, though urbanism and industrialization have affected the structure of the Puerto Rican family, studies overwhelmingly indicate that its members continue to play a vital function in the delivery of assistance to older Puerto Ricans residing both on the island and on the mainland (Sánchez, 1999, 1989, 1987; Sánchez-Ayendez, 1998, 1986; Dávila and Sánchez-Ayendez, 1996; Delgado, 1995; Delgado and Tennstedt, 1997; Cruz-López and Pearson, 1985).

The Puerto Rican family continues to retain many aspects of its ethnic Hispanic identity and cultural values. One such value, known as *familismo,* places a great emphasis on family unity, supports family integrity, and gives shape and direction to the behavior of its members. Attempts to instill a sense of family pride and obligation begin early in a person's life and are nurtured throughout. Most Hispanics are socialized to believe that the needs or welfare of their family as a whole or of other individual family members—particularly the very young or very old—should take precedence over one's own needs. It is within the family context that Puerto Ricans are taught the value of cooperation over competition, mutual assistance above individual problem solving, and sharing as opposed to withholding resources for oneself. Because they are family centered, members feel an obligation to relatives and a duty to serve them in times of crisis.

In the Puerto Rican community, the family is a source of strength for individuals of all ages. The Puerto Rican cultural heritage emphasizes the family's responsibility to care for those in need. This tradition means that the family is a significant primary provider of services. In accordance with cultural norms and values, and as a practical necessity, the extended family is still of great importance. For instance, as previously stated, many Puerto Rican elderly share a household with a child or other relative (Sánchez, 1989; U.S. Census, 1990a). The fact that they are more likely to live in multigenerational households is a function not only of the value system of their community but also of economic necessity. The shared household is one way poor families are able to meet their housing needs. In addition, grandparents often take care of young children for the increasing number of single parents, or when both parents work.

In addition to familismo, Puerto Rican culture places a high priority on the concept that life is a network of interpersonal relationships. The value of *personalismo* is central for Puerto Ricans. Though it is a form of individualism that focuses on the inner importance of the person, it is rooted in the family. As such, it is "an extension of the person[s]," thereby fostering a network of obligations. (Fitzpatrick, 1981: 211). This cultural theme encourages interpersonal relations and social interactions where individuals deal with each other as caring, complete persons rather than as impersonal players in segmented roles. The emphasis is on those inner qualities that constitute the uniqueness and fundamental self-worth of each person, regardless of social, economic, or political status (Lauria, 1972). Personalismo stresses the building of trust *(confianza)*, respect *(respeto)*, pride *(orgullo)*, and dignity *(dignidad)*.

Thus, basic to the values and lifestyle of the Puerto Rican elderly is interdependence between and among the generations. For instance, the relationship between grandparents and grandchildren has traditionally been one of great affection and interaction and is a clear example of reciprocity between generations. Grandparents are an essential part of the Puerto Rican family for the multiplicity of social roles that they fulfill, including providing financial assistance to adult children when feasible and, more often, caring for their grandchildren when parents are working or for orphaned children (Sánchez, 1999). Through the strong association between grandparents and grandchildren, cultural traditions and values are transmitted. Elders also are a source of strength, as they serve to unify the family and guard it against external forces.

As a result of family interdependence and reciprocity, older people expect their children to take care of them in old age. At the same time, children perceive such assistance as their duty, particularly in times of illness or crisis, as reciprocity for the care that their parents provided while they were young or any help they were given during their adult years. Contrary to various opinions about the demise of family supports, the evidence suggests that Puerto Ricans and Hispanics in general utilize kinship networks in a very significant manner (Sánchez, 1989; Padilla, Carlos and Keefe, 1976).

Research on informal support of older Puerto Ricans on the mainland and the island indicates that is generally women who carry out the role of principal caregiver to the elderly (Delgado, 1995; Sánchez-Ayendez, 1986; Sánchez, 1989, 1987). When the elderly couple is still functional, the daily support offered by offspring, generally daughters, tends to be secondary. However, when one of the spouses is forced to live alone because of death or divorce or when the older person's health deteriorates, adult children tend to assume a more active role, with female offspring serving as the primary caregivers. The support that these women offer and the services they render are taken for granted owing to cultural definitions of female roles and family expectations (Sánchez-Ayendez, 1986). Elder care responsibilities are so common among Puerto Rican women that sometimes it appears to be a stressful but normal situation for them. Since women have moved into the labor force in large numbers in past years, many are faced with the combined responsibilities of working, raising children, and caring for one or more elderly family members.

The findings of research conducted by Sánchez-Ayendez (1998) on middle-aged women as primary caregivers to the frail elderly provide insight into the dynamics of gender and elder care in Puerto Rico. She found that sex and birth order were closely linked to the obligation to assist dependent parents: whether the only daughter among several male siblings or the youngest or oldest daughter in the family, females were expected to provide the care. The majority of respondents indicated that their primary motivation for providing assistance was familial obligation and reciprocity. Moreover, some of the women clearly stated that it was indeed their responsibility as a woman to assume the caretaking role.

Although historically women have been the primary, and often the only, caregivers, nevertheless there is evidence that growing numbers of men are taking on the task as they are called on to assist, augment, or replace the efforts of women. In a study of Puerto Rican sons serving as primary caregivers of elderly parents, Delgado and Tennstedt (1997) found that the sons assumed the caregiver role out of a sense of responsibility and because there were no other potential caregivers who lived nearby. As a result of structural changes in Puerto Rican families and geographic mobility, daughters may not be able to assume fully the culturally dictated role as caregivers, and sons increasingly may have to take on this responsibility.

An important aspect of familial support in Puerto Rico is what happens when the elder becomes impaired and the family has to provide intensive assistance. To what extent are adult children able to furnish such care and, in the light of fast-paced modern life, assume the burden of caring for an ailing parent?

With more people surviving into old age, younger generations have a larger number of elderly relatives than in the past. The trend toward increased longevity among the elderly Puerto Ricans means that more families will extend to four living generations (e.g., middle-aged adults who are already grandparents will have elderly parents). In many Puerto Rican families there are already two or three generations of older members—for example, parents in their mid-sixties, grandparents in their eighties, and great-grandparents in their late nineties.

The actual and potential increase in the number and proportion of dependent, frail older people has serious implications for family care of the elderly. Clearly, filial responsibility remains strong in Puerto Rican society; it is the primary motivation for responding to a parent in need and one that is independent of any anticipated rewards. Yet, increasingly, middle-aged adults in Puerto Rico are expected to take care of their parents and grandparents as well as their own children. In the past, the middle-aged were more likely to be the oldest generation and consequently did not have the obligation of caring for their aged relatives. These structural changes make obsolete many of the traditional expectations of filial responsibility. Current generations have few role models to follow as they find themselves burdened sometimes with several chronically ill family members.

The physically and mentally impaired elderly are a subgroup in Puerto Rican society whose special needs are not being adequately or appropriately met. In spite of the extensive interest in avoiding institutional care, there are relatively few community alternatives to nursing homes. The present system of long-term care for the elderly on the island provides minimal funding for community-oriented supportive services. Not only is there a lack of appropriate and affordable services, but also elders and their families are reluctant to use those that are available. As a consequence, some families may be so overwhelmed that they cannot provide adequate care. Where there is a family history of conflict, some adult children may become enraged that they are forced to provide care, thus leading to ineffective assistance and even abuse.

The Informal Support Network

Interdependence and reciprocity are grounded in the web of relationships that surround Puerto Rican elders and their family members. Most older people in Puerto Rico are tied into a network of social supports in which not only families but also friends and neighbors provide for their care. While adult children occupy the key role in the informal support system of the elderly, other relatives serve as a reservoir from which other kin can be drawn, as needed. The mix of family, friends, neighbors, civic organizations, and religious groups constitutes the major sources of assistance for Puerto Rican elders.

Fictive kinship in the form of adoptive or special friends extends the obligations, responsibilities, and privileges of family, becoming part of the informal support system. These fictive kin are close friends and neighbors who, over a period of years, have proved willing to engage in family matters and events. Networks that extend beyond the immediate family are particularly important where familial supports are unavailable or have weakened. This natural support system also helps maintain that aspect of Puerto Rican culture that emphasizes the importance of interpersonal relationships beyond the nuclear family (Sánchez, 1992).

Research continues to show the importance of the informal system in the Puerto Rican community, both in Puerto Rico and on the mainland (Sánchez, 1989, 1987; Cruz-López and Pearson, 1985; Calderón, 1984; Lopata, 1978). Delgado (1995) emphasizes that in Hispanic communities the informal support system serves to minimize the use of formal resources. He states that the Puerto Rican elder's natural support system is a broad network that includes four key components: the extended family, including friends and neighbors; folk healers; religious institutions; and social clubs. These provide assistance (instrumental, informational, and expressive) on an everyday basis as well as in times of crisis, and they represent the Puerto Rican community's capacity to help itself. Religious institutions and ethnic community organizations are particularly important parts of this support system in the Hispanic community. They are available to all age groups, and, in addition to some direct services, they provide emotional support (affection, respect, trust, loyalty, and mutuality). Weeks and Cuellar (1981) also point out the importance of these informal support systems among Hispanics, who, they argue, show a great reluctance to turn to professionals for help. If family is not available, they turn to friends, neighbors, or community groups.

Sánchez (1989) documented the particular importance of the informal support system on the well-being of elderly widows. Her study showed that it provided mostly emotional support, followed by practical assistance, economic aid, and liaison with agencies. Daughters and then sons, sisters, and other family members were principally involved in direct care; friends and neighbors provided mainly emotional support, which included visits, telephone calls, and advice.

Similarly, the research and group support program for Hispanic caregivers conducted by Sánchez (1987) found an extensive informal support system among elderly Puerto Ricans in New York City, composed mainly of friends and neighbors. Daughters, daughters-in-law, sisters, grandchildren, spouses, friends, and neighbors of the Hispanic elderly took primary responsibility for elder care. These activities involved a variety of services ranging from emotional support, instrumental activities and financial assistance to linkage services. Emotional support emerged as the most frequent activity performed by the caregivers, followed by instrumental activities such as shopping, meal preparation, light housecleaning, laundry, and personal hygiene. One of the most significant aspects of this project was its documentation of the strong communitarian tradition among Puerto Ricans, especially as it relates to the care of the elderly. In addition, the study showed that families do not diminish or give up their responsibilities when formal services are available.

Social Services

Participation of the family in the care of the Puerto Rican elderly also has been related to factors other than cultural ones. An important influence is public policy on the island regarding services to older people. For example, Puerto Rico Public Law 121, enacted on July 12, 1986, established certain guidelines and promulgated a Bill of Rights for the Aged. This piece of legislation is of great importance in terms of social provision for the older population. According to the act, "This government has proposed to do whatever is under its control to improve the living conditions of the aged person, as long as the resources allow it. The Older Adults' Bill of Rights and the Government's Public Policy regarding the aged are a decisive step in guaranteeing the elders' welfare" (Leyes de Puerto Rico, 1986: 399). The intention is to keep older people in the community by preventing or postponing nursing home placement for as long as possible. However, actual resources and services are limited, and the government does not expect to assume total responsibility for frail elders. Rather, the law aims to promote a shared and complementary relationship between the family and the government. Consequently, such public policy indirectly imposes responsibility on the family for care of its older relatives. A lack of affordable alternatives and inadequate public resources thus are additional forces that promote family care in Puerto Rico.

Conclusion and Policy Implications

Clearly, the older Puerto Rican population both on the island and on the mainland will continue to grow in the next decades. In Puerto Rico, older adults will represent 19 percent of the total population in 2030. In other words, there will be a person sixty-five years old or older for every five inhabitants. The enormous rise in the proportion of Puerto Rican elderly during the first and second decades of the twenty-first century, especially those in the oldest age groups, will affect the political, social, and economic order of the island and the United States in general. Moreover, decreases in fertility rates will reduce even further the potential number of children available to support chronically ill older people in the future. Changes in family structure that have taken place in the Puerto Rican family will have a serious effect on elder care as well. The presence of more female heads of household, together with a higher participation of women in the labor force, will result in a reduction of available time for helping and taking care of dependent parents. Consequently, the formal system will have to assume more responsibility for the aged, particularly those who lack children or close relatives. This situation could be improved if better and more extensive collaborative efforts are made between the formal and informal systems.

Sound planning must begin with the recognition that the aging experience for Puerto Ricans, as well as other groups, is heterogeneous. Our health and social services must therefore satisfy the demands of fragile and high-risk elderly who suffer serious and disabling chronic health problems as well as the needs of those family members who are willing and able to help them. Service providers need to be aware that most families want to help their aged members but may need substantial and varied types of support to do so adequately. Families whose older members require continuous and special care are likely to experience stress, which could lead to mistreatment, abuse, or negligence in some family settings.

At present, elderly Puerto Ricans who need long-term care rely heavily on their families for assistance, more so than do other elderly people. The tendency for the Puerto Rican elderly to live with relatives means their kin have even greater burdens than do many other families in American society. The effects of the economic, physical, and emotional strains borne by Puerto Rican adult children have not been fully documented. Undoubtedly, however, formal services must stress in-home assistance to caregivers as well as elders and should include respite care. Ethnic social and community groups also should be strengthened if we are to provide a better quality of life for Puerto Rican older people and their kin.

When one looks at the situation of ill and impaired older people and what they need in order to remain in their community, it is obvious that they must be provided with an array of supports and services: financial help, clothing, shelter, personal assistance, emotional support, and social activities. Families, friends, and neighbors (the informal support system) cannot take full responsibility for dependent elders and must have some assistance from the public sector. Moreover, the ill and impaired elderly do better if they have both family and formal organizations available to them. For example, most Puerto Rican families cannot provide all of the financial resources their elderly parents require, but they do give them extra money. While both public pensions and family aid contribute to the older person's standard of living, the latter serves to articulate family devotion and responsibility.

Inherent strengths exist in the Puerto Rican informal support system. For this reason, formal service providers should not undermine the existing system of informal care, which can serve as one model of how ethnic groups manage to support frail, older members despite all the constraints they encounter in modern American society. At the same time, however, policymakers must not use the informal support system as an excuse for cutting public programs and services.

It is important for all of us—particularly professionals, practitioners, researchers, and government officials—to understand that the growing ethnic diversity in the United States, including the large and growing number of vulnerable Puerto Rican elders, will require a more systematic appreciation of cultural variables. This will be essential if we are to assure that services will be more accessible, more sensitive, and therefore more effective in serving older Puerto Ricans and their families now and in the future.

8

Urban Elderly African Americans

Peggye Dilworth-Anderson, Ishan Canty Williams, and Sharon Wallace Williams

The growth of the American elderly population in general, and more specifically of minorities, suggests a need to examine both existing and future resources to address their needs. It is projected that in the near future there could be more persons who are sixty-five and older in this country than those fourteen or younger (U.S. Census, 1996a). Further, the "middle series" projections from the Census Bureau predict that the elderly population will more than double between now and 2050 (U.S. Census, 1995).

As the population is growing, the nation also is becoming more racially and ethnically diverse; there are increasing percentages of groups such as Latinos, African Americans, Asian and Pacific Islanders, and American Indians. African Americans represent the largest minority group (13 percent) with a total population of 34.9 million in July 1999. Between April 1990 and 1995, the number of African Americans increased by 4.4 million, or 14 percent, while the total U.S. population grew by only 10 percent (U.S. Census, 1996a).

According to 1996 census population survey data, people sixty-five and older represented 11.9 percent of all Americans. However, owing to such factors as higher fertility rates and lower longevity than the non-Hispanic white population, the percentage among African Americans is somewhat lower, at 7.8 percent. Nevertheless, the older black American population is increasing more rapidly than older whites, from 2.7 million in 1995 to around 3.4 million in 2010. By 2050, it is projected that the total number of elderly in this country will include 52 million non-Hispanic whites and 8.6 million African Americans.

The majority of all elderly people in this country live in urban areas, and their numbers are expected to rise in future years. The Census Bureau defines "urban" as comprising all territory, population, and housing units in: (1) places of 2,500 or more persons incorporated as cities, villages, boroughs (except in Alaska and New York), and towns (except in the six New England states, New York, and Wisconsin), but excluding the rural portions of "extended cities"; (2) census-designated places of 2,500 or more persons; and (3) other territory, incorporated or unincorporated, included in urbanized areas (U.S. Census, 1996a). In 1990 there were 21 million whites and 2.1 million African Americans aged sixty-five and over living in urban areas, as compared to 7.2 million white and 404,000 African American elders in rural communities.

The census reported that 8 percent of white and 43 percent of African American urban people aged sixty-five and over had less than a ninth-grade education. Thirty percent and 17 percent, respectively, had a high school diploma. Among rural elders, 27 percent of whites and only 8 percent of African Americans graduated from high school.

Among urban elderly African American households there were 399,000 married-couple families and 668,000 individuals who lived alone, as compared to 97,000 and 115,000, respectively, in rural places. In addition, 61 percent of urban African American elderly couples and 96 percent of those who were single earned less than $25,000 in 1989. Most of the elderly living by themselves were in poverty, whether in urban areas (77 percent earned less than $10,000) or in rural areas (89 percent earned less than $10,000). In rural communities, 68 percent of married-couple families had incomes of less than $15,000 (see table 8.1).

The Great Migration North and Urban Life

As discussed above, the demographic profile of African American elders shows that the majority live in urban areas. Most live alone and have limited education and income. Their current situation has a long history that reflects the plight of urban African Americans generally, especially in the North, dating as far back as the first great migration north (1910–1920), followed by the largest one in the 1940s. These migrations represented the greatest exodus of blacks moving from southern rural to northern urban communities. Although it provided most blacks with moderately better jobs, housing, education, and political power than they previously had (Franklin, 1997; Johnson and Campbell, 1981), their social, economic, and political conditions were still very challenging and difficult.

Some people have argued that economic disadvantages and persistent discrimination in the urban North were major contributors to family disruptions among blacks. As Tolnay (1997) reported, such family disruptions were fostered by an inner-city culture that devalued the traditional black culture and customs of their southern life. Frazier (1939: 245), for example, declared that "family desertion has been one of the inevitable consequences of the urbanization of the Negro population."

Although black families who migrated north experienced somewhat less segregation and discrimination than those who remained in the rural South, real equality eluded them in almost all areas of their lives (Franklin, 1997; Jones, 1985). In fact, not only were whites and blacks segregated, many northern blacks disliked the arrival of recent southern migrants to their cities. These long-term

**Table 8.1 Living Arrangements and Income Levels of
Rural and Urban Black Persons 65 and Over, 1990**

	Urban	Rural
Married-Couple Families		
Total Persons	399,405	97,616
Income		
Less than $5,000	17,477	8,193
$5,000–9,999	58,352	30,303
$10,000–14,999	67,721	19,894
$15,000–24,999	99,331	20,603
$25,000–34,999	59,615	8,913
$35,000 and over	96,909	9,712
Persons Living Alone		
Total Persons	668,746	115,562
Income		
Less than $5,000	244,112	68,473
$5,000–9,999	271,091	34,398
$10,000–14,999	73,973	7,274
$15,000–24,999	52,520	3,728
$25,000–34,999	16,440	918
$35,000 and over	10,610	671

Source: U.S. Census, 1990.

northern African Americans believed that the growing communities of blacks from the South threatened their hard-won social, economic, and political security (Tolnay, 1997). These tensions in northern urban areas added to the growing alienation between the black elite and poor blacks, helping perpetuate hypersegregation in the North.

Economic and social discrimination in the larger society was instrumental in creating housing segregation, thereby limiting the expansion of black neighborhoods and fostering concentrated areas of poverty (Franklin, 1997). Therefore, growing old in urban America for African Americans, especially in the North, has always been a demanding experience.

In this chapter we focus on the informal support provided by the family and black church. We believe that these two domains of care for urban older African Americans speak directly to their quality and length of life and general well-being. Census data show that twice as many older blacks as whites live with their relatives (U.S. Census, 1996b). Researchers also have found that institutionalization for African Americans is less than half the rate for whites (Belgrave, Wykle and Choi, 1993). Although the incidence of severe functional limitations among older African Americans (40 percent) is higher than among whites (27 percent) (U.S. Census, 1995), the former use far fewer social and health services (Caserta et al., 1987; Logan and Spitze, 1994). The needs of dependent urban African

American elders are met primarily through their extended network of family and church; both of these support systems are pivotal in understanding who cares for and assists them.

Family Relations and Support

The majority of research on family relations among elderly African Americans shows that they have strong support systems that traditionally have consisted of close and extended family members. However, according to Taylor (1986), the available network of family support is smaller in urban than in rural areas. Nevertheless, whether elders live in urban or rural communities, their family support networks are more likely to be collectivist (two or more people) than individual (Dilworth-Anderson, Williams and Cooper, 1999). Although some research suggests that larger family networks represent greater support (Burton et al., 1995; Miller and McFall, 1991), Lockery (1992) reports that size does not automatically translate into more available care.

Regardless of size, other researchers suggest that perceived support (what is believed to be available) is as important as received support (assistance that is actually obtained) (Dunkel-Schetter and Bennett, 1990; Sarason, Sarason, and Pierce, 1990). Low levels of both perceived and received support are similarly associated with negative consequences of family caregiving to the elderly, such as burden, depression, and social isolation. A high level of perceived support, however, is more often associated with positive outcomes, such as mental and physical health, than even received support (Dunkel-Schetter and Bennett, 1990; Fredman, Daly and Lazur, 1995; George and Gwyther, 1986; Wailing, Seltzer and Greenberg, 1997). Little is known, however, about differences between older urban African Americans and their rural counterparts in terms of their real or perceived family support systems. Further, researchers have not fully explored the range of factors that we believe can significantly influence family support systems of older urban African Americans.

Family Relations and Support

With respect to the larger family context that can affect who gives support, what type is given, and how much is provided, several important issues have been raised in recent literature on the family. It is argued, for example, that analysts and policymakers must establish culturally sensitive and relevant information when describing and explaining the family support of elderly urban African Americans. For example, some researchers (Burton and Jayakody, in press; Dilworth-Anderson and Burton, 1999; Jarrett and Burton, 1999) have suggested that in defining family support networks for older African Americans it is important to (1) identify actual and potential individuals who could be viewed as part of the family; (2) include family members sharing a household as well as those who are not; (3) assess support on the basis of the socioeconomic structure of the kin network (e.g., poor, homogeneous networks versus heterogeneous networks composed of economically secure as well as poorer members); and (4) examine the age distance between generations in family networks, thereby allowing us to better understand how families establish age hierarchies and boundaries when negotiating and exchanging resources (Bengtson, Rosenthal and Burton, 1990; Ladner, 1971).

It is important to assess how issues raised by researchers on family support to older African Americans generally relate to urban African American elders specifically. Evidence shows that because African American families have flexible and permeable family boundaries (Chatters, Taylor and Jayakody, 1994; Chatters, Taylor and Jackson, 1986), the support network may include those who actually give help and those who would or could do so, if needed. Also, because African Americans have a long history of sharing households and moving among them, urban elders may have numerous people available to provide care who may not get counted when researchers use coresidence alone as the indicator of help available. Although Miller and McFall (1991) report that elderly people living in larger households receive the most assistance, their study does not take into consideration that coresidence is not the only measure of household composition for African American elders. Jarrett and Burton (1999) maintain that it is the sharing of goods and resources among households that often speaks to the availability of care for dependent family members in the African American community.

The economic structure of the support network in African American families is another important issue to consider when examining the assistance older people receive from their kin. When family networks are homogeneously poor, regardless of whether or not they share a household, fewer resources are available to dependent older people. These economically poor networks also have very few ties outside the family that could provide additional help (Sanchez-Jankowski, 1999; Wilson, 1996). In contrast, heterogeneous networks that have a greater ratio of nonpoor to poor can distribute surplus resources to poorer family members who need them; the latter also tend to be linked to support systems in the larger society (Burton and Jayakody, in press; Dilworth-Anderson, Williams and Cooper, 1999).

Further, when the extended family network includes both young and elderly dependents, it is more likely to experience a depletion of resources before the needs of its elderly kin can be addressed. African American families, second only to Hispanics, have the highest fertility rate of all groups in American society (U.S. Census, 1999b). Therefore, an understanding of the network's age structure can provide better insight into the availability of family support to its elderly. Given the high level of needs among at-risk teens, HIV/AIDS patients, and poor children and parents; school and neighborhood violence; and drug problems in African American families living in urban areas, the needs of older people may go unmet. Thus, we argue, the older person may receive the least from these family networks.

Church and Social Support

Because of its long-standing record of providing stability, comfort, and a social service system in the African American community (Lincoln and Mamiya, 1990; Pattillo-McCoy, 1998), the black church has traditionally been a viable support system for older urban African Americans. Research findings show that the black church provides some health-based interventions and care for the elderly (Hatch and Jackson, 1981; Taylor et al., 2000). Further, because urban black churches are usually larger than those in rural places, they provide more programs and groups that can address the needs of the elderly. For example, Billingsley (1999) found that although fewer programs were offered for the elderly than for youth, urban churches provided more programs for African American older people than any other nonfamily source. Further, because African Americans may find services from the church easier to access and accept than those provided by formal organizations, the strong presence of the church in caring for, and addressing the needs of, the urban elderly is particularly important.

Additionally, the high level of spirituality found among African Americans provides evidence that church involvement can serve the spiritual needs of the elderly as well. Findings show that African Americans are among the most religious people in the world (Gallup and Castelli, 1989) and that they have a record of frequent church attendance and sizable church membership (Gallup, 1996; Ploch and Hastings, 1994). Researchers also have observed that church support contributes to feelings of well-being and better physical health among African Americans, including the aged (Walls and Zarit, 1991; Wilson-Ford, 1992).

The Role of the Black Church

In spite of the long-standing record of the black church in helping the needy and high levels of church attendance and spirituality among African Americans, our current study of older African Americans and their caregivers shows that the majority of them are not receiving help from the church (Dilworth-Anderson et al., in preparation). For example, in reference to a program that aids African American families providing care to demented elders in the Atlanta area, Williams (1992: 36) noted: "For the participants in our caregiving workshops, the church played a minimum role in providing information or assistance with the caregiving process. In fact, several caregivers complained that as the condition of the older person worsened, the visits and calls from fellow church members decreased."

Reports from a national study (Caldwell et al., 1995) indicate that only about 8 percent of churches addressed the needs of the elderly or their families; almost four times as many churches assisted children and youth. Because these findings at both the local and national levels show that few older urban African Americans and their caregivers currently receive services from the black church, its future role as a major support system may be problematic.

Presently, there are no definitive explanations as to why the black church is not able to address the needs of urban dependent elders at a higher level. Nevertheless, when examining the competing demands on the church in the African American community (e.g., at-risk teens, the rise of HIV/AIDS among young women, poor single-parent households, and drug problems), some inferences can be made (Billingsley, 1999; Wilson, 1999). As with the African American family, the black church may have diminishing resources available to dependent elders because of the growing needs of younger generations in their communities, especially in urban areas.

The Future of Family and Church Social Support

We believe the traditional perception of strong, resilient black families and church support systems that care for dependent members will continue to be challenged by the reality of competing demands among the several generations of African Americans. Demographic shifts in the African American family, including the high and growing number of poor women and women heads of household who are uneducated, living in poverty, and caring for very young children, suggest that families will have fewer kin and resources to care for the elderly than were available twenty-five years ago (U.S. Census, 1999b). However, we predict that because of its strong cultural grounding, the extended African American family system of support will remain intact in spite of these changes, although it may become smaller and more densely structured, with fewer distant and fictive kin. Unlike in the past, close family will be more responsible for elder care. Further, given the current concentration of poor families and what some researchers call the urban underclass (Wilson, 1987; Massey, 1990), the family support system on which elders in urban areas depend may have very limited resources and only a small number of caregivers to assist them. Critically, they also may have few, if any, connections with resources outside the boundaries of their immediate lives. They will lack what Granovetter (1973) describes as the "strength of weak ties" to reinforce existing resources. Such connections, as Burton and Jayakody (in press) report, can serve as conduits for linking elders with social, economic, and health-related assistance in the broader community. Without them, families become isolated in their poverty and in the limitations of what their immediate environment can provide (Sanchez-Jankowski, 1999).

We believe that the structural characteristics negatively affecting urban African American families also will have an impact on services and programs available through churches. Urban black churches most likely will be faced with diminishing numbers of employed young and middle-aged parishioners who have resources that they can share with the church to address the needs of older members and other dependent people in the community. If the present is an indication of what black churches will be able to provide frail elders in the future, more programs and services will not be available to them as compared to those that address the needs of younger families and children.

Conclusion and Policy Implications

The evidence shows that although elderly African Americans residing in urban areas live somewhat better socially and economically than those in rural communities, they too are overwhelmingly poor, widowed, and uneducated. Families provide their major means of social support. Though to a much smaller extent than kin, the black church also plays a role in assisting vulnerable elders. The level of support they receive from these two sources, however, will be challenged increasingly by the growing needs of younger generations.

Most important, urban African American communities, especially those in metropolitan areas, have a significant number of families that fall on the fringe of society—the urban underclass. These individuals and families often are young and middle-aged with a high degree of joblessness and few resources to offer older dependent family members. This situation, coupled with the extremely meager resources of the older generation itself, lessens the ability of many urban African American families to maintain their legacy of strength and resilience.

Despite such pressures, researchers suggest that several aspects of the urban African American family should be examined in order to explore the extent to which it can keep on assisting all of its members. These include identifying the number of actual and potential helpers; examining support across households; assessing the socioeconomic structure of the support network; and determining the extent to which different generations compete for resources.

In conclusion, even with limited resources in many urban African American communities, we believe dependent elders will continue to be cared for by their families and, to a lesser extent, their churches. However, families and churches will be faced with enormous social, economic, and emotional challenges in continuing to provide adequate care. Nevertheless, if history repeats itself, black families, as in the past, will continue in their attempts to meet the needs of the most disadvantaged in the urban African American community—the young and the old (Billingsley, 1999; Franklin, 1997). Clearly, as noted by some researchers (Franklin, 1997; Wilson, 1999), local and national governments as well as the African American community must assist these efforts.

9

Diasporic Aging:
Haitian Americans in New York City

Michel S. Laguerre

This chapter examines the process of social aging among the Haitian American population in New York City. It is primarily concerned with the first generation of older immigrants, which I divide into two groups because of their different aging experiences in the United States. In the first group, I place those who came earlier, worked for a living, brought members of their family from Haiti to New York, and are now at the age of retirement. The second group comprises those who were brought here by their children and have always lived with them because they are unable to run separate and independent households owing to low incomes and a lack of fluency in English as well as an inadequate understanding of how American society operates. They are less visible to outsiders and most vulnerable because of their complete dependence on their children.

There are about one thousand second-generation elders dispersed throughout the Republic, according to the 1990 census.[1] While this group has developed its expectations in the context of the subculture of American society it grew up in, the first generation has based its expectations on the cultural traditions of the homeland. The socialization of these first- and second-generation immigrants has been shaped by different cultural practices influenced most heavily either by the homeland, by the United States, or by both.

The methodological reason we focus our attention on the first generation is that the immigration of that cohort to New York is less than half a century old and a majority of the elders belong to that group. However, unable to pass the citizenship test because of lack of knowledge of English, the majority of these elders are not citizens. Concentrating on this immigrant group of elderly is one way to shed light on their plight and the issues they confront every day, so that the government can be sensitive to their needs and social service providers may have a better understanding of their problems.

The gerontological, sociological, and anthropological literature on the aging process has made great strides toward explaining the role of ethnicity in social aging. It recognizes that aging cannot be divorced from the cultural process where its meaning is deciphered. A number of studies that used lifespan paradigms developed in the study of older white Americans and that had been applied to explain the aging process among Mexican Americans, African Americans, Native Americans, and Asian Americans were criticized for their cultural bias (Jackson, 1980; McNeely and Colen, 1983). These studies, because they paid little attention to ethnicity and gender, tended to explain aging in terms of "disengagement" and "activity theory" seen through the prism of life processes or developmental phases. Disengagement was presented as "an inevitable process in which the individual and society make a gradual and mutual withdrawal," while activity theory stated that "morale and life satisfaction are a function of continued active participation in important spheres of life" (Colen and McNeely, 1983).

As a result of a greater sensitivity to ethnic issues, the subfield of minority aging has blossomed since the 1980s (Gelfand, 1982; Harel, McKinney and Williams, 1990; Gelfand and Barresi, 1987a). In this new area of focus, ethnicity, racial discrimination, racial assumptions of white researchers, and gender are among the issues raised. Ethnic groups are seen as having their own specific needs because of the historical period of discrimination during which they were incorporated into American society and the experience of social and geographical exclusion they had to endure in the social construction of their communities. While discussions on ethnicity and racial discrimination are paramount in this literature, the focus is still, in the majority of studies, on groups of people (African Americans, Native Americans, Asian Americans, and Mexican Americans) that have been here at least since the nineteenth century. As a consequence of this narrow emphasis, these works are limited in what they can offer to our understanding of current first-generation immigrant elders.

The literature on these first-generation immigrant older people is still in an embryonic phase. However, it provides some insights into the everyday life of the elderly. The studies focus primarily on issues of language and communication, the relations of the aged with children and grandchildren, lack of access to social services, minority status, and dependency (Omidian, 1996; Blakemore and Boneham, 1994; Fennell, Phillipson and Evers, 1988). Padilla (1958: 3) notes that "aging individuals who came to this country in their youth are the conservative remainders and reminders of the Old World immigrations." She further points out that "the aged Puerto Ricans . . . tend to live with their married children" in New York and that "in Puerto Rico old people are more respected" (93, 307). Queralt (1983: 57) reports in her review of the state of the Cuban elderly that "in many cases intergenerational differences become severe enough to force the elderly to move away from their children." She further adds that "for the sick elderly . . . inability to communicate effectively with health providers can be anxiety-producing" (58).

Kozaitis (1987: 188), who carried out research among Greek immigrants in Chicago, reports that "the single most serious problem reported by this group was the language barrier. As one man said, 'without language you are a nobody,'" a sentiment expressed by many. The communication problem of the elderly may be caused not only by displacement in a foreign land but also by illiteracy. Indeed, Gelfand and Barresi (1987: 13) note that "this limited ability in communication makes it difficult for the elderly to avail themselves of services and also creates problems for service providers. The problem extends beyond elderly persons who speak a foreign tongue, however, to include also those who are illiterate." Illiteracy, a common and major problem in Haiti, continues to plague the Haitian American elderly in New York.

While the old literature focuses on the local factor as the site where solutions to elderly problems are sought, here we connect the local with the homeland in framing the issue and in providing explanations that take the transnational factor into consideration. We place the issue inside the ethnopole, at the site of a diasporic community that displays both a local and transnational orientation.[2] We use the concept *ethnopole* instead of *ethnic enclave* precisely to underline this global factor. The diasporic ethnopole is by definition a transnational or even global community because it maintains primary relations with the homeland and secondary relations with other diasporic sites.

By and large, the literature on Haitian Americans has been silent on the plight of the elderly and concentrates on labor migration, that is, on the working class or the individual migrants of working age (Chierici, 1991). This is so because of the visibility of the latter while the elderly continue to remain an invisible crowd. They are the most neglected and vulnerable members of the community for many different reasons that we will explain below.

The members of the early wave of mass migration that began with the presidency of François "Papa Doc" Duvalier in 1957 are now at or approaching retirement age (Laguerre, 1998). This cohort of first-generation elderly Haitian Americans faces its own unique set of problems. They have been accustomed to a Haitian way of aging (respected by children; sought after by the extended family for their advice, wisdom, and folk medical knowledge; longstanding members of the community church; persons with well-established reputations and with predictable futures) (Comhaire-Sylvain, 1975) and were hoping to return to Haiti after the collapse of the Duvalier dynasty. Their informal plan had been to return to the island, use their pension funds or Social Security, and live a peaceful life far away from the snowy winter months and criminal activities in the mean streets of Brooklyn. That plan had been dashed with the return to the status quo in the years following the extravagant exile of Jean Claude Duvalier to France in 1986.

The best a few can hope for now is to move to Florida, where the weather is more suitable to retirement for those who grew up on a tropical Caribbean island. In the past three decades, the secondary migration of Haitian Americans from the Northeast to Florida has been minimal but constant. For these lucky middle-class retirees, Florida is still another experience, with its possibilities of street violence brought about by aggressive drug traffickers and the yearly devastating hurricanes that visit this lovely and sunny state. Migration to Florida means adaptation to a new place, disruption of relationships developed in New York over many years, and a retreat from a fast pace to a more sedentary way of life. But psychologically speaking, for elderly Haitian Americans it is a comfort zone, offering the consolation that one is a little closer to the motherland.

The migration experience from Haiti to the United States has been more traumatic for some of the elderly because it subverted the natural rhythm of events that would have led to retirement. For these individuals, retirement began too early, as they were forced into a situation of dependency while in their early fifties; this is premature even by American standards except for those who are sick or wealthy. This forced retirement was imposed on them not because they had reached an acceptable age to retire, had enough money to take care of themselves, did not want employment, or could not work due to chronic illness but because they were placed in a situation of withdrawal against their will. By forced retirement, I mean the process by which biological age is divorced from social age, whereby the retreat from wage labor is wholly based on external factors, brought about by migration itself, over which the individual has little or no control.

Forced migration tends to lead to an inability to fit into the new society: lack of legal immigration status if the person is an undocumented immigrant, lack of knowledge of English that impedes formal communication with the mainstream population, and inability to live by oneself. This state of affairs often happens because a person was forced by her or his children to migrate to the United States at an age when it is difficult to find employment because of age discrimination and lack of marketable skills. Children generally will sponsor a parent after the death of one of the spouses in the homeland. The surviving spouse is encouraged by the children to join the immigrant branch of the family in the United States. Of course, the parent is not expected to live alone.

The following cases give us a glimpse of the local and transnational experiences of these elderly. It is appropriate to let them tell their stories in their own voices. These cases develop similar and different themes as they identify key elements that allow us to interpret their various experiences. Not only do these vignettes tell us about the elders, but they also shed light on Haitian American family life in New York. As the elders are additions to the nuclear family, their very presence places some stress on the household and contributes to the reshaping of household relations.

Case 1

I was employed in Haiti and arranged for my wife to emigrate to Boston in 1970. I came to the U.S. in 1982 as a tourist, after the death of my mother, with the help of my sister. In a short period of time, I was able to become a U.S. resident. My wife was living with a boyfriend from Haiti.

Since I have children with her, I sponsored her for legal residence status. We do not live together. I was sick, dependent, and living on Social Security. Therefore, I thought I should help her with residence so that she could send for the children, which she did.

With financial aid from the state, I receive $500 per month and the government subsidizes my apartment. This helps me support the four illegitimate children (ages ten, sixteen, seventeen, and eighteen) I still have in Haiti (I had eight children with my wife). I send them $200 per month so that they can live well with their mother. I have some savings in the bank in case there is a major problem with my family in Haiti. This money can be used to solve any potential problem that occurs with them. When my children here are unemployed, I help them with what I have.

For my weekly food intake, the state gives me $50 in food stamps per month. I cook my own food. Each day of the week, we come to this center; we give a dollar and they serve us good food. On weekends, my children bring me food gratis.

Unable to speak English, when I go to see a physician I need a translator. That's why I prefer to see a Haitian nurse or physician. When I go to a hospital, it is a total embarrassment. There is sometimes an effort made to provide an in-house translator. One cannot speak directly to the physician. It is embarrassing to speak through a translator because sometimes it is private business; I would rather keep it between me and the physician.

I am sick with a heart ailment but I am unable to select which food is good for me. In Haiti, the selection was basically between rice and cornmeal. Here in the market there are so many canned foods, the choice is bigger and the type of food [hot or cold properties] is not known.

Several issues are raised in this vignette: binational family organization, transnational relations, dependence on others for translation, and problems with health and nutrition. This case illustrates the situation of marital disruption brought about by the migration of a spouse who, far away from her husband, began having an affair, as did he. While it would have been difficult to take such a drastic course of action if she were still in Haiti, migration to New York allowed her to do so because she was no longer restrained by local standards. The husband was able to come to the United States with the help of his sister rather than that of his wife.

The specific conditions of migration help us understand the experiences of some Haitians in the United States. For example, this man's situation, with a separated wife here and a common-law wife on the island, augurs the problems he will face in old age. One major dilemma he confronted was that since he could not move in with his wife and was not financially solvent enough to send for his common-law wife and children, he had to live alone. In addition, though he is not supporting his first family, he has dependents to care for in Haiti. Therefore, much of the money that he needs for himself is sent to his homeland.

His situation cannot be understood simply by focusing on the local factor; the transnational aspect is as important. He is involved in a transnational operational circuit: he helps and gets help from his children in the United States and uses part of that money to defray expenses incurred in Port-au-Prince. Yet he lives alone, with neither branch of his family, managing his relations with both local and overseas households by himself.

This case also reveals how the limited money given by the state for the welfare of the aged is sometimes used to care for other members of the family who have temporarily lost their jobs. There tends to be interdependence; at times his adult children in the United States depend on him for financial help so that they can pay their rent or mortgage.

The lack of fluency in English also shapes his experience on American soil: it prevents him from communicating with the mainstream system without an interpreter and forces him to find his place in the ethnopole. The inability to identify cold and hot properties of food sold in the supermarket adds to his uneasiness and discomfort. Such information was known to him in Haiti. His lack of familiarity with the vast display of products in the supermarket contributes to a concern over his health. Language also influences his preference for a Haitian doctor. He describes his embarrassment about having a translator in the room while he is speaking privately to the Caucasian physician. Elders may complain about Haitian American physicians being too expensive, but they continue to see them because they can speak to them in Creole and explain the nature of their condition.

The experience of illness also helps us understand other aspects of the lives of older Haitians. Although they seek medical doctors for complicated illnesses, they use folk medicine for common maladies like colds, headaches, and minor physical discomfort. They find the ingredients to make these folk remedies in Haitian and Caribbean American markets. Failing that, they order them either from Miami or from the homeland. They also use these remedies for chronic illnesses that they think they can cure by themselves, such as hypertension and diabetes.

Since they are the oldest and usually the sickest in the household, they experiment on themselves with new folk remedies they have learned from other Haitians in the ethnopole. In a sense, the household becomes a medical laboratory where they concoct healing agents in an effort to treat their illness and recover their health. They test medicines on themselves, which, if proven useful, may be used to cure others. Not only do they retain the old folk remedies, but they also add new ones to the New York household repertoire.

Case 2

We came to New York and lived with our children. She is my second wife. Their mother had died and I remarried. We had our own room and we did not pay for it. But the children did not want to take care of us. Eventually we were evicted from my daughter's apartment.

When we came here, the children were no longer the same. They insulted us, spoke back, and had no respect for us. We felt devalued. Children can disrespect you in English and you won't even know it unless they translate their words. When we have an appointment at the hospital, we need someone to take us there. Haitians do not trust Haitian American physicians. The children do not have time; they either go to school or work, and are not available. It is a problem.

We feel isolated from our children and society. I baby-sit for my son's children but cannot speak to or understand them because of my lack of English. My sense is that we have lost control here. We are treated like babies. We are Catholic but we go to the Protestant church because it has a van that picks us up, and offers activities for seniors.

We cannot rely on our children for help even though we need to have them around for assistance and support. We worry a lot about the future. We don't want to go to a nursing home; we would prefer to return to Haiti instead. We don't know what the future holds for us.

Several more issues are raised in this scenario, notably generational conflict, consciousness of worthlessness, isolation, lack of access to one's church, and language problems. The elders soon learn that their children do not treat them according to their expectations. Communication problems come about because the children have been exposed to American culture while the parents are still seeing things according to Haitian traditions. They often have tremendous difficulties communicating with their grandchildren who speak only English. The control they used to have over their children and grandchildren has disappeared in the United States.

We have found that several families have converted to Protestantism in New York. They do so because of the fellowship they find there among the brethren and the social programs of these churches. While the Catholic Church generally does not provide transportation to parishioners to attend Sunday services, some Haitian American Protestant churches do.

Case 3

I live with my daughter and feel that all the responsibility for running the house is on my shoulders. Although I help them, I do not feel appreciated. Sometime I cook for the family and someone will voice his or her dissatisfaction with my cooking. I am shocked by this. I wake up early to prepare breakfast for the children so that they can be ready for the bus to take them to school.

I work day and night in the house. Sometimes I am tired of working full time in the house by myself since everyone is away. And they expect a clean home when they come back from work or school. They expect the food to be ready for them as well—and they expect good food. I work hard because I do not want my daughter and son-in-law to think that I am lazy or that I am not helping them maintain the household.

I have a lot of problems because I cannot speak English. The children are not well educated; yet, they make fun of me. After a while, I become frustrated because of their lack of respect and also because I cannot talk to or understand them fully.

My life is limited to the apartment space. I don't walk outside because I am afraid of crime and that I might get lost. But inside the house is no better. I may watch a little bit of television, but since I do not understand what anyone is saying, it does me no good; actually it frustrates me more.

Elders often help with the upkeep of apartments or homes. For them, it is not retirement in the strict sense of the term. They contribute to the household not only with the money they may receive from the state but also with their labor—for instance, by baby-sitting and cooking. Some may resent these tasks but have nothing else to do since the rest of the family is at work or in school.

An examination of gender can shed light on the differential experiences of elders. The older father is less likely than the older mother to be assigned a specific task in the household; generally, the latter ends up being responsible for cooking, cleaning, and baby-sitting if the younger couple works or attends school. For females, retirement comes with daily, unpaid responsibilities. This free labor keeps grandma busy during the day and allows the host adult children to save money. The presence of grandma contributes significantly to the smooth operation of the household. However, the elder woman may not be able to play this role because of illness. Moreover, since women tend to live longer than their husbands, they are more likely to become frail and dependent on the host household.

Since the grandmother in this scenario is the chief cook, her presence will keep family culinary traditions alive. With time she even may be able to teach the children some Creole, especially when they are young. This may be a cause of conflict if the parents don't want their children to learn their traditional language.

At times, elders become the dynamic center of the household. Grandma may end up being the best friend of the youngest children in the apartment because they spend more time with her than with their parents, especially when she is the main baby-sitter. But once the children start going to school, she sometimes becomes a folkloric fixture who behaves strangely. For example, she may order them to do things in a nondemocratic, authoritarian way, as is done in Haiti.

When the older person lives in the household, she may develop her own discourse on morality based on Haitian culture and a parallel one on the actual behavior of the family. She spends a good deal of time comparing the situation in the United States with that in the homeland. The aged mother may fault her adult daughter for not educating the children properly and even complain incessantly, whether anyone wants to hear her or not. Her critical comments stem not from lack of love for her family but from a comparison of their actions here with what she would expect to occur in Haiti.

Grandma tends to be a key proponent for aid to loved ones in the homeland. She constantly reminds her daughters and sons to send money. From the meager pension she receives, she often saves some for family and friends in Haiti. Without the presence of old parents in the apartment to plead for poor relatives, the size and frequency of remittances mailed to the island probably would be greatly reduced.

The household with seniority status among the extended family is the one in which the elderly parents reside. Their presence is a clear sign that this family plays a leadership role over the others. It is the site where other members of the family come to visit with grandma, where family reunions are held, and where major decisions concerning the extended family are made. This is the new headquarters household of the Haitian family.

However, any perceived authority of seniors is more symbolic than real. They are figureheads, with little power or means to enforce their will. Their dependence stems from the language problem, their financial situation, and their lack of familiarity with the American system. Generally, it is only in the area of "Haitian knowledge" that they are still considered the experts of the household. They are a major source for transmission of wisdom and folkways from the homeland to youngsters. They are the culture specialists to whom one turns to remember things from the past or for an expert opinion on Haitian matters. Lun (1983) has found a similar pattern among Asian Americans when he notes that "the transmission of ideas, customs, skills, and the arts and language of various Asian countries from the elderly to successive generations is a major value and goal."

Their opinion is rarely sought on anything outside their insights on Haiti. A good portion of the negative aspects of the island (poverty, diseases, violence, excesses of voodoo secret societies, political instability, and human rights abuses) is transmitted by elders, and this may be precisely the reason why some of their adult children prefer to associate themselves more closely with American culture. Older Haitians often complain about their isolation from the rest of society. That isolation is exacerbated by language difficulties: they cannot understand television or read newspapers. The next best thing is to listen to the Haitian radio programs such as Radio Soleil d'Haiti for news, comments, and the latest gossip. Because they stay at home and listen to the radio, elders can become a source of news and commentaries for the rest of the family. When other members of the household return from work, grandma is the first to break the Haitian news and to add her comments and spice to it. Since Haitian radio is in Creole, the family usually does not question the accuracy of her reportage; such news also is shared with grandma's informal network and may be the predominant topic of conversation for weeks. This is one area where she can speak with some authority. For information from the national networks, which is in English, she must rely on other members of the household.

The life of the elderly is embedded in an informal network of friends and relatives. This constitutes the social environment in which they manage their day-to-day existence. This network is made up of old-timers (that is, friends and relatives from the old country and the village or neighborhood in which they lived before their migration to New York); friends of the host family who may be living in the same building or who are employed at the same place; and new friends the elders may meet at church or senior centers. The members of this informal network have one thing in common: they all speak Creole. This is precisely why those friendships are considered so precious. Through this network, the elders learn about neighborhood news in Haiti and new folk remedies as well as services and programs for which they are eligible.

In fact, because grandma is so tied to the Haitian community, her presence in the household may complicate the possibility of her children relocating to better quarters in a suburb. As long as they remain in the ethnopole, grandma can listen to Haitian radio programs, access ethnic shops, visit with old friends from the island, attend church services in Creole, and get help from neighbors in case of an emergency. In the suburbs, these services and facilities may not be available.

The New York experience can be traumatic for the Haitian elderly in many different ways. During the month of November, elders are reminded in a painful way of their diasporic situation. This is the time of year when they are somber because the important Haitian tradition of remembering the dead cannot be duplicated here. In Haiti, during the early days of November it is customary to visit the cemetery, clean the tombs of loved ones, and pay a fee so that the local priest can stop in front of these graves to say a prayer. In America, this cannot be done for parents and other relatives whose tombs are in the homeland.

They also suffer from a double loss of status: first, vis-à-vis the larger society, they are considered second-class citizens; and second, vis-à-vis the ethnopole, their former reputations are not transferable. In New York, one is not known and there is no community recognition. One becomes simply an insignificant member of the crowd. In terms of social status, it is a step backward; one moves from being a national/majority member to being an ethnic/minority member. Many individuals also must form a new identity heavily influenced by the dominant sector of society, often resulting in internal conflict.

Conclusion and Policy Implications

The experience of elders is played out in the context of transnationality because they interpret life here through the prism of the cultural traditions of their homeland. They feed themselves with news from Haiti, which they get by listening to Haitian radio programs. They request from Haiti over-the-counter French medications and folk remedies (herbs, leaves, roots), and they send money back to the homeland. In some cases, they continue to hold on to their property papers, for which they must pay annual taxes to the Haitian government. Perhaps the most significant aspect of this transnationality is the fact that they are physically here but their minds are in Haiti. Those who are in good health make yearly trips to Haiti to visit family and take care of property left behind.

In this chapter, we have attempted to describe the situation of the Caribbean elderly living in American society by paying attention to cultural expectations from the old country and the contextual conditions in New York City. We argue that aging is experienced differently by divergent diasporic groups and even within each one by specific generations. However, because of the similar experiences of migration and the location of these Haitian immigrants in the ethnopole, they seem to mesh into a diasporic class of dependent individuals. The differences among them are more in degree than in kind.

Notes

1. The Haitian American elders that appear in the 1990 census are the offspring of the cohort that came to New York during the first U.S. occupation of Haiti from 1915 to 1934. Many of them resided then in Harlem because of the persistent practice of racial discrimination and housing segregation. See, e.g., Reid, 1939.

2. For a definition of an ethnopole, see Laguerre, 2000: 19.

10

American Indian and Alaska Native Elderly

Mona Polacca

> The old ones, full of years.
> The wise ones, the storytellers, the teachers.
> The almost ancestors.
> —*Almost Ancestors,* T. Kroeber and R. F. Heizer

The cultures and histories of the numerous American Indian and Alaska Natives (AI/AN) tribes and communities differ significantly, as do the attitudes of individuals toward traditional values versus acculturation. To further identify these differences, health professionals may seek information about specific groups with whom they work by consulting the specific tribal council in their area. While such variations should not be ignored, a few key observations, which generally apply to elderly AI/AN, will be reviewed in this chapter.

Demographics

It is more difficult to discuss AI/AN elderly than some other groups owing to the lack of solid information. Research on AI/AN elderly has been limited, and public information often fails to include or provide separate information about them. The U.S. government defines an American Indian as anyone who is one-fourth or more of Indian blood. The blood quantum must be from a tribe that is recognized by the federal government, and the individual must be acknowledged and enrolled on a tribal census.

To understand the uniqueness of the AI/AN in relation to the provision of health and social services in general, and more specifically elderly services, one must first examine the trust relationship they have with the federal government. Various tribes are sovereign AI/AN and possess a distinct and special political relationship with the U.S. government based largely, but not exclusively, on treaties agreed to by the two parties. This relationship was founded upon a trust responsibility that is unique in that it provides for rights and privileges that no other Americans or groups possess. Because of these special rights, a body of laws, policy, and regulations has developed that relate solely to the AI/AN and that dictates the provision and delivery of health and social services to AI/AN communities. Given their special status, AI/AN are citizens of three sovereigns: (1) the United States, (2) the state in which they reside, and (3) their tribal government. Therefore, they should have the rights and privileges afforded by each.

There are 507 federally recognized Indian tribal governments, which include 197 distinct AI/AN villages in Alaska. Indian reservations and Alaska AI/AN villages comprise 52 million acres of tribal trust land provided through acts of Congress and executive orders continuing into the 1970s. According to the Office of Technology Assessment's report *Indian Health Care* (1986), no single variable or socioeconomic indicator encompasses the diverse characteristics of AI/AN. Yet, mainstream society often perceives Indians as a homogeneous group with the same appearance, customs, and language. As with other groups in American society, AI/AN are in transition; all of them are changing, and some are changing faster than others.

According to the U.S. Census and the Indian Health Service, from 1980 to 1990 the elderly AI/AN increased more rapidly than the sixty-five-and-over age group overall. The general elderly population increased by 22 percent as compared to 59 percent for AI/AN. The proportion of elderly within the AI/AN population has grown faster than in other minority groups. Between 1980 and 1990, their numbers rose by 35 percent, a rate twice that of white or black elderly.

About 114,000 (6 percent) of the AI/AN population are over sixty-five. Of these, 37 percent are age seventy-five or over. Among AI/AN ages sixty-five to sixty-nine, there are 85 men for every 100 women. At age seventy-five and over, the sex ratio declines to 58 men for every 100 women. The marital status of AI/AN is comparable to that of the white population—the majority of AI/AN women are widowed.

About one-quarter of AI/AN elderly live on Indian reservations or in Alaskan AI/AN villages. Over half are concentrated in the southwestern states of Oklahoma, California, Arizona, New Mexico, and Texas. The remainder live in states along the Canadian border.

Older AI/AN have less access to government assistance than other groups, which increases their risk of substandard housing, poverty, malnutrition, and poor health. Only 40 percent of AI/AN over age sixty receive Social Security, a lower rate than for other ethnic minority groups. Less than one-half receive Medicare, and fewer than 40 percent receive Medicaid.

There is an important distinction to be made between AI/AN living on reservations and those residing in urban areas. Individuals and families living on federally recognized tribal reservations are eligible for a variety of government programs and benefits that are usually not available to those who move off the reservation. Though all elderly AI/AN can participate in Medicare and Medicaid, it is difficult for those living off the reservation to gain access to these benefits by themselves. This distinction is crucial in terms of the availability of health care and other services for the elderly.

AI/AN elderly have been educated almost exclusively within U.S. school systems. The quality of that education, both on and off reservations, has been poor. The cohort of elders sixty years of age and older are products of a federal system of education that was designed to uproot AI/AN from their culture. MacGregor describes the process:

> Children were virtually kidnapped to force them into government schools; their hair was cut, and their Indian clothes thrown away. They were forbidden to speak their own language. Life in the school was under military discipline, and rules were reinforced by corporal punishment. Those who persisted in clinging to their old ways and those who ran away and were recaptured were thrown in jail. Parents who objected were also jailed. Where possible, children were kept in school year after year to avoid the influence of their families. (cited in Simpson and Yinger, 1965: 145)

From the late 1800s until the late 1970s, U.S. government policy toward the AI/AN emphasized forced assimilation into the white world. The Indian boarding school was designed to remove children from the influence of their parents and tribe and create a new social environment where they could be "civilized." The AI/AN response was to drop out or sometimes even refuse to go.

About 22 percent of all AI/AN have graduated from high school, but nearly 12 percent have no formal education at all. Without any schooling, many of the elderly find it hard to understand benefits, rules and regulations, and application procedures for federal or state programs, which are a part of America's complex social welfare system. AI/AN are clearly victims of cultural estrangement. Efforts must be made to bridge the gap between the elderly rooted in their traditional lifestyles and the complicated, confusing programs designed for a highly technical society.

Low levels of education also may account for the high unemployment rate, which is 48 percent or more for all reservations. Of those employed, only 24 percent earn more than $7,000 annually. Significantly, more AI/AN than whites continue to work after age sixty-five. However, nearly twice as many AI/AN elderly who are actively seeking work are unemployed. The median income for AI/AN men age sixty-five or over is $9,967, as compared to $14,775 for their white counterparts. For women in this age group, the median income is $6,004 and $8,297, respectively.

Overall, 20 percent of AI/AN sixty-five years or older live below the official poverty level. In urban areas, 14 percent are in poverty; for those living on reservations, the proportion is even higher: 24 percent in 1990. Of those AI/AN elderly who receive Social Security, the majority depend on it as their sole means of support.

Health and Social Services

Indian Health Service figures for 1990 show average life expectancy at birth for AI/AN to be only sixty-seven years, eight years less than that of whites. The leading causes of death among AI/AN elderly are heart disease, malignant neoplasm, cerebrovascular disorders, pneumonia, influenza, diabetes mellitus, and accidents. AI/AN are ten times more likely to develop diabetes than whites. The other major health problems of elderly AI/AN are tuberculosis, liver and kidney disease, high blood pressure, pneumonia, and malnutrition. The majority of AI/AN elderly rarely see a physician, primarily because the elderly needing medical assistance often live in isolated areas and lack transportation. AI/AN traditions of ritual folk healing and the spiritual aspect of disease have also deterred reliance on a strictly scientific medical community.

These factors are often neglected and overlooked by health care professionals, including those making government policy related to the aging. For instance, in 1961, the First White House Conference on Aging was held. As a result, the Older Americans Act was developed and signed into law in 1965. A budget of $7.5 million was appropriated and allocated to the states for the provision of social and nutritional services to assist older Americans. However, since many state governments believed that they had no responsibility for the provision of health or social services to AI/AN whose reservation communities lay within their boundaries, much of this funding was not available for a large number of older AI/ANs. The Second White House Conference on Aging, held in 1971, addressed the special needs of elderly AI/ANs for the first time.

As a result of a strong lobbying movement by AI/AN organizations and tribes, in October 1978, Congress amended the Older Americans Act to establish Title VI, which provided for direct funding to "federally recognized Indian Tribes." Title VI was to be implemented within ninety days after Congress appropriated $6 million for the program. Owing to difficulty in developing the regulations, Title VI did not become effective until July, 1980. In the spring of 1980, Title VI applications were sent to the then 480 federally recognized tribes. Out of 86 formal applications submitted, 85 were funded. As of 1999, 212 Administration on Aging Title VI grants have been made directly to tribes.

Social indicators suggest that there is a great need for services among AI/AN elderly. Yet, they are seriously underrepresented in national programs. For example, while 11.4 percent of AI/AN adults are veterans, according to the 1989 Veterans Administration report *Native American Veterans*, less than 1 percent are participating in Veterans Administration programs. In Arizona, fewer than 10 percent of Medicaid-eligible frail AI/AN elderly are receiving long-term care services financed under that program. This is primarily due to the lack of nursing home facilities and certified home-care agencies in reservation communities.

Selected Aspects of American Indian/Alaska Native Culture

The AI/AN population is made up of many unique cultures, each with its own history, geography, language or dialect, and beliefs. In addition, AI/AN vary from those who are comfortable only with traditional ways to those who are completely acculturated and have accepted the lifestyle of the mainstream culture. In this complex circumstance, cultural sensitivity is mandatory. To realize success in serving AI/AN, it is vital that traditional values and beliefs be seen as tools for creative service provision rather than as hindrances to be eliminated.

Historically, the status of the aged in AI/AN tribes was one of honor and respect. Elderly people had certain rights, such as making their opinions known. Elderly people often held positions of authority in the household and in the ceremonial life of the tribe. In many AI/AN societies the aged are still a needed and highly respected segment of the community, which contributes significantly to a sense of well-being among them. The elderly remember who was related to whom, both present and past. As a group, they make up a tribal data bank that has accumulated information and knowledge on all aspects of AI/AN life.

Families are important in the lives of AI/AN elderly, who are four times as likely as their white counterparts to live with their kin. At least 17 percent of reservation households are three to four generations deep, although many AI/AN elderly live alone or only with a spouse. While a large number of elderly AI/AN provide support for their children and grandchildren, the significant poverty experienced by AI/AN families limits the extent of economic assistance.

Most vulnerable elderly remain in their home communities and are cared for by family and relatives. Recent studies indicate that 67 percent of AI/AN elders live within five miles of relatives upon whom they depend for assistance in shopping, transportation, and other needs of daily living. However, research also indicates that the AI/AN elderly are suffering from diminishing family support. While AI/AN are in many ways the least assimilated American ethnic minority in the United States, profound changes in the AI/AN family and all aspects of the social system have been brought about by continuing urbanization and adaptations to the mainstream culture. Though relatives traditionally have taken care of their aging family members, many of them, already and increasingly overburdened by competing obligations, have been forced to reduce their elder-care roles. Consequently, a growing percentage of frail AI/AN older people find themselves without any kin to provide care or support.

Moreover, the fear of crime is rising in AI/AN communities, particularly among the elderly. Elder abuse and financial exploitation also add to the problems of older AI/AN. In some cases, the safest alternative is institutionalization, mostly in facilities outside the reservation. However, as with many other groups, AI/AN families view placement of elders in nursing homes as the last option.

Today's AI/AN elderly are a generation who have met with numerous negative incidents throughout their lives. As children, they were forcibly removed from their homes to attend government boarding schools or Christian mission schools, institutional environments that were foreign to them. They were given Christian names, stripped of their traditional clothing and hairstyle, and fed foods that were unfamiliar to them. Now, once again at a crucial time of their lives, some AI/AN older people are reexperiencing the trauma of separation, being removed from their familiar environment and being placed in a nursing home far away from their reservation. These elderly, many of whom do not speak English, often become depressed, lonely, and isolated. Language barriers, along with a lack of awareness, respect, and/or tolerance of AI/AN cultural practices and beliefs on the part of non-native service providers, can interfere with the delivery of quality care. For example, certain behaviors may appear alien to nursing home aides, such as the AI/AN preference to sit on the floor or sleep in their everyday clothing.

The following is an illustration of one such miscommunication:

> An elderly Apache Indian woman, upon admission into a nursing home, was instructed to put on a hospital-type gown instead of her traditional dress. She became very distressed. When asked why she was so upset, she told the aides that she wanted her own clothing back. Although a tribal social worker intervened and she was allowed to wear her traditional dress, she discovered that it had been cut down the back. This time she became extremely agitated. The nursing home staff eventually discovered that the Apache believe that cutting clothing means death.

It would appear crucial to place AI/AN elders in facilities that have other AI/AN residents. Some tribes will even arrange special trips, bringing the ambulatory elderly from the reservation to visit. Moreover, the negative attitude of AI/AN toward nursing homes is reinforced by the fact that, as one elder puts it, "friends and relatives leave the reservation not to live at a nursing home but to die." Therefore, to ease their fears, it is important to include frail AI/AN older people in the long-term care decision-making process, providing them with as much information about the facility as possible.

Traditional Healing and Spirituality

Spirituality is a highly important aspect of AI/AN life. It is the belief and practice of interaction and communication at a level beyond the physical and intellectual. AI/AN have highly organized traditions that provide for spiritual, moral, social, physical, and mental guidance. A primary purpose of traditional AI/AN spirituality is to facilitate the maintenance of harmony and balance among the individual, other people, nature, and the spiritual world. Practicing spirituality helps to maintain stability and to give a sense of cohesion to an individual's life; it is not separated from health care as it is in most Western cultures. Indian medicine refers to a traditional or specific cultural approach to health and life for a person, rather than medical treatment of a disease or illness alone. Therefore, in working with the AI/AN elderly, it is important to consider their spiritual needs, which are often overlooked in our highly technological society.

It has not always been easy to address issues related to Indian medicine or native healers, but attitudes are beginning to shift. For example, in 1977 the World Health Organization adopted a resolution urging governments to encourage the use of traditional systems of medicine (native healing practices). The American Medical Association revised its code of ethics in 1980 and gave physicians permission to consult with, and make referrals to, practitioners without orthodox medical training, including AI/AN medicine people (Krippner, 1995).

AI/AN elderly often use two health care systems, depending on whether they view the disease as an "Indian" or "white man's" disease. If the cause is deemed to be spiritual, indicating that it is an Indian illness, they employ traditional medicine, such as healing and cleansing ceremonies. They use Western doctors, through the Indian Health Service medical care system, when the ailment is seen as resulting from Western influences.

Death rituals and taboos vary between groups, as do attitudes about touching the body. The Omnibus Reconciliation Act of 1987 and the Patient Self-Determination Act of 1991 were enacted to protect patient rights. However, AI/AN cultural beliefs may conflict with some of their provisions, including whether medical intervention is desired in a particular case and the extent of aggressive treatment such as resuscitation and intubation. Another consideration is that an open discussion of death and dying is not accepted in some tribal cultures and therefore could harm the patient psychologically.

Although healing practices differ among AI/AN they usually include purification of the patient, smoking or offering religious tobacco, gentle massage, small sacrifices, and prayers. Other traditional approaches to health care are herbal remedies and bonesetters. Some patients take traditional medications such as herbal teas in large doses. Medical care providers must be careful to avoid any lethal interactions between traditional and Western medications and to instruct AI/AN elders on appropriate use of prescribed drugs.

Communication

The communication patterns of an AI/AN reservation reflect the history, cultural practices, and attitudes of the community. Each community possesses its own idiosyncrasies and norms, which are reflected in both verbal and nonverbal language.

Elderly AI/AN generally are exceedingly reluctant to share personal, especially intimate, information, even under circumstances that require it in order to receive assistance. Older AI/AN need more time than whites to establish relationships and will share intimate information only when there is a foundation of trust. Intimate information for an AI/AN could include family history, beliefs and values, health, or financial matters (e.g., annual income or how much land he/she owns).

The concept of reciprocity is very important in establishing rapport. Trust relationships can be established by *not* insisting that information be revealed and by demonstrating a willingness to listen and just "be there." The elderly person may initially test the worker's genuineness by asking him or her to perform some task, such as assistance in filling out forms. This pattern reflects the AI/AN value of cooperation or exchange. Humor is one technique frequently utilized by the AI/AN to get more information, strengthen relationships, or demonstrate affection.

The nonverbal communication patterns of silence and eye contact are important when relating to AI/AN elderly. They are comfortable sharing physical space (simply sitting together) without engaging in verbal conversation. This silence should not be interpreted as a lack of interest or comprehension; silence is one way the elder processes information and internalizes suggestions. Most AI/AN minimize eye contact, even though they are listening intently. It does not mean that they are unassertive, depressed, or lacking in self-confidence. One useful guideline is to look at their chin rather than directly at the eyes. As always, one must rely on the other person's response, especially his or her body language, as a guide.

Dietary Practices

Dietary practices of the AI/AN vary from region to region, according to the natural food supply in the area. The contemporary AI/AN diet combines indigenous natural foods with modern processed commodities. Game and fish, where plentiful, are important food sources. Fruits, berries, roots, and wild greens are highly valued but scarce in many places. When indigenous foods are not available, the daily diet consists of packaged goods and produce donated by the U.S. Department of Agriculture or purchased at stores. Even then, fresh fruits and vegetables are not always available or may be too expensive, unless locally grown. Distance from grocery stores and problems with transportation also limit the consumption of fresh meat, milk, fruits, and vegetables. Consequently, nonperishable foods tend to comprise the bulk of the AI/AN diet; their meals may lack variety and be marginal or deficient in key nutrients but high in refined sugar, cholesterol, fat, and calories.

One factor to consider when preparing meals for AI/AN elders is that there are many culturally related aspects to their consumption of food. Corn is a sacred product for many tribes and is used in ceremonies such as weddings. There also are many dietary taboos among different tribes. For example, some Plains Indians won't eat any fish at all.

Long-Term Care

Unfortunately, planning for long-term care of the AI/AN elderly is less often discussed among policymakers and is even more uncoordinated than for elderly members of the general population (Manson, 1989). A related problem is access to available services. Several recent reports amply document numerous barriers to long-term care, institutional as well as noninstitutional, that are experienced by older Indians. These include lack of information about programs, apprehension over application procedures, transportation problems, discomfort with telephone contact and/or inability to hear well, and general fear of program staff (Kramer, Polisar and Hyde, 1990; National Indian Council on Aging, 1981; U.S. Senate, 1987). Nursing homes, both skilled and intermediate care facilities, are extremely rare in AI/AN communities. For the most part, they are located far from these areas.

Problems for elderly Indian nursing home residents and their families include distance and orientation to non-Indian populations. Visiting by friends and family occurs less often as a consequence of difficulties in transportation. The average age of the institutionalized population is eighty-two. Cognitive disorders are the most frequently cited explanation for institutionalization of older adults in the United States, conditions that are relatively infrequent among Indian nursing home residents. The three most common diagnoses for AI/AN patients are diabetes mellitus, alcohol abuse, and stroke (Mick, 1983).

There are only ten reservation nursing homes, which range in size from twenty to ninety-six beds. Admission criteria vary from exclusively Indian with tribal preference to unrestricted admissions. Seasonal patterns of admission have been noted by a number of nursing home administrators: occupancy rates are higher during winter months.

Attitudes about Aging among AI/AN

> Um wuyomi uqatsiy naavokyawintani;
> *You shall experience the fullness of life to old age*
> Qa o opultikyangw
> *Never experiencing infirmity.*
> Um [wu'taqw] [wuti'harz kye] vuwvani
> *You shall pass away into sleep, an old [man] [woman];*
> Niikyangw, um yan maatsiwni;
> *And you shall be known by the name* _____
>   —Naming liturgy given by the paternal
>   grandmother of a newborn Hopi Indian

In a rural mental health project, funded by the Administration on Aging, interviews were conducted among five southwestern tribes. When they were asked how they feel about growing old, the participants reported a number of both positive and negative factors. Poor health and physical problems were seen as major disadvantages, as were limitations on activities and concerns about dependency. They also experienced stress and depression; frustration with the state, federal, and tribal governments contributed to their anxieties. In addition, respondents identified lack of access to medical care and concern over the future of their children and grandchildren as major problems in their lives.

On the other hand, happiness was related to feeling healthy, keeping busy, and being productive. In particular, caring for, and enjoying the company of, children, grandchildren, and great-grandchildren, as well as helping others in the community, are important sources of life satisfaction and well-being. The respondents pointed to talking with people, laughing, and being with their family as their major coping mechanisms. Whether confidants are relatives or friends, they must be people with whom one can be open and honest. Singing, dancing, and listening to a "good drum" can also lift the spirits of the AI/AN elderly. They stress the importance of religion and spirituality in their lives. According to one participant, "I pray a lot, and knowing God loves me keeps me strong."

Conclusion and Policy Implications

Several problems have emerged as a result of the lifelong inequities experienced by today's AI/AN elderly population. For example, most have been employed in low-paying jobs that lacked both pension and health care coverage. Despite the enactment of legislation and policies that are geared to improving employment opportunities and earning power among the general elderly population, high levels of unemployment, low-wage work, and poverty are ongoing problems for AI/AN elders. Since they are underrepresented in the policymaking process, underserved in programs, and unrecognized with regard to their historical past and cultural heterogeneity, many of their needs continue to be ignored.

The National Indian Council on Aging (NICOA) has identified a number of areas that must be addressed if the AI/AN elderly are to be better served. In addition to more services, the federal and state governments, including the Bureau of Indian Affairs, should increase funds for training so that long-term care providers can become more sensitive to the special needs of the AI/AN older population. The council also advocated community-based education for caregivers.

Housing was identified as a particularly crucial problem. In particular, NICOA suggested that the Department of Housing and Urban Development's Section 202 program should set aside independent and/or supervised housing specifically for AI/AN elders as well as lower the age of eligibility from sixty-two to fifty-five to conform with criteria set by the Bureau of Indian Affairs.

The growth of the AI/AN elderly population, along with an increase in life expectancy, will create a demand for more at-home services, hospices, and nursing homes. Future efforts must take into account their specific problems, issues, and needs discussed in this chapter. We also must ensure that current AI/AN elders are not subjected to the same disenfranchisement and displacement that they experienced during their younger years.

11

Mormon Elderly

Bruce L. Campbell

"The elderly are not a constituency group for us."
—Mormon welfare official

The elderly, especially those who are frail, are not a central focus of the Mormon community. The record indicates that Mormons are concerned with meeting the needs of their aged, but the community as a whole has not developed a unique set of programs specifically designed to provide long-term care for its growing older population.

In fact, there is almost no published, scholarly material on the subject. Therefore, in some cases this chapter utilizes findings on the state of Utah to create a general impression of trends among the Mormon aged. I also rely on church documents, official addresses (talks and articles) by Mormon leaders, and personal correspondence. Where possible, Mormon attitudes toward the elderly are presented in the language of Mormonism.

There are several reasons why the elderly are not an important constituency group for the church. First, because Mormons have sustained historically high fertility rates, baby boomers are not going to produce the tidal wave of elderly the larger American society will experience over the next several decades. Second, maintaining faith and affiliation with the church is not as problematic among the elderly as it is for children and adolescents. As a result, the focus of the church has been to produce strong families that tie children and adolescents to the church and its practices, which may divert time and energy from the issues of the elderly (Duke and Johnson, 1998). Third, present church programs generally meet the needs of the Mormon elderly. And fourth, the aged are not evenly distributed throughout the wards and stakes of the church: new wards in the up-scale suburbs have few elderly members, while those in older sections of urban centers may be populated mostly by older people. (A stake is an organization of several wards in a local area and may include a few thousand members.)

Developing an entire church response to the aged and their issues may not be as effective as allowing local leadership to organize programs to meet local needs. Local leaders often develop effective responses to problems in their wards, stakes, or even missions that are subsequently adopted by the whole church. Thus, in the future we may see local initiatives designed to respond to the needs of the elderly bubbling up from the wards and stakes to become churchwide programs.

The Elderly in Conference Talks

One way to gauge the relative importance of the elderly in Mormonism is to analyze the official discussions about them and their issues in the talks given by the General Authorities at General Conferences. General Conferences are televised to the membership at large and are later printed in the *Ensign,* the official church magazine. Over the last three decades there have been about a few dozen conferences, talks, or articles published in the *Ensign* focused specifically on the aged and their issues.

In 1989, President Ezra Taft Benson, in perhaps the most direct communication to aging Mormons by a president of the church, presented eight suggestions to follow for aged Mormons to make the most of their senior years (Benson, 1989). These included performing temple work, being involved in missionary service, accepting church callings, taking on leadership in the family, serving others, and keeping physically fit and active. Benson acknowledged that in spite of their best efforts some elderly will not be able to care for themselves and might need help from family, the community, and church resources. He also cautioned bishops and others to be sensitive to the physical, spiritual, emotional, and financial needs of older people. Benson (1987: 7) said, "[W]e must fulfill these duties without reluctance or hesitation." Other church leaders expressed similar sentiments (Alder, 1987; Oaks, 1991; Pinnock, 1979; Dunn, 1983).

One of the constant themes of official Mormon comments is the loneliness of the elderly, especially of widows (Monson, 1981; Tingy, 2000). Barbara Smith, president of the Relief Society (the church's primary women's organization), focused on the problems of the disabled (frail) elderly, discussing such issues as nursing home placement and caring for caregivers (Smith, 1987). While the Mormons have not ignored the issue of the elderly among them in these official pronouncements, older people have received much less attention than children and families, missionary work, temple work, and, of course, doctrinal and behavioral expectations. An examination of these sources reveals little sense of urgency from the church about being overwhelmed by its growing aged population, nor is there any mention of special programs for the elderly. The emphasis is on self-reliance in preparing for one's senior years, coupled with the responsibility of the family to provide care for its aging members.

Demographic Issues

Utah has the lowest proportion of baby boomers in the United States, with 24.3 percent of the state population in that age cohort compared to 29.4 percent in the nation as a whole. It also has the highest fertility rate, the largest percentage of the population under five years of age, and the highest percentage of five-to-seventeen-year-olds. Moreover, Utah has the next to lowest percentage of the population who are sixty-five and older. However, the state will experience a greater rate of growth in its elderly population than much of the nation in coming decades (Wright, 1998).

The dependency ratio can be defined as the number of dependents (including children under eighteen and adults over sixty-five) per hundred persons of working age. With the highest dependency ratio in the nation, Utah also has the lowest number of elderly included in it. Therefore, working Utahans support more dependents than the national average, but the vast majority of them are their children, not aging parents. While these data are not precise descriptions of the Mormon population per se, they indicate that for Utah, which is largely Mormon, the elderly are a growing population but not a dominant age group. Moreover, the future impact of baby boomers on the Mormon community will be mitigated by its ongoing high rate of fertility and emphasis on large families (Wright, 1998).

Health and Longevity

Even though its rank had slipped from third to ninth by 1997, Utah has one of the healthiest populations in the nation (Wagner, 1997). In 1990, life expectancy for males was 79.1 years and for females 84.5, rates much higher than the national average. One Mormon bishop, when I asked about the elderly in the church, said, "By and large, we are talking about sisters [women] when we are talking about the elderly in the wards." There is also some indication that the elderly in the western states are more likely to die at home or spend relatively little time hospitalized before death ("Where You Live," 1997).

Preventive maintenance is a key aspect of the Mormon response to issues of aging. While often effective, this approach is not based on an awareness of the specific needs of the elderly or on initiatives tailored to meet them. Rather, it is focused on overall church programs from which the elderly incidentally benefit. The success of this strategy is based in part on a fundamental aspect of Mormonism: the Word of Wisdom. Adherence to this commandment, which forbids the use of coffee, tea, alcohol, and tobacco for all Mormons, appears to result in high levels of physical health over the life cycle, including the senior years. It also may result in fewer disabled elderly and/or briefer periods of frailty among them.

A number of studies have documented relatively low rates of cancer among

Mormons, especially tobacco-related cancers (Gardner and Lyon, 1982; Lyon et al., 1976). Enstrom (1998) studied a group of Mormon men (high priests) and their wives who have been active in the church and have obeyed the Word of Wisdom by never smoking. High priests are not clergy, but most of them would have been lay leaders of the church as bishops, branch presidents, or stake leaders. These men and their wives were found to have very low levels of cancer, heart disease, and other illnesses, even lower than those of nonsmokers in general. "Indeed, this population is currently achieving the 50 percent reduction in cancer mortality that the National Cancer Institute has set for the year 2000" (Enstrom, 1998). The high level of social support found within the church among the high priests was suggested as another possible reason for their excellent health.

Every Member a Missionary

President David O. McKay elegantly stated a central mission of the Church of Jesus Christ of Latter-day Saints when he proclaimed "every member a missionary." Since its inception, Mormonism has been a missionary church, and it is very difficult to understand Mormonism without appreciating the unique and central role of the missionary in its culture. The recent inclusion of the elderly as potential missionaries has significantly altered the place of older people. It is a recognition of the experience, skills, wisdom, and devotion of its aged members and the vast talents they can bring to missionary work. The potential benefits for the aged themselves are also great.

Not all young men serve as missionaries, but fully 32 percent do so (Peck, 1992). Because the church has no clergy, all offices in the local congregations are staffed by lay members, and returned missionaries make an important contribution to the operation of the church in these roles. Community leaders tend to be men who were missionaries; they often report that their missionary years were the best times of their lives. Stories of missionary work and promotion of faith—sad, exotic, and humorous—are the common parlance of Mormon life.

The missionary work of the church depends heavily upon the young men and, increasingly, the young women of the church who serve for two years at age nineteen or twenty. However, without the leadership provided by successful middle-aged men in the church—mission presidents—the system could not work. It is considered a high honor to be asked to serve the Lord as a mission president, who, along with his wife and family, travels anywhere in the world that the church has a need. In this spirit, thousands of men and their families take time in mid-career to serve as mission presidents.

The church recently has developed an important place for the elderly in its missionary system. In fact, in his talk to the elderly in a General Conference, Benson (1987) stressed this potential role. A California Mormon whom I interviewed provides an example of lifelong devotion to missionary work:

My father served his own mission in Argentina when he was a young man. After a career in the army, he was called to be a building missionary by the church in Argentina. He took my mom and the rest of us to Argentina for three years while he helped build chapels across Argentina and South America. After that mission, we returned to Lake Arrowhead, where dad worked as a building contractor.

After his seven children were grown up, he was called by the church to help set up the Missionary Training Center in Mexico, where Mormon missionaries for Latin America would come for two weeks of training before going to their specific missions. After that, Mom and Dad moved to Arizona, where he continued to work in construction into his sixties and seventies. Right now, at seventy-eight, he and Mom are finishing a temple mission in Chile. His life has been dedicated to missionary work.

Even among Mormons such a mission-centered life is unusual, but it is becoming less so. The church has seen the service that the middle-aged and elderly could provide their worldwide constituency and has moved to develop missions that take advantage of their skills and experience. While few older Mormons are expected to proselytize, many of them are called to help establish smooth-functioning church organizations around the world. Men and women who have served in church callings throughout their lives can provide enormous support for Mormon congregations populated largely by recent converts. Older couples as well as singles, including widows and widowers, can elect to serve on missions ranging from a period of six to eighteen months. In contrast to the younger missionaries, the church allows them to select specific calls that are posted in the chapels. Some work in genealogical offices or temples, while others serve as doctors, farmers, nurses, and the like. However, the elderly appear to be allowed a wide latitude in developing their calling within their mission. The church has worked hard to accommodate the mission experience to the needs and desires of the elderly in order to make it attractive to them.

Of course, not all Mormon elderly are capable of serving on a mission. They must be physically fit and are expected to pay their own living expenses. Others are not viewed as worthy to serve because they do not live the commandments. However, for committed, healthy elderly, the church has created significant opportunities for service. Even in retirement, missionary service provides important opportunities for older people.

In many cases, elderly missionaries make great sacrifices. They often find it difficult to leave their children and grandchildren. A few of them find the work overly demanding or the environment too unhealthy; some of the elderly become very ill or even die as a result of the rigors of their mission call. However, as one missionary couple said, "We want to dedicate our lives to the work of the Lord. We have loved these years as missionaries; it is not time to leave yet. We want to serve until we die."

Although going on a mission as an elderly couple or as an individual is not a vacation, many find the experience personally beneficial. For example, another couple remarked, "Our decision to go on a mission brought new vigor, new emotions, new friends, new places, new challenges—new spiritual growth instead of spiritual retirement" (Monson, 1981). In fact, missionary work may be another example of how Mormon life helps maintain the health and vigor of its senior members. The frail elderly do not usually serve as missionaries, but some are called locally to missionary service designed to provide them an opportunity to serve no matter how limited it might be.

Welfare and the Elderly

The Mormon Church is widely known for taking care of its own through its welfare system. While the program was not developed primarily to support elderly Mormons (it was a response to the Great Depression), when in need they can depend on it helping them, as can any other member of the church. In fact, the Mormons have developed and administer an extensive and unique church-run system that includes vast farms and ranches, canneries, an elaborate storage and distribution system, an employment service, and Deseret Industries, which collects, repairs, and distributes used clothing, furniture, and other useful items. Goods and commodities not given to the poor are sold to the general public, and the funds are returned to the system (Fisher, 1978; Chen and Yorganson, 1999).

However, welfare is not an entitlement; it is a temporary safety net rather than comprehensive long-term services. For Mormons, there are important Gospel truths at work in the welfare program. They believe strongly in self-reliance and expect members to be industrious, defer immediate gratification, obtain education or skills to make themselves employable, develop a business, run a farm, or take any job to produce family income. Elder J. Thomas Fyans (1979: 86) captures the dual nature of the self-reliance/generous-giving obligations of Mormons:

> Let us be ever mindful that the greatest blessing of the welfare system is derived by the givers and that each of us should work to be independent and self-reliant as families in order to be in a position to help our less fortunate brothers and sisters. Stated in plainness, each family unit's personal and family preparedness activity is every bit as important as this vast and marvelous welfare system. The real strength of the Church does not ultimately lie in the financial and commodity reserves of the Church, rather it rests in the reserves and strength of every household.

If, in spite of their best efforts or through some misfortune, church members are not able to care for themselves, they are expected to turn to their extended families for social and economic help. If the family cannot meet their needs, they can receive support from the church welfare system. The expectation is that the assistance is temporary and that the recipient will work in some way for the church while receiving aid. Thus, Mormon elderly who do not have sufficient economic resources and have no family to help them can receive assistance from the church.

Home Teaching

The elderly benefit from another Mormon program designed for other purposes: the home-teaching program of the church is an important part of providing for the spiritual and temporal needs of its members. The male priesthood holders (practically every man) are assigned as groups of two to visit all members of the church each month. The home teachers are expected to ascertain if anyone in their ward is in need of assistance—spiritual, emotional, social, or physical. The women in the church, through the Relief Society, also have a visiting-teachers program similar to home teaching. Reports of need from either source will trigger an immediate response from the bishop, who has the responsibility to make sure no member goes without food or other important needs. Home teachers and visiting teachers have become an important source of contact and support in times of need. Home teachers visit three or four families each month to develop trust. They are expected to inform the bishop of any problems they encounter. This is an important key in how well the welfare system works. If the home teachers/visiting teachers are doing their job, the frail elderly should receive prompt help, if needed.

The Bishop

One of the unique features of Mormon welfare is the great latitude and power given to the bishop to help the needy. He determines eligibility and the amount of aid to be offered. Members can expect help, but they are not automatically entitled to some specified amount of goods at a given level of income or need. This is to be worked out with the local bishop, who is expected to know his members and their requirements. His goal is to provide temporary support so that they can become productive again. He can give food, clothing, shelter, payment for physical and mental health treatment, or practically anything he determines would help the member become self-reliant. He is not restrained by bureaucratic rules but is governed by what he thinks will actually aid those in need. And, of course, divine inspiration is expected to play a role in this determination.

As suggested earlier, the elderly are not a special constituency of the church welfare program. Just like other members, they can expect that when their needs are reported to the home teachers or the bishop, they will receive assistance. In theory there are no hungry Mormon elderly. In practice, however, one former bishop interviewed for this research said that the system does not always work effectively. Some home teachers fail to make their monthly visits or do not build sufficient rapport with elderly members, thereby discouraging them from mentioning their needs. Some Mormon elderly are embarrassed to ask for aid or do not feel worthy to receive it because they are not living the rules of the church. Still others have distanced themselves from the church and its leaders and actively shun help offered them.

The second pillar of the welfare program is the fast offerings, which were an early part of the church's response to the Great Depression (Arrington, Fox and May, 1976). Members of the church are expected to fast for two meals the first Sunday of each month and contribute the potential costs to the poor through the local ward bishop. This money is kept by the bishop to buy goods and services for needy members. However, it is important to remember that Mormons expect to be self-sufficient or rely on family help. Most would do anything they could to avoid receiving church assistance. The average stay on welfare in Utah is eighteen months, while the national average is thirty-six months; the stay on church welfare is about four months (Peck, 1995).

I interviewed several bishops, and all agreed that if an elderly member was not self-supporting and had no family to rely on, the church could support that member, even to the extent of placing him or her in a nursing home. But they make it clear that this occurs only under unusual circumstances. Moreover, like any other member receiving church assistance, the elderly would be expected to work, if fit, so that they would not be undermined morally.

Just how much church aid is received by older people is difficult to determine. The Mormons keep records but do not publish the data. However, the average for church aid overall is between eleven and twelve weeks at an approximate value of $300 (actual money is rarely, if ever, given) (Van Biema, 1997). It would appear that the level of economic support for elderly Mormons from the church is not very high. However, because of the power of the welfare system, if the bishop determines that an elderly member needs substantial help, it can be provided.

In the local congregation, the women are expected to provide "compassionate service" to others, while men's priesthood quorums and teen programs have service projects as part of their mission. The elderly are often the focus of these services. A church member interviewed for this study describes one such effort:

> Every year in our ward the Aaronic Priesthood young men would have a service project to help one of the needy families in the area. There was an older couple, a brother and sister, if I remember right, who lived in a home heated by a woodstove. We called the man "Step-and-a-Half" for the extremely long gait he employed while walking with his cane. Looking back now, it must have involved some hip disorder, but for us young people it was just strange. Every year right after we got out of school at Christmas, we would go to their yard and cut their winter's supply of firewood.
>
> There would be about twenty of us ranging in age from twelve to eighteen hacking away with enthusiasm and frivolity. Given our generally low level of maturity and lack of skill with an axe or saw, this must have been the Lord's work, or we might have hurt ourselves. But we were preserved.
>
> After laboring in the cold winter air, we would have a party—playing sports and eating lunches we brought and shared. While this couple was the ostensible beneficiary of this project, the satisfaction we received from this service always tipped the balance in our favor. So did the sports and party afterwards.

Many Mormons could report experiences of service to an elderly person or couple in their ward. In many cases, the elderly do receive help from their local congregation. However, the system is not perfect, and some needy older people slip through the cracks.

The Mormons, of course, do not neglect the spiritual or religious needs of the aged. If an elderly person cannot make it to church, priesthood members will go to his or her home and conduct a worship service, including the administration of the sacrament.

For those in nursing homes, there are several different responses. In some cases, if there are enough Mormons in the facility who are fit, the church might establish a branch (like a ward without a full complement of programs) in the home and call the elderly to serve as branch president and other officers. In other cases, the ward in which the institution is located has the responsibility of providing church meetings for the elderly. Every Sunday, church services are held, and members of the ward visit the elderly as home teachers. However, on an informal basis, the bishop and others from the former ward continue to visit and treat the older person as a member of the ward family. This is a significant contact for many elderly because the ward often has the closeness of family and the bishop is often viewed as a warm, loving father figure.

The Family

If the elderly are not a constituency group for the Mormons, families and children clearly are. Church programs are so geared to meeting the needs of families with children that Mormons who are single often feel left out of church activities (Raynes and Parsons, 1982). Two of the three official church magazines are devoted to issues related to children and youth. Family home evening was designed to help fathers focus on their role as family leaders. Sunday school, Primary, Mutual, Boy Scouts, and released-time seminary are all programs devoted to children and families. Many conference talks and official admonitions in the *Ensign* and from the pulpit focus on the family. The church has built an education program, including Brigham Young University (BYU at Provo, BYU–Idaho, BYU–Hawaii) and hundreds of other sites near high schools and colleges across the western United States, that is estimated to be worth $1 billion (Van Biesma, 1997). This extensive system serves the needs of young adults to acquire a more complete church education as well as to associate with other marriageable Mormons. The church also has chosen to be politically active in support of the traditional family. It opposed the Equal Rights Amendment as antifamily (Johnson, 1981) and has even more strongly opposed marriage for gays and lesbians (Miller, 2000).

Mormon temples are at the heart of the essential, sacred nature of the Mormon family. The temples are designed to tie the extended family unit together eternally. One potentially important role for elderly Mormons is that of temple worker; many of them play an essential role in helping the temples function. For some, retirement provides an increased opportunity to become more involved in the temple.

Temple work can be a time-consuming commitment, and it is not for all Mormon elderly. Only those who had lived righteous lives would even be considered worthy of this calling. Temple workers must satisfy stringent standards of moral rectitude that many Mormon elderly cannot meet. Others do not have easy access to a temple. However, for older Mormons who are worthy, capable, and interested, temple work offers a role central to their personal salvation and a means to serve others as they take their eternal vows. It can be an important source of self-esteem and prestige in the Mormon community.

A second important family role is that of genealogist. Mormons are expected to trace their families' genealogy as completely as possible so that temple work can be completed for their ancestors who did not have an opportunity to be baptized into the church. Frequently, an elderly member of the family will become the genealogy leader for the family. Genealogical research can be time consuming and exacting and requires a commitment to develop the expertise necessary to trace obscure family lineages.

For older Mormons, temple work and genealogical research are important family-centered activities. However, while many elderly Mormons find satisfaction in them, they are not the exclusive preserve of the elderly, nor were they designed primarily as a response to the issues of aging. Although they provide important roles and activities for some aged Mormons, they are not likely to do so for the vast majority. Because these roles can be physically demanding, neither is likely to be pursued by the frail elderly.

Conclusion and Policy Implications

While the Mormons have yet to develop programs designed specifically for the elderly, their culture contains noteworthy programs that others might emulate. First, Mormon health teachings, including the Word of Wisdom, appear to point the way to preventing many health problems in the church's aging population. Second, Mormon programs appear to offer important opportunities to help others after retirement. Serving on missions, for example, may greatly increase life satisfaction for many elderly Mormons and may contribute to a more vigorous aged population. Temple work and genealogy may have similar results. Third, in many cases, the Mormon welfare plan offers substantial help to its aged population. Fourth, Mormon practices of thrift, self-restraint, self-reliance, and financial planning may be useful for others to emulate. Fifth, the latitude given the Mormon bishop may suggest a new approach to helping others. Because his hands are not tied by red tape, he can often meet the actual needs of his members and move many of them rapidly to their former state of self-reliance. Sixth, the church provides significant support for its members in a variety of ways. For example, in their study of recently bereaved Mormons and non-Mormons in Utah, Lund,

Caserta and Diamond (1988) found that the former had a larger social network, knew that network longer, and received more visits per month than the latter. Interestingly, however, despite the large social system, the authors noted that the Mormons did not seem to have a significantly better adjustment to the death of a spouse.

Yet there are some problems with the Mormon Church's welfare program. First, the present level of success in helping its members may blind Mormons to the need for a more focused response to older people. Because of the welfare plan, Mormons may believe that the church provides most of the services needed by the elderly. A review of the programs offered by the government in Utah suggests that this is not the case (Wright, 1998). Mormons are not as self-reliant as they believe. Second, the emphasis on young families and children may leave few financial or emotional resources for the care of the elderly, especially those who are frail. Third, the focus on educating young adults may distract from the real needs of the elderly. Finally, there is the possibility that many members of the Mormon community who do not feel worthy of church welfare are not sufficiently provided for, and those who reject Mormon association entirely may not have adequate services.

Despite a sense of closeness with family members and frequent contact with them, many older Mormons are worried about where they will live when they can no longer take care of themselves. Some wish nursing facilities had a greater Mormon orientation (Gelfand and Olsen, 1979). Many vulnerable aged Mormons have had to turn to government for support. Moreover, in some aspects, the Mormon welfare system duplicates national, state, and local government programs instead of working with them, thus further reducing total aid available for the very old.

The frail elderly are not yet an important constituency for Mormons. However, given its ability to discover problems and a strong desire to help those in need, the church may yet develop creative and effective programs for its vulnerable aged population.

12

Mutual Aid and Elders in Amish Society

Lee J. Zook

Elderly people in the Amish culture are venerated because of their age and valued for their contributions. The traditional method of caring for elders consists of the elders' moving into a *Grossdaadi Haus* (grandfather house) on the family farm. Usually this takes place at a point when one of the sons in the family gets married and begins to manage the farm. Typically this occurs when the elders are still in good health and continue to participate in farm-related activities. Grandparents live in a separate dwelling, as privacy for both the nuclear and the extended family is viewed as important in the culture. The younger generation provides the elders with material and social support. In general, elders are looked after while maintaining a sense of freedom and independence (Miller, 1950). Older members continue to contribute to the life of the family and community according to their ability and inclination, providing leadership and help with farm and family work.

Care of the elders in the Amish community is based on informal mutual assistance that developed during the Anabaptist movement of the sixteenth century, an extension of the religious reformation of that time. Much of the Amish way of life, including the assistance given to all members of the community, reflects that time period (Hostetler, 1992). The Amish church dates from 1693, during a time when Anabaptists were persecuted; mutual assistance within small communities was not only commonplace in the society as a whole but also a matter of survival for them.

The practice of mutual assistance was, and continues to be, based on religious belief. Durnbaugh (1974: 9) points out that "several aspects of mutual aid and Christian community may be summarized under these somewhat overlapping categories: brotherly love, material support, admonition and discipline and concern for outsiders." Other writers also note that mutual aid was only a part of the larger system of religious belief (Klassen, 1963; Hostetler, 1992; MacMaster, 1992).

Related to the practice of mutual aid is the rejection of most of the modern welfare state. Hostetler points out that the Amish tradition of self-sufficiency and mutual aid is their answer to government programs such as Old Age Insurance, Social Security, and other programs this country has for its elders (Kraybill, 1989). While Amish people do pay income, property, and sales taxes, they are exempt from participating in the Social Security program, primarily because they believe that contributing to the system would "undermine their own stable community and their form of mutual aid" within their community (Hostetler, 1992). This would especially affect older retired people, creating less interdependence with their extended families.

Thus religious belief and historical tradition are two of the reasons often given for the Amish's extensive use of mutual aid within their communities. This system of informal mutual aid explains much about care of the elderly in Amish society.

Migration of the Amish: An Ongoing Phenomenon

Migration for the Amish is an ongoing phenomenon. They have a long history of leaving places where they felt uncomfortable or were actually persecuted for their religious beliefs. They first came to this country around 1737 after suffering two hundred years of hardship in Western Europe: their religious beliefs, an outgrowth of the Reformation of the sixteenth century, had brought persecution in the form of imprisonment and even execution. The Amish culture has a long memory; these events are kept alive by verbal storytelling and the *Martyrs Mirror,* a large book often found in Amish homes, documenting the atrocities in text as well as with graphic pictures (Oyer and Kreider, 1990; van Braguth, 1984).

Historically, the Amish are a part of the Anabaptist tradition, which believed that the changes brought about by the religious reformation of the sixteenth century had been inadequate. Their convictions, while rather benign today, were viewed by the church-states of Western Europe as controversial and even threatening. These beliefs included the separation of church and state, separation from the larger society, nonviolence in all matters of life (including not participating in any military organizations), and adult (rather than child) baptism into the church (Hostetler, 1992).

When invited to migrate to this country by William Penn, who himself had been persecuted as a Quaker, the Amish gladly accepted the offer. A more progressive Anabaptist group, the Mennonites, often assisted them in their passage. Because of their practice of mutual aid, they came here in better financial condition than many other people who arrived at the time. This first migration took place in the mid-1700s. They flourished in Pennsylvania and began moving west, as did other immigrants. There was a second migration during the nineteenth century, with immigrants often settling in Ohio, Indiana, and even as far west as Iowa as soon as they came to this country, joining others who were also moving westward (Hostetler, 1992).

More recently the Amish have been relocating because of the pressures of urbanization and modernization they face in the eastern states where their population is largest. These states include Pennsylvania, Ohio, and Indiana. They have been moving to states where no Amish settlements existed before, many times to the south and west of the older settlements.

Amish Attitudes toward Aging, Elders, and Care of Elders

As Hostetler and Huntington (1992: 34) suggest in their discussion of the Amish, "the care of the aged does not depend on a single institution; it is part of the total way of life." Care for frail elders is typically provided by close relatives. It is the responsibility of the younger generation to make sure their needs are met appropriately. Further, many of the problems associated with aging in modern society do not occur with the Amish. For example, "inactivity of retirement, economic insecurity, prestige loss, social isolation, loss of health, and death" are not real problems with this subculture (Hostetler and Huntington, 1992: 34).

Retirement is not mandatory; rather, it occurs within the context of family decisions about when to move into the Grossdaadi Haus and have a younger son or son-in-law take over the family farm. Even after the elders move to the Grossdaadi Haus, life and work continue in much the same way as before. Taking residence in this dwelling is a normal, expected way of "retiring" in the culture. Men and women have more time for other activities that they want to pursue. As long as they are healthy, they seek to help others in the community, attend funerals and weddings that last all day, and take care of obligations for other elderly in the community, such as visiting those who are sick or bereaved.

Prestige actually increases with age in the Amish community. This is most obvious in families where there are grandparents living in the Grossdaadi Haus; they are asked for advice, though it may not always be followed. Old people are seen as having knowledge about many things that they have stored in their memory and are often asked for such information. They are consulted on numerous issues from the economic health of the farm operation to problems in the family or church.

Independence is very important to Amish elders. In general, they continue to function as autonomously as possible while accepting what is necessary from those around them. The following story exemplifies this sense of independence. An informant's cousin was planning to take over his father's farm. The widowed grandmother lived alone in the Grossdaadi Haus, and now his father and mother would move there while he and his wife moved into the farmhouse. Instead of living with either household, the grandmother insisted that the woodshed attached to the Grossdaadi Haus be converted into a dwelling so she could have her own living quarters. Her wishes were granted, creating a situation where there were three attached dwellings inhabited by four generations of the family.

Church structure and traditions also indicate that age is respected. Typically, in an area where there are many church districts and bishops, the eldest bishop is looked to as the person with the most authority. The office of bishop is the highest leadership position in the community. Individuals are usually not ordained at a young age. Typically they are ordained as ministers first and only after years of service in that capacity are chosen as bishop. There is no retirement from being a bishop, minister, or deacon; rather, these positions are held until death. Since such roles are for a lifetime, age does not isolate these individuals from their community. Additionally, elderly lay people in the church are sought out for advice on many public matters (Hostetler, 1992). Older people are given the best seats during the church service; in some areas, chairs with backs are provided for elders while the rest of the people sit on backless benches. In some places, the elders sit in the very back row of the room so they can lean against a wall during the service.

Aging is accepted with dignity. It is expected that the elderly may not be as physically strong as younger people. Illness related to aging is assumed to be a natural part of life. If people become sick, they have support from the whole community. For example, if someone is too ill to go to church, others will be aware of this and the situation will be discussed at length.

As elders become disabled or simply grow feeble, they work less and become more dependent on other people for their care. Relatives who are living in the adjacent house are the first to be aware of this need and to increase aid. For example, if an elderly woman has arthritis, the female in the farmhouse may cook some meals for the older couple and bring the food to their residence. Or, if either of the grandparents needs help in hitching up a horse to go to town or visiting, the people in the farmhouse will help.

Both women and men are involved with aid to the elderly, but most of the care is associated with female roles and therefore provided by women. Men and women have rather prescribed roles in Amish society, which is generally quite patriarchal (Hostetler, 1992). Men tend to assist the aged in ways that are usually viewed as male tasks. For example, they are involved with helping severely disabled elderly transfer from bed to chair. They also help in other types of activities where physical strength is seen as important or in areas that are perceived largely as the male domain. Women, on the other hand, are typically the primary caregivers for the sick or disabled. In addition to making sure that they have food, clothing, and a clean living space, women are involved with making decisions about when doctors should be called and other health-related issues.

Often, the need for care of elders increases at about the same time that married adult children have teenagers who do much of the physical work on the farm. This allows the parents to spend more time with the care of grandparents while maintaining control and management of the farm and household operations. Amish often marry in their early twenties and begin to have children soon after. Thus, it is possible for a teenager to have parents who are forty or younger and grandparents who are in their sixties. By the time young Amish people are in their middle teens, they are typically expected to take on a great deal of work and responsibility on the homestead.

One informant related how his grandfather had a debilitating stroke that left him unable to walk, get out of bed, or do other activities of daily living on his own. He lived in the Grossdaadi Haus with his wife. For two years, until his death, the extended family cared for him. Every evening relatives would visit, get the grandfather out of bed, set him in a chair while they were there, and return him to his bed before they left. This informant said that he was asked by his parents to go along to help his father, as two men typically did this task. As a teenager, he did not exactly enjoy doing this, but since it was expected of him, he complied. In addition, the grandmother was assisted daily by one of the relatives in other chores, such as bathing and feeding the grandfather. Female kin typically helped the grandmother with these everyday activities. The adults in the family did not seem to find the work associated with assisting the grandfather objectionable. In fact, often more than one son or daughter would be visiting at the same time. The grandparents' residence became the gathering place for the entire extended family.

Ober (1988) reports in her study of attitudes toward Amish elders that the "gerontocracy" of the Amish does not to seem to produce the type of resentment usually associated with such social arrangements. Further, she states that the negative attitudes toward the elderly prevalent in the larger, more modern society have not affected their views.

In addition to the family of the son or daughter who lives in the farmhouse, other relatives and neighbors assist the elders. These people help in small ways, especially during a time of crisis or when there is a need for increased labor to accomplish some task. They share garden and farm produce, help with transportation, visit, and in general continue the face-to-face relationships that existed before the elder became frail. Of course, life changes upon retirement and when Amish elders become disabled, but not to the extent that it does for persons in the larger culture.

The arrangements described above are typical for farming couples. When the Amish have nonfarm occupations, the pattern is quite similar. Elders still live near one of their married children and enjoy the benefits of both helping the younger family and knowing they have assistance when they need it. In these situations the grandfather is often employed part-time, possibly doing seasonal work for some of his relatives or neighbors or working in the cottage industry operated by one of his younger kin.

Old age is seen as a time when life is to be enjoyed, travel is more frequent, grandchildren are appreciated, and the good of the community can be a concern. In Amish society, grandchildren play important roles in the intergenerational homestead. It is clearly the responsibility of parents to care for their children, but grandparents are also involved in their upbringing. Each extended family works out its own arrangements, but there is some indication that grandparents are not expected to be baby-sitters for the young couple (Hostetler, 1992). In short, elders are not socially isolated but are involved with family and church. At the same time, they can retreat to their own home and remain by themselves when they wish.

Economic issues are not typically a problem for Amish elderly. There may be income from some aspect of the farm where the elders continue to work and/or from the rent or mortgage payments the younger farmer makes to them. There is also typically some savings to rely on.

Moreover, each church has a deacon whose role includes ensuring that church members' basic needs are met. He has the responsibility of being aware of those who require help and of gathering the appropriate resources to aid them. Most elders will not find it necessary to rely on the deacon and the church for sustenance. However, they serve as a safety net for everybody in the community, including the elderly.

View of Death in the Amish Community

Death is not feared in the Amish culture; it is hoped that one will have a better life in the hereafter. Amish folks do not want to be in a hospital when they die; they typically die in the home with people who know and care for them. When death occurs, the patterns that are in place in the Amish community take over, and individuals know what roles to play. Most Amish use the services of a funeral director only to embalm the body but do not use the funeral home facility itself. Rather, visitation and services occur in the home where the person lived and died.

One informant who had Amish relatives but was himself not Amish describes the funeral of his Amish uncle in some detail:

> It happened that I was home visiting my mother when Uncle Israel's funeral occurred. My wife, who had never been to an Amish funeral, went with me. I remember as a young boy having been to several Amish funerals; the most vivid was that of my grandfather. When we arrived at Uncle Israel's homestead, there were literally hundreds of people in the yard and house. We were not the only non-Amish folks there, but we were certainly in a minority.
>
> We were welcomed by one of my cousins [whom] I had not seen for some years. He ushered us into the house and told us where to sit. He allowed my wife and I to sit together, though the Amish men and women sat in different rooms. Both the farmhouse and the attached Grossdaadi Haus were full of people. There was a door that opened between the two houses so everybody could hear what the ministers were saying. There was an open casket in one of the rooms. It was basically a pine box that one of the Amish men had made for the occasion.
>
> After the funeral service, which consisted of prayer, Scripture reading, singing, and a sermon, everybody filed out of the house past the casket to have a last look at the deceased. Some people went home at this point, but many stayed and went to the cemetery that was only several miles away from the homestead. The funeral procession moved very slowly as there were mostly horses and buggies, with only an occasional car. A special horse-drawn wagon with the casket led the procession.
>
> At the cemetery more prayers were said, Scripture read, and comments made by the minister. Finally, the casket was lowered into the grave and covered with earth. When the service was finished, I visited with several of my relatives. I fondly re-

member visiting with one of my aunts [whom] I had not seen for some time. She looked so much like my grandmother when she was alive. I told her so; she seemed accepting of my comments.

We all went back to the homestead where a meal was prepared for the mourners. By now it was noon, and to send Amish folks away in a horse and buggy with miles to go without food would just not be the appropriate thing to do. People ate in shifts, sitting on benches that had been used for the service and makeshift tables that had been put together for the occasion.

The food was simple—bread, sandwich meat and cheese, a casserole, and several sour condiments. People ate quietly, bowing their heads in silent prayer before and after the meal. Then we left the table and went into the yard while others filed into the house to eat. We visited with more relatives and left.

Amish Attitudes toward Government Programs and Welfare

Amish attitudes about formal public welfare and government programs of any kind are quite clear: they want to have as little to do with the government as possible. An ideal situation for them is to be left alone, unencumbered by any government regulations. Of course this is not possible in modern society, but it is the prevailing ethos that permeates the culture. This preference is based on the principle of separation from the "world," which includes the state. Separation from the state is one of the original tenets of the early Anabaptists. Accepting any kind of help from the government would fail to uphold that principle.

The most cogent example of this negative attitude toward taking help from the government and how it has caused problems for the Amish is the difficulties experienced in regard to Social Security, including the Old Age and Survivors Insurance and Medicare programs. The Amish strongly believe that participation in the Social Security system would be problematic. While they pay other taxes, this particular program threatens their way of life, especially the role that mutual aid plays in their culture. While their reasons may include an aversion to contributing the high percentage of income that self-employed persons must pay, much more important is the fear that any financial involvement eventually could lead to some members of the community demanding benefits as well. Drawing money from the program would be seen as a direct violation of their separation stance and would make mutual aid and family care of elders less important. Such changes would alter intergenerational relationships, thus slowly undermining the culture in many ways.

Rarely is the local *Ordnung*, roughly translated "rules and order," of an Amish church published. Rather, these rules are verbal and unwritten, intimately understood by members. However, in *Amish Roots* several such lists are printed. In one, the very first line reads, "No worldly insurance or Social Security benefits" (Hostetler, 1989).

In short, drawing benefits from the Social Security program would go against the religious beliefs of the group, even though certain Amish individuals may not see this as a problem per se. The issue is that any participation in the public pension system potentially could lead to larger problems for the community. Thus, the Amish seem to be advancing a slippery-slope argument of the kind often used by Amish and non-Amish alike when confronted by change.

Up until 1955 the Social Security issue was not a problem for the Amish, as most of them were self-employed farmers and the program exempted this class of workers. However, in that year self-employed farmers were required to pay into the system, and the Amish were faced with a double bind. While the Amish think they should obey the law, pay their taxes, and generally attempt to get along with the government and outside world, they saw this tax as violating their religious beliefs, and they refused to participate in the program. This brought on a clash between them and the Internal Revenue Service that culminated in 1961, when IRS agents took an Amish man's horses after he had refused to pay the tax for some years (Ferrara, 1993).

The outcry from the general public about this incident was intense and steady. The IRS and the Amish met in Washington, D.C., to work out a solution. For a time, the Amish considered suing the IRS but dropped this idea because they believe it is inappropriate to use the court system to settle disputes. Over the course of several years, they requested an exemption from participation in the system and actually lobbied Congress to that effect. Finally, in 1965 a waiver was granted for self-employed persons belonging to any religious sect that found the system to be contrary to their beliefs. However, since the government did not want to include groups of people who just did not want to pay Social Security taxes, the exemption was made to fit the specific religious concerns of the Amish (Kraybill, 1989).

Since that time there have been several other problems with Social Security. The Amish attempted to expand the exemption to people who are not self-employed. In 1988, after considerable difficulty, it was extended to Amish employees but only if they work for Amish employers.

This opposition to the Social Security program exemplifies the general Amish attitude toward state-supported welfare. However, because Social Security is funded by a tax levied solely for the purpose of social insurance, no other tax or welfare issue has created such an intense reaction.

Finally, the Amish believe that it is inappropriate for them to have any insurance policies. They view these contracts as a way out of the responsibility they have to themselves and other members of the community. They also regard them as evidence of insufficient trust in God. Amish communities have their own form of formalized mutual aid that acts as an insurance policy. However, they refer to these plans as something other than insurance. Amish Aid raises money, assessed by their own people, for such problems as fires or natural disasters. These funds are used for buying materials to rebuild any houses or barns destroyed by fire or storm. The community works together to provide the labor for such projects.

Other forms of formal mutual assistance include Amish Liability Aid, which protects against accidents by outsiders on an Amish person's property. Amish Church Aid assesses members for hospitalization costs, though many of the more traditional Amish do not believe this is an appropriate use of formal mutual aid. Rather, the more traditional churches use a less formalized system of raising money to support a member when he or she is hospitalized and needs help with medical bills.

Elders Who Do Not Have Children

Most Amish adults marry and have children. However, there are some childless couples and a few individuals who remain single and thus do not have children to look after them when they are old. Typically, childless couples will have a reciprocal relationship with a nephew or niece in much the same manner that parents have with one of their children. How particular nephews or nieces are chosen is not well known, but it is an informal decision and emerges from long-standing relationships. Amish farms and households are difficult to operate without the labor of children and teenagers. Thus, many childless couples will have nephews or nieces working for them and even living in their homes part-time. These children tend to be from a large family where a close relationship has existed between their parent and aunt or uncle since childhood.

There seem to be more single women than single men in Amish communities. Unattached women generally double up together or live alone in a Grossdaadi Haus–type setting on a farmstead, often on the one where they grew up. Sometimes these dwellings are built specifically for the person who is alone. Because of this arrangement, some homesteads have three dwellings: the farmhouse, a house for the grandparents, and a residence for the single person. More often than married women, those who are single engage in work that brings them cash income. Their employment ranges from teaching Amish school, managing a store from their home, producing crafts such as quilts, or serving as a maid for some young Amish family. As with childless couples, they often have special relationships with young nieces and nephews, who often become their primary caregivers if it becomes necessary. Many times, older, single women marry men who have been widowed. Remarriage after the death of a spouse is encouraged within the Amish community and happens quite frequently.

One informant told me of an instance where an Amish farmer retired and his children were already established or did not wish to farm, a rather unusual occurrence. He and his wife moved into the Grossdaadi Haus adjacent to their eldest daughter's homestead and rented their farm to a relative. In this case, two elderly single sisters occupied the Grossdaadi Haus on the original farm. This is just one example of the informality and flexibility of elder care in the Amish community.

There are very few single, never-married older men in the Amish community. These men often will work for others as day laborers or have a craft they engage in for cash income. Their living arrangements vary from living with a sibling or an extended family member to living alone. However, they are less likely to live by themselves than are single women.

Conclusion and Policy Implications

Care of the elderly in Amish society is a part of their informal system of mutual aid, which permeates the entire culture and is a routine part of everyday life. Thus, while mutual-aid activities often focus on particular problems, they also occur regularly when work situations require large groups of people.

This informal network of care is effective only because a substantial number of people in the Amish community have flexible time as independent farmers or craftsmen. For informal mutual aid to work effectively, people must be both willing and able to attend to one another's problems as they arise. Kraybill (1989) suggests that in the future the Amish way of life will be threatened as more and more of the younger generation pursue nonagricultural employment. However, as cottage industries increase within the Amish community, mutual aid and elder care could continue unabated, since these enterprises are operated in a similar fashion to farming. Patterns of elder care among those who have taken up cottage industries have remained the same.

The Amish way of taking care of their elders reflects the beliefs and value system by which they live. Assisting the elderly helps to continue a society the Amish view as biblical and appropriate. Yet it has other advantages for the Amish as a group. The persistence and stability of Amish society today exists in part, I argue, because of how they care for their elderly.

Their approach to elder care is important for a variety of reasons. First, it exemplifies the veneration and respect granted to older people. They have considerable authority within Amish culture, greater than elders generally have within the larger society, and their treatment is related to respect for that power and rank. Maintaining their informal system of care helps the Amish to be mindful of traditional values and preserves the differences between their society and the outside world. It is partially what allows them to be separate from other cultures.

If elders were cared for outside the community or by those who are not Amish, their isolation would be eroded in a number of ways. Home health care professionals from other cultures would be in and out of Amish homes. An Amish person living in a modern long-term care facility would encounter modern conveniences, such as radios, televisions, telephones, and other devices that they reject. For most Amish people, living in a long-term care facility would be a total change of lifestyle. Further, their family would not be close by for visiting. Given their veneration for elders, the Amish would find nursing homes entirely inappropriate.

Second, mutual aid and care of the elderly help preserve cohesion among the Amish. Informal mutual aid usually involves face-to-face contact. Such connections are maintained in many other ways within the Amish community, but helping and receiving help from others is a reciprocal process that automatically bonds them together; the joys and sorrows of life are shared without much thought or discussion. Actions in Amish society are more important than words, and mutual helping behavior increases solidarity.

Third, mutual aid helps preserve a sense of tradition and family. Intergenerational assistance is common among the Amish; such interdependence and responsibilities of one generation for another enhance the preservation of their time-honored practices overall. Change comes about more slowly when younger people are closely associated with elders. Three generations are often in close contact in the Amish homestead, creating a situation in which customs and values are constantly passed on. Moreover, parents living in multigenerational households will in all likelihood raise their children somewhat differently from those who have little contact with, or responsibility for, their own parents.

Finally, the informal system of elder care is also an economic benefit to Amish people and their communities. By not paying into the Social Security system, an Amish household has about 12 percent more income to use when they are raising their family. Since elders live on homesteads with their adult children, they do not have to pay rent, and other household expenses are minimized. When elders are sick, relatives and neighbors help out by bringing food and other items. Even payment of large medical bills is shared informally among Amish people, and there are no health insurance payments. From an economic viewpoint, there is really no comparison between the low costs of having a frail elder living in a Grossdaadi Haus and the exorbitant expenses associated with nursing homes or other formal long-term care options used by the larger American society.

The way the Amish care for their elders helps preserve the communal society, or *gemeinschaft*, they continue to value. This communal society stands in stark contrast to the individualism of the twentieth and twenty-first centuries, in which each person calculates what is in his or her best interest, thus setting up competitive, contractual relationships and a society that is governed extensively by law and bureaucratic regulation. In contrast, the Amish seek to preserve cooperative relationships and informally agreed-upon rules, most of which are unwritten and sometimes even unspoken.

13

Jewish Aged:
Diversity in Need and Care Solutions

Zev Harel

This chapter reviews the diversity that characterizes the Jewish aged, factors that contribute to family relations and informal care in later years, and the development and organization of programs and services in the Jewish community. Jewish aged sixty-five years and older, estimated at nine hundred thousand in the United States, represent a highly diverse cross section of individuals and families. Though these Jews share common ancient and contemporary histories and subscribe to many similar norms and values, they also reflect age, gender, socioeconomic, religious, and other differences.

In the United States, the majority of the aged are U.S. born to first- or second-generation immigrants. However, significant numbers are first-generation immigrants from various corners of the world. Most Jewish aged perceive themselves as American Jews, yet a sizable proportion, especially those who immigrated here, retain some relationship to their national origins as well. Recognition of the diversity in the Jewish aged is important for understanding their informal care as well as their need for, and uses of, long-term care services.

The United States is a pluralistic society, and affiliations and membership in Jewish institutions have to be acquired. For these reasons, national origins and ethnicity may have different meanings for the affiliated and the unaffiliated Jewish aged. Generally, ethnicity may function advantageously. Persons with higher levels of integration into ethnic groups may be more inclined to contribute to Jewish institutions and to practice self-reliance and engage in self-help and mutual-help efforts. These ethnic aged may also have more extensive and meaningful social relations and informal social support networks and look to Jewish agencies for help in times of need.

Following the review of the nature and long-term care needs of the Jewish aged, this chapter examines the diverse approaches to long-term care affected by cultural values, attitudes, and behaviors related to service options. Next, the chapter examines the social, political, and economic context in which elder-care decisions are made. The social and political forces at the national level and at the Jewish-community level account for the variations found in current programs and services. The chapter also discusses the values and goals among the frail elderly and their caregivers and the social, political, and cultural factors encountered by planners and service workers that are of critical importance in the use of services. The chapter concludes with the changing challenges faced by Jewish agencies in their efforts to better understand the nature and needs of vulnerable Jewish aged and develop the services needed to assure their security and quality of life in later years.

Jewish Diversity: People, Needs, and Care

Jewish aged count among their ranks a number of highly respected, visible, and prominent individuals. These include political leaders, Nobel Prize winners, jurists, academicians, scientists, financiers, business leaders, journalists, artists and entertainers, novelists and playwrights. At the other end of the continuum are the severely vulnerable aged who live in poverty or near poverty, having difficulty meeting their daily basic needs. In between these two extreme groups, however, the overwhelming majority of older Jews are found.

The Jewish community in the United States has been aging more rapidly than the overall U.S. population, having a larger share of people aged sixty-five and older. As in the general older population, the older age groups have higher percentages of women, and the majority of poor Jewish elderly are also women. Because of differences in life expectancy and marital patterns, older men are more likely to be married while older women are more likely to live alone.

At any given time, the majority of Jewish aged live independently, as is the case generally for the aged of diverse ethnic and racial ancestry. They care for themselves and contribute to the well-being of others. About 20 percent of Jewish aged are frail and vulnerable; they either live in nursing homes or are cared for by their family members because they cannot, on their own, meet their basic needs.

The diversity in the Jewish aged cannot be understood solely by an examination of the sociodemographic and socioeconomic indicators typically employed in sociological analyses of the aged. The consideration of national origin and ethnic background, religiosity, and affiliation patterns will add considerably to our understanding of the characteristics and needs of the Jewish aged in the United States. While many view Jews as a monolithic group, Jews themselves consider national origins, ethnicity, and affiliation with religious and civic groups as important for differentiation in social relations and, to some extent, in civic, economic, and political activities.

In the United States, parents and grandparents of the Jewish aged have come from all corners of the world. However, the overwhelming majority today are native born, either second-, third-, or fourth-generation descendants of immigrants. The migration patterns of Jews during their history, and especially in the twentieth century, have been affected by two major forces. Anti-Jewish hostilities, and especially the Holocaust, pushed them out of many countries, primarily in Europe and the Middle East. The opportunity structure in the United States attracted and brought them here.

The single most important factor characterizing the American Jewish elderly at the turn of the twenty-first century is that most of them are American born. By both country of birth and lifestyle, they resemble other Americans much more than they resemble their immigrant parents. In fact, 86 percent of the elderly in 1990 were born in the United States, a striking change from the 1970s, when nearly 60 percent were foreign born (Glicksman and Cox, 1994).

It has been estimated that in 1990, the elderly made up 16.5 percent of the American Jewish population, a figure somewhat higher than the 12.5 percent of older persons in the overall U.S. population. In 1970, the proportion of elderly was 12 percent among Jews and slightly less than 10 percent in the nation. From 1970 to 1990, while the U.S. population grew at a rate eleven times that of the Jewish population, the rate of growth in the proportion of elderly was greater among the Jews by nearly 50 percent (Glicksman and Cox, 1994). In 1990, the largest group of older Jews, 42 percent, lived in the northeastern United States; 26 percent resided in the South (including Florida); 9 percent in the Midwest; and 23 percent in the West (Glicksman and Cox, 1994).

Physical mobility and its consequences have been central themes in Jewish history from the very beginning. The Jewish population overall is more mobile than Americans in general (Glicksman and Cox, 1994; Kahana and Kahana, 1984). This mobility, which reflects the greater willingness of many American Jews to move to achieve economic and professional success, affects the social integration of the Jewish elderly. Not only does it create distances between older people and their adult children, but also many of these younger Jews are moving to smaller communities with fewer resources to care for the aged (Kahana and Kahana, 1984).

Educational attainment, occupational status, and income of Jewish aged are somewhat higher than for the general U.S. older population (Kahana and Kahana, 1984). Overall, the current generation of older American Jews is better off financially and educationally than the generations of American Jews who preceded them. Sixty-three percent own their own homes and 37 percent rent their living quarters. This is the most mobile generation in American Jewish history, having experienced significant social, economic, and educational changes in their lives. Of the elderly who relocate, the majority in the highest age group (seventy-five and older) are widows moving to be near their children (Kahana and Kahana, 1984). For many of the elderly this is not their first move; many of these Jews changed locations frequently during their lives (Kahana and Kahana, 1984). Older Jews who take up residence in the Sunbelt, as well as those who move to Israel, are more settled in their own lives, more likely to be American born, and more likely to be risk takers than those who do not move. They are in some ways part of the elite of the Jewish elderly.

The Jewish elderly include several groups that deserve special mention. These are Holocaust survivors, Jews from the former Soviet Union who recently immigrated to the United States, and those who are unaffiliated with Jewish organizations. It should not be assumed that these are the only special or unique populations among the current or future generations of Jewish elderly. Elderly Sephardim (from the Middle East) are a separate population, and within this sector there are different groups, such as elderly Turkish or Syrian Jews. There are also aging former Israeli citizens who have lived in the United States for many years. Another group consists of Jewish aged with non-Jewish spouses, and individuals who are considered to be Jewish by descent according to the Reform and Reconstructionist movements but not by Jewish law as accepted by the Conservative and Orthodox religious movements (Glicksman and Cox, 1994).

Some of these aged persons may have high ethnic identity, low socioeconomic status, no informal support system, and limited knowledge about, and access to, services. They may be, therefore, among the most vulnerable among the Jewish aged and are likely to experience the most extensive degree of unmet service needs. This segment of the aged Jewish population may rely less on agencies than those aged who are aware of procedures and policies of Jewish service agencies. Foreign-language communication by agency staff is essential for conveying information about benefits as well as providing direct services effectively. In addition, special outreach efforts may be important to reach this population and address their needs.

Special attention also needs to be directed to the needs of non-affiliated Jewish aged persons—those who do not belong to Jewish groups or organizations. Unfortunately, they tend to be invisible to the planners and the Jewish community service system and thus are generally underserved. This group is likely to include a significant number of elderly Jews who have limited economic and social resources. For example, one study (Huberman, 1986) found that in New York City, 13 percent of the Jewish population was poor, half of them elderly. Yet 62 percent of this indigent population did not report contact with Jewish agencies. In Chicago, 15 percent of the Jewish population was economically disadvantaged; close to half of these individuals were aged. These situations pose serious challenges for Jewish Homes for the Aged and Jewish social service agencies. Some Jewish elderly who are hidden and are not capable of militant advocacy on their own behalf may become isolated, both physically and mentally.

Survivors of the Holocaust also require special attention. They are, in some ways, like other first-generation immigrants from Europe only more so. Many of them are affiliated with fellow survivors and survivor organizations but are not integrated into the mainstream of the organized Jewish community (Harel, 1990; Kahana, Harel and Kahana, 1988). A significant number are likely to experience difficulties as a consequence of the interaction of declining health and functional losses with intrusive imageries of their Holocaust-related experiences. Some may even face anti-Semitism here in the United States. Efforts on behalf of unaffiliated Holocaust survivors are especially important, as only the Jewish community and Jewish professionals are likely to be interested in, and capable of, meeting their needs. Holocaust survivors bring into old age traditions from their countries of origin as well as memories of the terrible experiences they endured in Europe. This may result in special psychological challenges in old age, especially in nursing homes. Holocaust survivors often experience difficulties in institution-based long-term care because of the memories of the concentration camps (Harel, 1990).

Another population, which is unique in the sense that its members arrived in the United States in more recent years, is elderly Soviet Jews. Many of them came when they were older and may reside at a distance from their family members or lack a viable informal support system (Glicksman and Cox, 1994). They often experience declining health and functional status in an environment to which they have minimally acculturated, and they have limited knowledge about ways to seek out and secure the resources they need.

As in the general older populations around the world, the highest growth within the aged population is projected for the oldest age groups. While, on the one hand, it is expected that future cohorts of elderly are likely to be healthier and command better economic resources, on the other, evidence also indicates that the higher age groups will consist of the most vulnerable older persons. Severe vulnerability is characterized not only by poor health and functional status but also by limitations in personal, social, and economic resources (Harel and Noelker, 1995). These Jewish aged will require more assistance at the time when informal support is declining. More women who have been the primary caregivers are entering the labor force both by choice and by necessity. In addition, the number of never-married, divorced, and childless elders among Jews is on the rise. In the face of reduced informal support, these aged will require more services in the future.

Among the Jewish elderly, as is true of other aged in the United States, it is estimated that about 20 percent are severely impaired and in need of long-term care. Slightly more than 5 percent are in institutions; the others are cared for in the community (Harel and Noelker, 1995). Three times as many severely impaired elderly individuals live at home as in nursing homes because family caregiving has become the norm (Brody, 1985). Often these family caregivers, primarily women, are described as "the sandwich generation," caught in the middle between caring for parents and their own lives, including children, spouses, and careers. In recent decades, the number of older people with severe vulnerabilities who need long-term care has been on the rise and will continue to increase in years to come.

Among Jewish aged, the fraction of severely vulnerable elderly is slightly higher than in the general older population, with a slightly greater percentage found in nursing homes or receiving paid care in their own residence. In part, this can be accounted for by the substantial mobility of both younger and older generations as well as their desire to maintain separate residences. Fewer Jewish aged live in multigenerational households than other groups; 30 percent of all older Jews live alone, and another 55 percent reside in two-person households, mostly with a spouse. As in the general older population, women represent the overwhelming majority of those receiving services at home or in institutions, as well as those who provide the formal care.

The Jewish community and Jewish professionals have historically served the needs of the Jewish aged. They have adapted to the changes in consumer characteristics and used national resources to develop and refine health and social services. They continue to be aware of changing preferences and needs on the part of Jewish aged. Interest, expertise, and professional resources in the Jewish community will continue to be needed in the development of effective ways to meet the service needs of all Jewish aged in their homes, at service sites, and in long-term care settings.

Values and Attitudes Related to Care and Services

The element of religion distinguishes Jews from other ethnic groups defined largely by national origin and/or language; consequently, Jews may be considered a religioethnic group (Gelfand and Kutzik, 1979; Kahana and Kahana, 1984). Religious commitment or identification contributes to the influences of historical background on the lives of Jewish aged in the United States today.

There are multiple bases of integration in the Jewish community. Generational continuity in religious affiliation and identification is one of these bases, as is ethnicity. The notion of generational continuity implies a high level of consensus between and among generations in lifestyles, interests, kin networks, economic linkages, values, and norms (Goldscheider, 1986), all characteristics that may be associated with ethnicity. While the extent and nature of religious and organizational affiliation may have changed in recent years among the Jewish aged, it is still a very important factor in the development of care solutions and in receiving care and services.

Generational continuity in contemporary society suggests that a complex and dynamic perspective of ethnicity must be developed if we are going to understand how it influences the process of aging and the characteristics of Jewish communities in the United States. On the one hand, cultural differences among Jews (for example, Sephardim versus Ashkenazim, or German Jews versus Russian Jews) provide norms, values, and resources that make the experience of aging different for each ethnic group as well as different from the dominant culture. Cultural similarities among Jews, on the other hand, provide critical converging norms and practices allowing for the development of formal as well as informal support structures that benefit aged individuals and the communities in which they reside.

Consideration of the national origins, ethnicity, and religious backgrounds that characterize Jewish aged is useful for identifying strengths and resources available in Jewish communities for planning, organizing, and delivering services. Recognition of the importance of ethnicity among Jewish aged and its interaction with historical and contemporary experiences may help distinguish needs of the Jewish aged. Some may be consequences of traditional patterns in the countries of origin, while others have emerged in response to challenges faced in the host country (Harel, 1990; Gelfand and Kutzik, 1979). Appreciation of the ethnic and racial diversity present in the United States has been increasing in the field of social gerontology. As Markides and Mindel (1987) have pointed out, the early development of the field of aging during the post–World War II period occurred without special attention to racial or ethnic origins. Since the 1960s, however, gerontological literature and research increasingly have focused on race, national origin, and ethnicity (Gelfand and Barresi, 1987; Gelfand and Kutzik, 1979; Harel, 1986; Rosenthal, 1986).

It is now generally accepted that a better understanding of the function of ethnicity on the lives of the aged would enhance the planning and delivery of more effective services for older individuals and their families. This awareness has fostered an increasing emphasis on the need for ethnically sensitive practice in various fields. Such an orientation recognizes the role and importance of ethnicity as it interacts with other factors and shapes the definition of problems for which services and resources are sought and/or needed. Moreover, along with their acculturation, a significant number among the Jewish aged in the United States have been in the forefront of the development of Jewish institutions and are major supporters of these institutions today.

Ethnicity in the lives of the aged in the United States may be conceptualized as an ongoing phenomenon. Ethnicity no longer simply describes a traditional immigrant model of obstacles to acculturation and assimilation. Rather, gerontological researchers and professionals in applied fields of health and human services have begun to explore systematically the ways in which ethnicity may act to perpetuate ethnic life and culture. This research also provides important data for understanding the impact that ethnicity has on service needs and use among elderly members of different ethnic communities (Gelfand and Barresi, 1987; Harel, 1986; Rosenthal, 1986).

When considering the effects of ethnicity, it is important to differentiate between the defining elements of ethnicity (e.g., ethnic affiliation, ethnic identity, and ethnic practices), factors that contribute to the perpetuation of ethnicity, and the impact or consequences of ethnicity (Harel, 1986). Ethnicity has been defined and measured in a variety of ways. It has included referents such as membership, traditions, culture, beliefs, identification, experiences, behaviors, and practices (Gelfand and Kutzik, 1979; Rosenthal, 1986). Furthermore, ethnicity or ethnic identity may be related to, or influenced by, historical, traditional, social, cultural, religious, and language characteristics. All of these are evident both in the characteristics of Jewish aged and Jewish communities in the United States.

It has been suggested that elderly persons who enjoy a strong association with their ethnic groups may have more sources of informal support than those having

a weaker or no association (Gelfand and Kutzik, 1979). A strong ethnic affiliation, therefore, would benefit the Jewish elderly. At the same time, unacculturat-
ed members of the Jewish community with limited economic resources may be
unaware of the available benefits and services to which they may be entitled. Furthermore, some Jewish aged may not utilize agency services since they lack
knowledge about how to obtain them or because their attitudinal predisposition
precludes relying on need-based benefits. These persons may overburden informal sources of support or go without the assistance that they need (Harel, 1986).
In summary, it appears important to clearly differentiate between the defining elements of ethnicity, factors that determine ethnicity and ethnic connectedness,
and the consequences of ethnicity, especially as these affect care and services for
Jewish aged. It is equally important to recognize conventional factors that are
found to be determinants of service use in the general aged population.

Jewish Aged, Informal Care, and Service Use

The status of the Jewish elderly in the family is affected by a desire to maintain
close familial ties, which conflicts with the equally important value of professional success. Achievement in the United States means both socioeconomic and
geographic mobility, and either can create strain between generations. The vast
majority of the Jewish elderly, as with the elderly in the United States as a whole,
are not abandoned by their children but are cared for and receive a wide variety
of support. Research indicates that a majority of the Jewish aged receive some
care from their adult children. There tends to be a preference for the latter to have
legal responsibility for their impaired parents, and there is close contact between
the generations (Glicksman and Cox, 1994). While a minority of Jewish aged parents would prefer that their children not move far away from them, a higher fraction state that mobility is important (Kahana and Kahana, 1984; Rosenthal,
1986). Older Jews often feel an ambivalence, a mixture of pride and grief, over
children who live at a distance (Myerhoff, 1978).

Evidence indicates that while older Jewish parents and their adult children prefer to live near one another, they do not want to live together (Glicksman and Cox,
1994; Rosenthal, 1986). These feelings are generally mutual. Autonomy, described in some works as independence, is intimately associated with privacy, and
the loss of one is usually accompanied by the loss of the other. The desire of most
elderly is to live independently but in a reciprocal family bond. The best predictor of positive contact between older Jewish parents and their adult children is a
warm relationship over the life span (Kahana and Kahana, 1984; Rosenthal,
1986).

A review of the literature reveals that Jewish caregivers generally provide
fewer hours of caregiving themselves and secure more hours of paid help than
other caregivers. They have been found to employ paid sitters for twice the number of hours as members of other groups (Glicksman and Cox, 1994). This may

be accounted for by the fact that American Jews have developed a sense of the importance of using "professionals" in various aspects of their lives, including care for their aging parents (Glicksman and Cox, 1994).

To better understand the issues related to service use among elderly members of the Jewish community, it may be useful to review the commonly found predictors of such use. Research indicates that in addition to sociodemographic status and health and functional capacity, knowledge about, and access to, benefits and services play important roles in the prediction of utilization (Biegel and Harel, 1994; Harel, Noelker and Blake,1985). Not all older people are likely to have adequate information about the various forms of assistance that might enhance the quality of their lives. This lack of knowledge tends to reduce the chances that the aged individual will search for and find help.

Research reveals that the availability of informal help and the interface between formal and informal support systems are important determinants of service use among the elderly (Biegel and Harel, 1994). Families are more likely to provide assistance with emotional requirements, personal care, and household management. In contrast, the formal system of public and voluntary agencies provides entitlements to housing, education, safety, and transportation, as well as health and social services (Biegel and Harel, 1994). The better integrated and acculturated Jewish aged are more likely to pursue services on their own or with assistance from family members. Many immigrants, the poor, and those with less than a college education, who have the greatest need for social services, tend not to use them (Huberman, 1984). Because they are likely to refrain from reaching out for assistance, some Jewish elderly, especially those who were left behind by their culturally and geographically mobile children and those who have not acculturated to the mainstream of American life, may become isolated both physically and mentally. This isolation could lead to a worsening of their condition, and some may find themselves in a hazardous situation. However, the majority of the Jewish aged, some with assistance from members of their informal support system, are likely to find the services they need.

In addition to family members and friends, synagogues, civic groups, and other organizations play significant roles in the lives of elderly members of the Jewish community. Jewish and non-Jewish associations alike provide opportunities for involvement and affiliation and are important sources of information and support. Service agencies are increasingly aware of, and rely on, informal sources of support in care for the Jewish aged (Harel, 1990).

Social, Political, and Economic Forces
Shaping Programs and Services

The many factors that shaped the development of policies and programs for all aged in the United States also have had beneficial effects for the Jewish aged. They, along with members of other ethnic groups, gain significantly from programs that have taken a major responsibility for the security and health care of older people. The Social Security Act of 1935 provides a very important basis for income benefits. Medicare (1965), Medicaid (1965), the Older Americans Act (1965), and Title XX of the Social Security Act furnish the major funding for health and social services (Monk and Warach, 1994).

The Jewish aged in the United States also have enjoyed services over the years that have evolved with their ethnic religious legacies. From the days of the first Jewish settlement in New York City, through the traditions of charity—*Zedakah*—and contemporary health and social service initiatives, the commandment "Honor thy father and thy mother" guided the successive efforts to assure services for needy persons, including the aged (Monk and Warach, 1994).

In the United States, each successive wave of Jewish immigrants made its unique contribution. The Sephardic Jews created synagogues whose *Bikur Holim* (visits to the sick) and charitable benefit funds were the predecessors of the Jewish Family Service agencies. The German Jewish immigrants, following the traditions of their origins, established the hospitals, homes for the aged, settlement houses, and family and welfare agencies that carry on to this day. They also founded the community-wide fund-raising organizations, federations, and welfare funds that became the dominant force in Jewish philanthropic endeavors and social planning. The indigent and dependent aged benefited from these charities, including financial help to cover food, clothing, and medical expenses (Monk and Warach, 1994).

During the first half of the twentieth century, centralized philanthropic fund-raising for the charitable agencies of the Jewish community provided the major source of support for service agencies. Since then, government funding of health and social services increasingly has replaced voluntary philanthropy as the means for basic support. Key leaders of the Jewish community were in the vanguard of the advocates for passage of the federal and state legislation that remains the foundation for funding the social insurance and health and welfare programs for the aged in the United States today (Monk and Warach, 1994).

Since the mid-1960s, with the advent of Medicaid and Medicare and the concurrent rise in the cost of services, all voluntary agencies serving the aged in long-term care and social services have benefited from governmental support. Many Jewish Homes for the Aged have been fundamentally transformed into long-term care complexes, established in suburban areas, to serve the new generations of Jewish aged (Raichilson, 1994). In addition to institution-based services, some of these facilities now feature independent housing units as well as day-care centers and offer home- and community-based service programs. Financial support of Jewish Homes for the Aged from Jewish Federations has declined substantially since the passage of Medicaid. However, Jewish philanthropic contributions to Jewish homes, in the form of annual, endowment, and building-fund gifts, have actually increased. These facilities have been beneficiaries of substantial legacies, and some now have sizeable endowments. Persons with limited income or whose resources have been depleted and who can prove need or hardship may also apply for economic relief to the federally administered Supplemental Security Income (SSI) program and to Medicaid for health and long-term care (Monk and Warach, 1994).

Jewish Family Service agencies adapted to the array of public funding. Initially they helped older persons gain access to programs and entitlements through information and referral and, in recent years, developed case management, counseling, transportation, and home- and community-based services. There was no predetermined pattern concerning which agency ministered to what specific needs of the Jewish aged. Some Jewish Federations launched long-term planning initiatives and established multifunctional and interagency coordinating committees, and several communities fostered the creation of autonomous multifunctional agencies to provide direct services for the Jewish aged.

The Federation of Jewish Philanthropies of New York organized the Jewish Association for Services for the Aged (JASA) in 1968. Chicago similarly established the Council for the Jewish Elderly in 1970, and Washington, D.C., followed suit a few years later with the Jewish Council for the Aging (Monk and Warach, 1994). In other large urban communities three separate Jewish agencies address the service needs of corresponding segments of the vulnerable aged: Jewish Homes for the Aged; Jewish Family Services; and Jewish Community Centers (Monk and Warach, 1994)

Organizational reshaping and the creation of community-based long-term care have taken place primarily in large cities. However, the provision of social services and support to Jewish elderly who reside in the community has been a standard for every Jewish community of significant size in the United States. Jewish Community Centers have diversified their programs and now offer education, recreation, travel/vacation programs, and socialization and nutrition programs to a growing market of senior adults. Jewish Family Service organizations have diversified and provide a range of service products for the elderly, including homemaker services, housekeeping, and case management. Jewish community-sponsored senior housing is often a provider of social services. In many areas, senior housing organizations have assumed responsibility for coordinating the provision of housekeeping and socialization services. Although already providing a large number of discrete services, the long-term goal for the Jewish community has evolved into offering a continuum of care, integrating health and social services.

Every Jewish locale in the United States is confronted with the challenge of allocating funds among competing demands. There is generally a consensus that the aged require special attention to assure that their service needs are met. But the questions of how much funding and for what purposes continue to be discussed by diverse constituencies within these Jewish communities.

Jewish Federations have been allocating funds for services to the elderly for many years (Tobin, 1994). The relatively higher percentage of older persons, particularly those at the more advanced ages, has led Jewish communities not only to develop services sooner than other places but also to create programs and services that have become prototypes for other organizations. Many innovations evolved from the necessity to respond to an increasing aging population in which generations often reside in separate locales (Tobin, 1994).

Homes for the aged illustrate the transformation of services that has occurred over time. These facilities have become nursing homes for the sickest of Jewish elderly individuals, who average eighty-five years of age. They now have adjacent residential options and assisted living residences for the less functionally impaired, day-care centers, and services for impaired aged residing in the community. Jewish Family Services have developed an array of home- and community-based access, nutritional, and social services. Jewish Community Centers have expanded their offerings to accommodate the functionally limited elderly in senior adult programs, furnishing congregate meals and special social programs. The centralization in planning and coordination of service provision, in contrast to decentralized autonomous and strong service organizations, reflects the relative power of the Jewish Federations vis-à-vis Jewish agencies (Weismehl, 1994).

As the number of frail elderly kept increasing over the years, supportive and protective services were added to maintain the aged in their communities of residence. These included housekeeping, homemaker and home-health services, and home-delivered meals. To finance these programs, agencies had to acquire fund-raising skills. Government funds tended to cover service areas explicitly designated by legislative enactments. Foundation and private funds were more discretionary. They enabled agencies to experiment with innovative approaches as well as cover the gaps left by the public sector, particularly administrative costs. Jewish service organizations tended to intensify their reliance on public funding in those service areas where the voluntary sector alone could not cope with either the incidence or the severity of emerging needs (Monk and Warach, 1994).

Since 1965, public funding of nursing home care has made it possible for Jewish homes to serve increasing numbers of poor aged. The number of beds in Jewish-sponsored facilities, however, could not expand enough to meet the increasing demand, and more older persons are placed in secular, private, and for-profit facilities. Jewish-sponsored voluntary agencies and nursing homes have increased their efforts to secure philanthropic contributions directly from the public (Monk and Warach, 1994).

The Jewish Family Service agencies and Jewish Community Centers, while serving a significant number of Jewish aged, could not meet the needs of all older Jewish people. An increasing number of elderly, therefore, are using the nutritional and home-care services available at community service agencies. Jewish service agencies retain, for the most part, a distinctive religious and cultural profile; but, like all sectarian facilities that benefit from public funds, they cannot discriminate on the basis of religion, or for that matter on any other grounds (Monk and Warach, 1994), and therefore serve diverse aged individuals and families.

Social, Political, and Cultural Factors in Services

As agencies have taken advantage of public funding and insurance payments for services, consumers of their services have changed, and with it the Jewish mission and character have been reduced in emphasis. At the same time, a more Americanized population of non-Jews as well as Jews has raised the question of what is specifically Jewish in Jewish nursing homes and at Jewish Family Services agencies. These kinds of issues are not only complex but also sensitive ones that pose challenges and require ongoing attention (Tobin, 1994).

Because Jewish service providers are likely to be perceived as more understanding of the needs of Jews, as well as having greater expertise, a sufficient number of staff must be Jewish. In addition to maintaining the Jewish dimension in services, including sensitivity to Jewish historical experiences, lifestyle, and religious rituals, agencies have offered new programs for specific Jewish groups, such as recent Soviet immigrants and Holocaust survivors. In Jewish Family Service agencies and Jewish Community Centers, the content of most services may not be particularly Jewish, but the comfort level for older Jews using them may be higher than with public services generally. Regardless of religious orientation, facilities can be expected to celebrate Jewish holidays in traditional ways and offer specific Jewish cultural and social activities.

As these service agencies rely increasingly on public funding for access, nutritional, and home-based long-term care services, both the staff and service consumers have been changing to include other than Jewish persons (Tobin, 1994). Jewish service agencies have been employing professional and paraprofessional staff of diverse ethnic and racial backgrounds, which necessitates that consumers and employees learn about each other and be respectful of their differences. In nursing homes and in community-based service agencies, employees work for low wages and their benefits are often limited, leading to high staff turnover. Some agencies have developed new benefits such as child care on the premises and offer transportation to and from work. With employment conditions in the United States continuing to improve, agencies will have to be creative in structuring their work environment to maintain a quality workforce.

Conclusion and Policy Implications

The growing number of older persons, coupled with changes in the family structure and publicly available benefits and services, will continue to challenge the general and professional leadership of the Jewish community in efforts to meet present and future needs of the Jewish aged. As with the general older population, the highest growth within the Jewish aged is projected for the oldest age groups, which include the most vulnerable people. The leadership of the Jewish community will continue to be challenged in the mobilization of needed resources as well as in the planning, organization, and delivery of services.

Professionals planning for, and working with, Jewish elderly persons will have to persist in their advocacy for more adequate health care and long-term care benefits. They also must continue to plan, organize, and deliver effective services; develop innovative education and information-dissemination strategies; create appropriate linking mechanisms among benefit offices, service agencies, and the Jewish elderly; enhance support for informal caregivers in the community; improve the responsiveness of Jewish non–service organizations in meeting spiritual, cultural, social, and recreational needs; and identify and meet the needs of the unaffiliated elderly, especially those who do not have the benefit of an informal support system.

Because of the diversity that characterizes the Jewish aged population, it is important to consider various attitudes toward, and preferences for, services by older persons and members of their informal support system. On the individual level, the older person has a right to determine and participate in the planning and choice of services. On an aggregate level, this information is useful to planners in the development of "demand-responsive" community service systems. Also, it is essential to identify patterns of self-help and informal care available and offer support to caregivers among all Jewish elderly, both to reduce heavy reliance on agencies for assistance and to facilitate the use of professional services when they are needed (Biegel and Harel, 1994; Tobin, 1994; Weismehl, 1994).

While all Jewish communities play an important role in efforts to meet the demands of their members, there is a great deal of variation in the resources and expertise available to them. The development of appropriate and adequate services for the Jewish aged will continue to challenge planners and service providers in the future. Some Jewish communities simply do not have the expertise and resources to provide sufficiently for their elderly members. They require assistance with all aspects of care, including assessment of needs, planning efforts, and the organization and delivery of services (Biegel and Harel, 1994).

Care for the vulnerable aged must take into account the array of services offered at agency sites and in the older person's home, as well as those available in congregate living environments. Many of the fundamental efforts required to meet the needs of Jewish aged at present and in the future are already in place and will continue to be of highest priority for the Jewish community. However, attention must be directed toward the identification of changing needs and preferences, coordination among Jewish agencies, broader community representation on planning boards, and greater involvement of older consumers of services in decision making.

Research indicates that the utilization of services is also affected by organizational characteristics. Jewish elders and their families may have difficulty in penetrating the boundaries of bureaucratic health and social service organizations. They may also have problems with the fragmented service system that requires consistent and active pursuit of services. In this context, future activities should incorporate efforts to enhance knowledge about, and access to, community programs, along with discussions on attitudes toward the use of services. Respect for, and understanding of, the diversity, needs, and preferences of older consumers, coupled with effective communications with them and members of their informal support system, will continue to be essential in working with all aged, including those who are Jewish.

Finally, special effort needs to be directed to encourage an appreciation of diversity and ethnically sensitive practices. Jewish agencies employing and serving persons of different religious and ethnic backgrounds must offer educational and staff-development programs that will enhance understanding of, and respect for, people working and residing in various Jewish-sponsored settings. Both residents and staff also must have opportunities to celebrate and enjoy their holidays and maintain their religious and cultural practices.

14

Growing Old in an Arab American Family

Hani Fakhouri

Knowledge regarding aging and the aged population has been gradually and steadily increasing during the past three to four decades; however, interest in ethnogerontology as a subfield within social gerontology began to emerge during the 1970s. Information about certain ethnic and racial groups is still meager by comparison to the accumulated knowledge and information regarding the dominant groups.

Since only limited factual data are available on the Arab American elderly population in the United States, the study reported in this chapter was undertaken with the objective of evaluating the continuities and discontinuities of traditional cultural traits that early and recent waves of immigrants brought with them from the Arab world. The chapter first will examine cultural traits that reflect the social organization of the family and kinship groups, in particular the elderly's roles and affiliations in that social network. Second, it will investigate the impacts of socialization and social interactions and their viability as social, economic, and emotional support systems in old age. Third, the chapter will explore the process of adaptation of Arab Americans to aging and retirement. Finally, it will assess the conditions, needs, and problems of aging and the aged among the Arab American population.

The Community in Historical Context

Arab Americans are viewed in this chapter as a distinct ethnic group within American society. It is an ethnic minority that reflects a heterogeneous group with a broad cultural background in terms of its national origins in the Arab world. The vast majority of Arab American immigrants came from Lebanon, Syria, Jordan, Palestine, Iraq, Yemen, and Egypt.

Immigration from the Arab world to the United States began during the later part of the nineteenth century. During the 1990s, the size of the Arab American community was estimated to be from 1 million to the most frequently cited figure of 2.5 million to 3 million people (Suleiman, 1999).

As with other ethnic groups in the United States, the Arab American community is not immune to the effects of modernization and rapid cultural transformation. What will be the impact of evolving social, cultural, and economic needs on traditional norms and values as they affect the life situation of the Arab American elderly population? Any changes should be viewed in light of increasing longevity, especially with respect to the increased number of years spent in retirement.

Research Methodology

This study is based on a survey that was conducted in four counties in Michigan, where more than 300,000 Arab Americans reside. The first part of the survey was conducted in Flint, Genesee County. The second phase of the study took place in the metropolitan Detroit area, which includes Wayne, Oakland, and Macomb Counties. Since it is difficult and time consuming to locate elderly people by a random selection process, and even more so when seeking specific ethnic groups, the principal investigator obtained names from community leaders, social clubs, churches, and mosques. This analysis is based on 230 individuals of Arab American affiliation who were sixty-two years of age and older. Face-to-face interviews were conducted in both English and Arabic.

The Arab American family reflects both continuity and change. By continuity we are referring to the preservation of some of the traditional characteristics that have been brought by the earliest immigrants from the Arab world and continue to be strengthened by recent waves of newcomers. Furthermore, the institution of the family has experienced changes as a result of modernization and acculturation. The continuity of certain traditional values is reflected in the social structure of the Arab American family specifically and in the kinship network generally. The following analysis will focus first on the conjugal-extended family and second on the kinship network.

The Arab American family is a tightly knit social unit that defines roles and performs certain functions for its members. The norms and values that members of the Arab American family acquire through the process of socialization define the relationships and obligations within that social unit.

Love, respect, and support for parents are emphasized and are reflected in children's behavior toward their parents, grandparents, uncles, and aunts. Similar norms and values also can be detected in the parents' and grandparents' behavior toward their children and grandchildren. This mutual feeling of love and respect among children, parents, and other members of the family is maintained through the different stages of the life cycle.

Table 14.1 Household Composition, Arab Americans

	Percent
Elders living alone	20.1
Elders living with spouse only	34.8
Elders living with spouse and married/unmarried children	30.8
Widowed living with children	10.2
Elders living with sibling or relatives	0.4
Elders living in nursing home	3.7
Total	100.0

N = 230

Living Arrangements

The survey reveals that more than two-thirds of the households (76 percent) are made up of families that consist of two or more people related by blood or marriage (see table 14.1). Of the 34.8 percent of the elderly who live only with a spouse, about 90 percent have family members—children, siblings, nephews, nieces—living nearby. The other 10 percent have no immediate family members living in Michigan.

Two-thirds of the 20.1 percent of the elderly residing alone said that they live alone because they never married (3.0 percent), they are childless (6.0 percent), or their children live out of state (3.0 percent). The other one-third of the elderly population who are alone prefer to live independently of their children since the latter have moved into suburban areas. As long as the parents are healthy and maintain contact with their children, they are satisfied and content to live their retirement years independently in their own homes. Upon the death of the husband, it is common practice for a widow to move in with one of her children. However, when a wife dies, the husband usually is reluctant to reside with any of his children, unless his health begins to deteriorate.

Arab American families stress close contact with their members. This closeness is reflected in the maintenance of ties and the frequency of social interaction between parents and their children, especially when they are not living together (see table 14.2). More than two-thirds (71.6 percent) of the elderly parents who are not living with their children see them at least twice a week, if not daily. The 6.4 percent of elderly parents who visit with their children only on special occasions and during holidays do so because their children live outside the state. In addition, 1.7 percent of the elderly do not interact or visit with their children for personal reasons.

Living with their children provides elderly parents with more security than does

Table 14.2 Frequency of Visitation with Children Not Living with Parents, Arab Americans

	Percent
More than once a week	71.6
Often, but less than once a week (at least once every two weeks)	20.3
On special occasions (holidays, birthdays)	6.4
No visitation or interaction	1.7
Total	100.0

N = 230

living alone, and they can maintain daily contact with their children, grandchildren, and in some cases their great-grandchildren. Such family settings consisting of three to four generations promote social interaction, which is of great benefit to those within that extended unit. Grandparents play an active role in their grandchildren's lives, and a closeness often develops between them. They also can act as protectors of their grandchildren, especially when parents become too demanding. Furthermore, when parents are not at home, grandparents tend to baby-sit them.

The moral, social, and economic obligations expected of children toward their parents have been greatly emphasized in traditional Arab cultures. The ethic of filial piety requires children not only to show respect but also to assume their duty toward their parents, regardless of the burden. Filial piety has even been supported legally and religiously in the different countries of the Arab world. The following two verses from the Quran reflect on how parents should be treated according to Islam:

Thy Lord hath decreed
that ye worship none but him,
And that ye be kind to parents.
Whether one or both of them attain
Old age in thy life,
Say not to them a word
Of contempt, nor repel them,
But address them in terms of honor.
And out of kindness
Lower to them the wing
Of humility, and say:
My Lord! Bestow on them
thy mercy even as they
cherished me in childhood. (Quran 17.23–24)

These verses emphasize that parents deserve our reverence and services. It is a religious edict that affects the social and cultural aspects of the Arab American family, whether Muslim or Christian.

Among those interviewed were two female respondents of advanced age. The first, an eighty-six-year-old widow living with her son, is physically handicapped and relies on a wheelchair. The second, a ninety-two-year-old widow also living with her son, is disabled because of the loss of her eyesight fifteen years ago. Both women, who are well taken care of and satisfied with their lives, are members of families with four living generations. Several grandchildren who are living with one of them told us:

> Our *sittu* [grandmother] is a remarkable lady. We are fond of her. When we were children, she and grandpa always had something for us, a surprise. She was and still is fond of us, and we are of her. Our childhood memory of our relationship with our grandparents is a delightful one, even when we were teenagers. When our parents were angry with us, we always knew we could turn to our grandparents and they would be there for us. Now, since they are getting frail and old, we are here to help them in any way possible and to make their life a pleasant one.

The Arab American elderly are at the center of an extended family network, with a variety of important cultural characteristics that affect individual socialization, self-identity, and the feeling of belonging. They also influence social interaction beyond the nuclear family and the ethnic social network.

Children are taught to respect and care for the elderly. The traditional value system emphasizes parents and grandparents as well as uncles and aunts, the latter two terms including other elderly people who are members of the extended family and social network. Such relationships are evident in the usage of terms to address elderly persons as "uncle" or "aunt," even if they are not blood relatives. This linguistic interaction creates a sense of belonging among Arab American members that extends beyond the kin groups.

The sense of belonging among the elderly population in general is a significant contributing factor to longevity. It has been emphasized in gerontological literature as contributing to life satisfaction in old age (Atchley, 1997). Such life satisfaction is expressed by 87.4 percent of the elderly Arab Americans in the survey; they also share a strong sense of belonging with their kin groups.

The Arab American social network stresses close contacts with extended family members, as well as other individuals who are linked to their social network by marriage. These relationships are reflected in the frequency of contact between the elderly population and their kin. More than two-thirds (69.4 percent) of the respondents communicate with their extended family members regularly. Arab American immigrant groups have also developed a variety of ethnic social networks to promote connections beyond their kin groups, such as interacting with friends or affiliation with religious and cultural organizations. Almost all (96.5 percent) of the respondents have friends in the area where they live, and 80.5 per-

Table 14.3 Frequency of Social Interaction with Extended Relations and Friends, Arab Americans (for those with friends in area)

	Percent
See them once a week and/or talk with them by phone	82.5
See them often (once every two weeks) or talk with them by phone	9.6
Rarely see them	6.1
Stopped seeing them	1.8
Total	100.0

N = 230

cent interact with them weekly or biweekly (see table 14.3).

Religious and social organizations promote and contribute to the maintenance of many traditional cultural characteristics of the elderly Arab American community. The older population is included in cultural events, and their retirement doesn't discourage them from participating in social activities. For example, the Syrian Lebanese Association in the Flint area frequently invites the elderly to banquet dinners to reaffirm their link to the community and to honor them. In the interview, we asked respondents about their church and mosque attendance before and after retirement. Those who were less active or did not participate after retirement gave as their reasons poor health, lack of transportation, or loss of interest because of changes in their congregation.

The demographic characteristics of the elderly population, such as age, marital status, education, occupation, and income, shed light on the general lifestyle and later adaptation to aging. Moreover, race, ethnicity, and gender also have an impact on aging. Tables 14.4–14.8 show the demographic characteristics of the Arab American elderly population in this survey.

The median age of the sample is seventy-two years; nearly 35 percent are over seventy-five, and 65 percent are under seventy. Of the population surveyed, 57 percent are male and 43 percent, female. However, for married couples, only the husbands were interviewed; if their wives were included, the actual sex ratio of the total sample would be 67 males to 100 females. Significantly, nearly all of the men are married, whereas most of the women are widowed (see table 14.5). As expected, the proportion of widows increases in the higher age groups. Moreover, there has been an increasing life span, as reflected in the high percentage of the Arab American elderly population over the age of seventy-five. Improvements in health care and increasing awareness of good diet and exercise will contribute to even longer life expectancies in the future.

Over one-third (35.2 percent) of the older people interviewed were born in the United States, while the rest were born in various countries of the Middle East

Table 14.4 Percentage and Distribution of Respondents by Age, Arab Americans

Age	Percent	No. of Cases
62–64	13.0	30
65–69	30.5	70
70–74	21.7	50
75–79	15.3	35
80–84	13.0	15
Total	100.0	230

(see table 14.6). Of those who are not American born, 95.4 percent are naturalized citizens and 4.6 percent are permanent alien residents. The majority of the respondents have been residents of Michigan for more than ten years. Almost all (91.0 percent) intend to continue living in Michigan, only 1.8 percent plan to move to warmer climates, and 7.2 percent are indefinite about their future plans.

Over one-third of the sample were self-employed as owners and operators of grocery-store outlets or other types of service businesses (see table 14.7). This distribution reflects a representative pattern of employment. The unskilled workers include laborers and operators, especially in the automotive industry. The majority of the professionals are second- and third-generation Arab Americans who have been educated in the United States or in the Arab world. There appears to be a significant change in the type of occupation pursued, especially between the immigrant and second and third generations of Arab Americans, reflecting rapid upward mobility.

The Arab American family stresses the importance of education. This social characteristic was reflected in response to the question, "If you had to relive your life again, what are the things that you would change and why?" The vast majority of those who did not go to college stated that they would have attempted to attain higher levels of schooling. They felt that education was very important. An im-

Table 14.5 Marital Status, Arab Americans

Status	Percent	No. of Cases	Males	Females
Single	3.1	7	2	5
Married	52.3	120	90	30
Widowed	36.8	85	10	75
Divorced	7.0	16	4	12
Separated	0.8	2	2	0
Total	100.0	230	108	122

Table 14.6 Country of Birth, Arab Americans

	Percent
Egypt	3.3
Jordan	10.0
Lebanon	20.5
Palestine	21.0
Syria	5.0
United States	35.2
Yemen	5.0
Total	100.0

N = 230

pressive number have been fairly successful financially, but despite their achievements, they felt that their life would have been improved with more education.

Arab culture in general views education not only as a key to success for children but also as a source of achievement for the parents who educated them. The importance of education was also reflected in answers to the question, "What would be your advice to young people?" The majority stressed education as a key to success and the good life: young people should spare no effort to attain the highest educational level possible. Other advice emphasized the importance of the family as a social unit; caring for parents, grandparents, and siblings, with special emphasis on social interaction; and a clean life, such as staying away from drugs.

The quality of life and lifestyle of people are influenced and shaped to a great extent by the financial resources available to them. In general, when older people enter retirement, their income decreases. At the same time, their basic requirements remain the same, and the need for some items, such as health care, transportation, and housing maintenance, actually can increase. Employment status also affects the quality of life among the elderly.

Table 14.7 Occupation, Arab Americans

	Percent
Self-employed	35.9
Skilled worker	11.7
Never worked (housewife)	21.7
Professional (lawyer, professor, physician, engineer, teacher, manager)	12.7
Unskilled worker	18.0
Total	100.0

N = 230

Table 14.8 Monthly Household Income, Arab Americans

	Percent
$350–450	10.5
$451–550	11.0
$551–650	10.5
$651–750	8.0
$751–850	8.5
$851–999	11.5
$1,000+	40.0
Total	100.0

N = 230

This survey reveals that 20 percent of the elderly respondents are still employed. The majority of those are self-employed, that is, managing their own private and commercial businesses. Others are in professional occupations such as medicine, law, and education. Many of the respondents indicated that they intended to retire gradually, by reducing their hours of work.

The trend of early retirement during the past three decades that took place in the society at large, especially for those between the ages of fifty-five and sixty-two, is not apparent among the Arab American elderly population. Moreover, the majority of those who eventually retired (65 percent) have done so voluntarily. Most of the forced-retirement cases occurred prior to the enactment of the 1985 federal law that allowed people to work beyond the age of sixty-five. All of the respondents who have retired experienced a drop in their income, and some faced a financial squeeze for the first time in their lives. Nearly two-thirds (60 percent) are living on less than $1,000 per month (see table 14.8).

The economic resources of the respondents in our sample are derived from a variety of sources: Social Security, pensions, private investments, real estate, and bank savings. Over one-third stated that their income meets their basic requirements, while about two-thirds indicated that it does not. The latter were asked which areas represent their greatest unmet needs. Sixty percent reported deficiencies in health care, while 20 percent indicated inadequate housing.

In response to the question, "Who ought to provide for such needs?" 70.5 percent said the government, while 15.5 percent mentioned previous employers. Significantly, only 14 percent stated the family. The majority of the responses identifying the government as the agency that ought to provide for their needs reflects the national trend. The response is also based on the attitude that benefits are owed to them after a lifetime of paying taxes.

The elderly do not seem to seek or show interest in the services available from community agencies until they experience poor health, death of a spouse, or financial and other problems that force changes in their daily life. In the interview, we asked respondents about their need for such help as housekeeping, shopping, transportation, visiting nurses, and institutional care. Only 18.5 percent of the respondents expressed willingness to accept formal assistance, if offered. Those who are living alone and experiencing debilitating illnesses are more inclined to use services than those who are healthy and/or living with their families.

All of those receiving social services were unable to communicate in English. The Arab-American and Chaldean Council made arrangements so that providers hired from the community could communicate with elderly recipients in Arabic or Chaldean. These translators were limited to twenty hours per week at a rate of $5.25 per hour, paid for by the council.

When the elderly are no longer able to manage, whether because of rapid health deterioration, lack of family support, or depleted financial resources, many turn to the government for long-term care. According to the Arab-American and Chaldean Council, 10 elderly people out of 230 cases they surveyed were admitted to nursing homes under the Medicaid program. Seven of these Arab American elders had advanced Alzheimer's disease, and the other three were paralyzed by stroke. Sadly, in the three nursing homes where they were admitted, there were no native speakers to interact with them, and attendants used sign language to communicate basic needs. The only real social interaction for the residents occurred when a member of the family came to visit.

Nursing homes are not home settings for any patients, including those with dementia. As an elderly Arab resident of one of the nursing homes described it to me, "It is a dumping ground." Elderly Alzheimer's and other patients are languishing in these poorly managed facilities. The care is not adequate, and frail older people feel trapped.

The Arab American elderly in general enjoy good health. About 66 percent of the survey respondents viewed their health as good, and 20 percent as fair. Only 14 percent indicated that they experienced poor health or felt restricted in their movements.

The Arab American elderly population live in various types of housing. The majority (75 percent) live in single-family dwellings. Of these, 81.5 percent own their homes. Since half of these homes are more than twenty years old, they require continuous maintenance and repair. In fact, housing costs are cited as one of the greatest problems for many of the respondents. Despite their financial concerns, the majority felt adequately housed and were contented with their living arrangements. Such factors as good neighbors, conveniences, available services, Arabic food and shopping outlets, and familiarity with the area seem to play significant roles in their satisfaction.

Conclusion and Policy Implications

The Arab American elderly represent a heterogeneous group in terms of education, occupation, income, religious affiliation, living arrangements, and health conditions. In spite of such differences, they share similar values and attitudes, including the high motivation of their families to take care of them. The traditional filial obligation between children and their parents and the roles that the elderly maintain within their own extended families and kinship network manifest traditional cultural traits. However, many of these customs may not endure. For instance, more Arab American women are either working or seeking higher education to improve their economic and social status. Such changes will have an impact on the maintenance of traditional roles within the Arab American family, especially in the care of the elderly. Since most older Arab Americans and their families cannot afford full-time formal assistance, there is a widening acceptance of placing elderly parents in nursing homes, an acceptance that is fueled by the institutional bias of the Medicaid program. Subsidized home-care services would be more humane, and possibly less costly for taxpayers. Certainly such services would better meet the needs of the Arab American elderly—as well as other frail older people—during the last stage of their life cycle.

To conclude, I would like to stress that planning in Arab American communities must become paramount as needs for elder care become greater than families can provide. Local communities and social services agencies, with state and federal financial support, have taken only limited steps to remedy the growing shortages of services for older Arab Americans. A greater effort must be focused on at-home assistance. At the same time, the quality of life for those who must live in nursing homes must be improved substantially, including the provision of bilingual aides to communicate with the Arab American and other ethnic residents.

Note

The first phase of this study was partially funded by a Faculty Research Development grant and a PURA Technical Assistant grant from C. S. Mott Foundation for the International Institute at the University of Michigan, Flint. I would like to recognize the Arab-American and Chaldean Council in the Detroit metropolitan area for its help while conducting this research. I am indebted to those who volunteered to assist me in compiling names of, locating, and meeting with the elders of the Arab American community. Without them, this survey would have been difficult to accomplish. However, those who deserve the greatest credit are the Arab American elderly, who have cooperated in every possible way. Their support, advice, and constant sense of humor have sustained this project and made my task much easier.

15

Aging in Polonia:
Polish and Polish American Elderly

Celia Berdes and Mary Patrice Erdmans

Polonia: Its History, Character, and Conflicts

Polonia, the community of Poles living outside Poland, has a long history in the United States. While small groups of political émigrés arrived throughout the nineteenth century, the largest wave of Polish-speaking immigrants (roughly 1.5 million) began in the 1870s (from the Prussian partition) and crescendoed in the first decade of the twentieth century with the arrival of Poles from the Russian and Austrian partitions. By the time Poland gained statehood under the conditions set forth in the Treaty of Versailles in 1919, there were almost 2.5 million Poles and Polish Americans (American-born of Polish descent) living in the United States.

This large turn-of-the-century migration was mostly the movement of labor, as Poles left villages in Poland where there were few jobs and settled in the burgeoning industrial cities of the northeast, mid-Atlantic, and midwestern regions of the United States. The majority of immigrants were uneducated, landless peasants; in America they were often labeled immigrants *za chlebem* (for bread). But this wave also included Poles escaping religious, political, and cultural persecution from Bismarck's *Kulturkampf* in the Prussian partition and Russification programs in the eastern territories. These intelligentsia, revolutionaries, and clergy played a significant role in developing the institutional base of Polish communities in America, in particular the Roman Catholic parishes and large voluntary fraternal benefit associations (Brozek, 1985; Parot, 1981; Erdmans, 1998b). Chicago became the largest community and the organizational center of American Polonia. Other Polonian communities emerged in New York City, Detroit, Cleveland, Buffalo, Pittsburgh, and some smaller cities like South Bend, Indiana, and New Britain, Connecticut.

The Polish immigrant community of the early twentieth century matured into an ethnic community after World War I. Second-generation Polish Americans constructed a Polish American ethnic identity that helped them assimilate into the dominant white European society. Combatting racist eugenic theories that stigmatized "dumb Polaks" as inferior or "lesser-grade" whites, Polish Americans redefined themselves as hardworking, religious, and disciplined people who celebrated a cultural attachment to the folk culture of their ancestors but maintained a political loyalty to the United States. By World War II, Polonia was composed mostly of this second generation of ethnics, that is, Americans of Polish descent. By the 1940 census, 66 percent of the Polish "foreign stock" were born in America (Erdmans, 1998a: 32). Today, the Polish American elderly are descendants of this early immigrant cohort.

Polish Americans and the Roman Catholic Church

The Polish community was built around the Polish Roman Catholic Church, an important institution that provided for the immigrant's social and spiritual needs. The first Polish parish was established in Panna Maria, Texas, in 1854. By 1870 there were 10 Polish parishes in the United States; by 1900 there were 330; and by 1930 there were over 800 (Brozek, 1985: 45). For Polish Americans, religious and cultural identities were tightly intertwined. Jacobson (1995: 68) writes that "the vernacular of the Polish peasant Catholicism was frequently referred to as 'the Polish faith' just as speaking the Polish language was speaking 'in Catholic' (*po katolicku*)." The parish helped organize the community: parish clubs and organizations (of which there were often dozens) provided venues for social interaction, a structure for status attainment, and training for community leaders (Lopata, 1994: 59–64; Thomas and Znaniecki, 1958). The parishes formed the first mutual aid societies, which later became the nuclei of the large Polish fraternal insurance associations. Today, many of the old Polish parishes are located in central cities that experienced economic and social decline in the latter half of the twentieth century. Polish parishioners who have remained in the old neighborhoods are often the elderly who can not afford to sell their homes. Many of these old Polish American pockets have become trilingual communities, such as Saint Stanislaus Kostka in the Wicker Park neighborhood on the north side of Chicago. Wicker Park was the main Polish neighborhood in the first part of the twentieth century, and while today it is predominantly Hispanic, key Polish institutions such as the Polish Museum of America and the best Polish restaurants are still located there. Another way that Polish parishes survive is by incorporating new Polish immigrants. Chicago's Saint Hyacinth (Swieta Jacek) Parish is an example of an old Polish parish that still attracts the elderly Polish American population but serves primarily new Polish immigrants. The old Polish American parishioners jostle with the new Polish immigrants for leadership and "ownership" of the community (Erdmans, 1995; Blejwas, forthcoming).

Over 200,000 Poles arrived in America during and after World War II. Most were refugees of the war. Many of them entered the United States under the Displaced Persons Act of 1948, which admitted over 120,000 ethnic Poles *(Statistical Yearbook,* 1978: table 6E). Members of this cohort were pushed out of their homeland by war, border changes, and the repressive postwar communist regime. Most of these war survivors are in their eighties today and represent the old-old Polish-born elderly in the United States.

This cohort of post–World War II political émigrés differed from the earlier cohort of za chlebem (economic) immigrants. These émigrés came from a modern independent Polish nation rather than the partitioned rural Poland of the nineteenth century, and their experiences in World War II elevated nationalistic feelings. Most of them felt a fierce political loyalty to (precommunist) Poland. In addition, the war émigrés were often better educated, more urbanized, and of a higher social class than the early peasant cohort; their higher occupational and educational levels resulted in greater occupational mobility and faster assimilation (Janowska, 1975; Mostwin, 1971; Lopata, 1976; Blejwas, 1981). Finally, the new émigrés had a different cultural understanding of Polishness than the Polish American ethnics; they spoke a different version of Polish and appreciated different art forms (e.g., they did not dance the polka).

The newest cohort of Polish migrants, which began arriving in the 1960s and whose numbers peaked in the 1980s, is often referred to as the Solidarity wave because of its connection to the Solidarity movement in Poland. This group included three types of newcomers: permanent immigrants, temporary nonimmigrants (also known as *wakacjusze,* or vacationers), and political refugees. Between 1960 and 1989, over 201,000 Poles were admitted into the United States as immigrants, almost 1 million arrived in the United States on temporary visas, and nearly 43,000 were admitted into the United States as refugees (Erdmans, 1998a: 59, 64). These Poles, most of them highly educated, with professional and technical skills, emigrated from communist Poland for both economic and political reasons. With the collapse of communism in 1989, the raison d'être for Polish refugees was taken away, yet the number of Polish immigrants increased. Between 1990 and 1996, roughly 150,000 Polish immigrants were admitted into the United States, almost double the number admitted in the 1980s and more than triple the number admitted in the 1970s. In addition, more than 450,000 temporary visas were granted to those coming to study, work, and "vacation" (i.e., "visitors for pleasure" who work off the books).

The elderly in Polonia today are mostly Polish American ethnics of the second, third, and later generations from the early immigrant wave, but there are also Polish immigrants, the old-old from the World War II emigration, and elderly immigrants from the most current migrant cohort. We will see an increasing number of the elderly as more immigrants bring their aging parents to the United States and as the newest migrant cohort ages. Immigrants and ethnics differ in the foci and loci of their identity, needs, and networks. Immigrants have a dual locus of orientation—the country of emigration and that of immigration. Those who emigrated as adults (the case for most new Polish immigrants) continue to have real and sentimental ties to the homeland. Still, once abroad, they are mostly occupied with the business of learning the routines of the new country. Moreover, their housing, employment, education, and language-skill requirements are related to their newcomer status. In contrast, the needs of ethnics are linked to their generational distance from the homeland. The ethnic works to maintain a cultural identity rooted in the ancestral homeland but emphasizes an American identity. Elderly Polish immigrants have networks that extend back to the homeland, while Polish American elderly have an ethnic identity and network enmeshed in America.

The Demographic Face of Polonia in the 1990s

According to the 1990 census, 9,366,106 people in the United States reported some Polish ancestry (U.S. Census, 1992: 3), and 94 percent of this community was composed of native-born Polish American ethnics (U.S. Census, 1993: 59). There were 388,328 foreign-born Poles in the United States, and 70 percent of them had entered before 1980 (U.S. Census, 1993: 11).

The Polish population remains concentrated in the mid-Atlantic and east north central regions, where 60 percent of people reporting Polish ancestry live (U.S. Census, 1992: 9). The states with the largest populations have been, and continue to be, New York, Illinois, Michigan, Pennsylvania, and New Jersey. The established Polonian urban centers continue to pull in new immigrants: for example, in 1996, Chicago was the intended city of residence for 35 percent of new immigrant arrivals, while 19 percent listed New York City as their destination (*Statistical Yearbook,* 1996: 68). There has been, however, a slight geographic shift in Polonia over the last few decades. California now has the sixth largest population (578,256), and Florida has the ninth largest (410,666). The former is the result of general demographic trends in the United States as well as an increasing number of post–World War II and post-1980 immigrants settling in California. The Florida population represents the growing retiree resettlement.

Compared to the total white population in America, the Polish American ethnic community is aging. In fact, a larger percentage of the community is over sixty-four years of age than under fifteen. While 14.8 percent of native-born Polish Americans in 1990 were over sixty-four, only 12.8 percent of whites were in that age cohort; and while only 12.6 percent of Polish Americans were under fifteen, 21 percent of all whites were (U.S. Census, 1993: 59; 1997: 49).The population of foreign-born Poles in Polonia has a bimodal age distribution representing two immigrant cohorts: 39 percent were over sixty-four years old (mostly representing the post–World War II cohort) and 29 percent were between twenty-five and forty-four years of age (representing the post-1980 cohort) (U.S. Census, 1993: 11). Only 3 percent of the population of foreign-born Poles were younger than fifteen (because the children of foreign-born are automatically U.S. citizens if they are born here).

Recent immigrants as a group are younger than ethnics owing to the tendency to emigrate in the first half of one's life: between 1980 and 1993, only 26 percent of the immigrants were forty years of age or older (U.S. Dept. of Justice, 1997: table 3). In addition, there is some indication that Poles are now emigrating at an even younger age. According to Polish sources, the proportion of emigrants who were between eighteen and twenty-four years old rose from 11 percent in the 1980s to 17 percent in the 1990s (*Maly Rocznik Statystyczny,* 1997: 74). Despite the fact that new immigrants are a slightly younger population than the established ethnics, they make up such a small percentage of the total community that they do not shape its aggregate demographics. In summary, by the 1990s Polonia had become a large population of mostly native-born Polish Americans, the majority of whom still live in the old industrial Rust Belt region of the United States, with some migration to the West Coast and the Sun Belt. The community is an aging one, but immigration is bringing in not only new blood but also younger blood.

Aging in Polonia

Growing old in Polonia can best be understood by examining aging in Poland, among Polish immigrants to America, and among Polish Americans. The attitudes toward, and practices regarding, aging that have their roots in Poland are variously expressed by the Polish immigrant population in America and the Polish American ethnic population.

Aging in Poland

There is a significant literature about old age in Poland, the main theme of which is the tension between family and state responsibility for aging and how it affects the experience of growing old. Many authors use as the starting point for such analyses a landmark survey of elderly people in Poland conducted in 1967 by Piotrowski (1973). Worach-Kardas (1976), citing Piotrowski's data, reported that 47 percent of elderly people who have children live with an adult child. The comparable figure today is 28 percent (Laczko, 1994), but the multigenerational family still structures the roles, expectations, and dependency relationships of elderly people in Poland. For example, Worach-Kardas (1987) points out that, until advanced old age, elderly Poles provide more aid for their children than the other way around, primarily through child care and housekeeping. This *babuszka* (grandmother) role is more viable for women than for men, though it is slowly disappearing.

In Poland, dependence is the normal hallmark of old age. In fact, writes leading Polish gerontologist Brunon Synak, "Old age is defined as a period in the life course in which fathers or mothers depend to a large extent on their families. There seems to exist a 'norm of reciprocity' which is not perceived in negative terms, but as a natural state of family relations in later life" (Midre and Synak, 1989: 255). Moreover, the responsibility of children to their parents is formalized in Polish law. Reflecting traditional reliance on the family, Polish old people are entitled to state care only when family help is unavailable, and the range as well as the quantity of social and health services for the elderly is quite limited. Worach-Kardas's (1976) research showed that Polish elderly people were willing to apply for public help only when all other sources (family, friends, neighbors, workplace) failed them and that their application for assistance was accompanied by a sense of shame.

At a policy level, Synak (1989) believes, social and health care for the elderly reflect an incompatibility between the spheres of family and public care. That is, when public aid represents a failure of the family and is socially accepted only for people without kin, social services are seen as a fallback, emergency solution that achieves only a low priority in competition with other social needs. There has therefore been a lack of investment in such services, crippling the ability of the social care system to respond to present needs. Simultaneously, families are less able to meet the financial and care needs of their elderly members. Thus the matrix of social support for the elderly is failing in Poland. Synak sees cause for optimism only in the increasing role of the Catholic Church in the provision of social services, both because church-sponsored assistance will increase the quantity of services available and because they may be more acceptable to the elderly than public ones. He believes that Poles do not want social services to supplant the family but rather to supplement and reinforce it.

Morawska (1991), writing since the fall of communism in Poland, conveys the continuing pessimism that the Polish state and the Polish family will be able to cooperate in achieving even that modest goal. Owing to inflation, pensions (the only old-age entitlement) now consume more state funds than previously, leaving less for state-sponsored health and social services. No new nursing or retirement homes have been built since 1980, and disabled elderly who need such care must in many cases wait for years in hospitals, crippling in turn the ability of the latter to respond to acute care needs. Privately sponsored assistance agencies do not exist. Aside from ad hoc increases in pensions, no old-age policy initiatives have emerged from successive democratically elected governments. And families in the vise of the economic crisis are less and less able to respond to the financial and care needs of their elderly members. More than a million people (some 3 percent of the population) have emigrated from Poland since 1980 in search of work; 70 percent were less than thirty-five years old. Immigrant adult children are effectively unable to meet the other-than-financial needs of their elders. So the elderly in Poland today are vulnerable and not likely to become less so in the near future. Calasanti and Zajicek's (1997) analysis of the impact of economic transformation on Poland's elderly shows that the reciprocal concepts of "dependence" and "burden" have been socially produced by the transition from socialism to capitalism. Pensions are so low, compared to the cost of living, that retirees are compelled to seek low-wage jobs in the formal or informal economies. Small wonder, then, that even some of them are emigrating.

Polish Immigrant Elderly

A classic needs assessment undertaken by Roman L. Haremski (1940) of Polish immigrant elderly living alone in Baltimore is still relevant today because it illustrates the effects of immigration on the lives of the elderly. Haremski studied how immigration led to his immigrant elderly subjects living alone. He identified two salient factors related to immigration: about half of those who arrived in the United States as single people never married or remarried, and about half of those who arrived alone but as married people were never able to reunify their families in America. Further, few of those who had children had a close relationship with them or received any help from them. Some of the reasons cited were clearly connected to the immigration and are relevant even today: their children remained in Poland or had moved to other cities in the United States; had intermarried with non-Poles; were institutionalized in hospitals, mental hospitals, or prisons; or were experiencing an economic situation that prevented them from providing assistance. Haremski concluded that his sample of Polish immigrant elderly were geographically, socially, culturally, intellectually, and religiously isolated.

Guttmann (1979) and Mostwin (1979) studied elderly people of eight white immigrant/ ethnic groups in Baltimore. They found that Poles had the highest life satisfaction; that pre–World War II immigrants had significantly higher life satisfaction than postwar immigrants; and that life satisfaction also was correlated with activities, health, and feelings about ethnicity. Guttmann and Mostwin observed that postwar immigrants were helped by their children more than twice as often as prewar immigrants, and they suggested that this was because prewar immigrants came to the United States alone and postwar immigrants came as refugees with their families. Compared both to families in Poland and to earlier waves of Polish immigrants, fewer postwar Polish immigrants (about 30 percent) lived with their children.

More recent work by Kahana et al. (1993) indicates that the Polish cultural value of family solidarity and the expectation of family care persist among today's Polish immigrants. When a sample of Polish immigrant nursing home residents was asked about their future hopes, 40 percent said they anticipated leaving the nursing home. Paradoxically, however, family cohesiveness did not appear to support this expectation. The authors speculate that the high rate of intermarriage for adult Polish children may erode the motivation to provide care.

It is important to note here that in our experience, Massey et al.'s (1987: 284) observation of Mexican immigrants holds true for Polish immigrant elderly: "The issue of settlement versus return is never definitively settled within the migrant generation." Many Polish immigrant elderly—although they may have lived in the United States for many years, and even have accepted U.S. citizenship—keep open the issue of returning to Poland. And, in fact, many do go back. Historically, as much as 40 percent of Polish immigrants returned to their homeland at some point in their lives. Even today, the U.S. Social Security Administration pays out millions of dollars monthly to recipients living in Poland.

Polish American Elderly

As noted above, 9.3 million Americans claim Polish ancestry or identity. About 4 percent are immigrants; thus, Polish Americans of the second or successive generations predominate. Research on Polish American elderly confirms the idea that the expectation of family solidarity persists in the second generation (Polish Americans) but that the reality of support does so to a much lesser extent, and the perception of support to an even lesser extent. Lopata details the changes in Polish family life occasioned by immigration to the United States. Her studies in the early 1970s in Chicago "uncover[ed] an undercurrent or open expression of hostility of the elderly toward their adult children and grown grandchildren for 'abandoning them'" (1981: 26). Yet, adult children were identified as the only source of assistance, and Polish American widows tended to live with an adult child more often than non–ethnically identified women (Lopata, 1977). Paradoxically, Lopata's subjects also emphasized pride in their ability to be independent, reflecting immigrant women's gain in power within the nuclear family and an increase in independence from the extended family.

Lopata identifies these reactions as rooted, respectively, in two Polish cultural values: status competition and independence. The former, in Poland, is family dependent. You are born into a status, rarely can rise above it, and maintain that family status only by individual effort. Simultaneously, Poles are fiercely independent and unwilling to subjugate themselves to others or to ask for help. Thus in Polish Americans these two values conspire to produce high expectations of assistance from children and an almost vengeful independence when help received does not meet expectations.

Caring for Polonia's Elderly

In this final section of our chapter, we will share the information gleaned from three studies we have conducted in order to discuss and analyze the issues described above in greater detail.

Polish Immigrant and Polish American
Ethnic Elderly in Chicago

In 1991, Berdes and Zych conducted a survey of the quality of life of one thousand elderly Polish immigrants and Polish American ethnics living in metropolitan Chicago (for a fuller description, see Berdes and Zych, 1996; Berdes and Zych, forthcoming). The study was a replication of (and comparison with) an earlier study of Polish elderly conducted by Zych and Bartel (1988, 1990). There were many barriers to data collection. First, the study used a convenience sample, since there is no comprehensive list of immigrants and ethnics. Second, it became necessary to obtain the data in face-to-face interviews because the respondents' willingness to participate fell when we asked them to complete written survey forms. Third, we had to conduct the interview in the respondent's language of choice, eight hundred choosing Polish and two hundred English. Fourth, in seeking to include undocumented people, we had to overcome significant distrust. We worked with community institutions and organizations these immigrants trusted and, by working in those sites, "piggybacked" on that trust. Also, we recorded no identifying information about the respondents.

Our survey collected information about demographic characteristics including living arrangements, characteristics of migration, quality of life, functional capacity, and knowledge of community services. From this survey (unique in this community), we have learned that:

- The quality of life of Polish American ethnic elderly is significantly better than that of Polish immigrants, and the quality of life of Polish immigrants is significantly better than that of the elderly in Poland.
- Age (taking into account functional status, nursing home residence, and living with a spouse) was the most important variable in the quality of life of Polish American ethnic elderly. In contrast, variables associated with migration (age at immigration and time in the United States) were the most important variables in the quality of life of Polish immigrant elderly.
- By analyzing the date of first immigration, we can document in this sample the waves of immigration described earlier. Further, by comparing the class origin of Polish immigrants and Polish American ethnics, we confirmed the class distinctions among immigration cohorts described above.
- By comparing the living situation of Polish immigrants and Polish American ethnics, we see that Polish American elderly are much more likely than Polish immigrant elderly to live with a spouse but much less likely to live with or near their children. Thus, immigration has an isolating effect, preventing or disrupting the marital bond in the first generation of immigrants and loosening the intergenerational bond in subsequent generations.
- When asked what services and facilities there are for elderly people in the United States, 29 percent of our respondents were unable to name any service or facility, and an additional 41 percent were able to name only one service or facility. Therefore, information about services for the elderly seems to be very low among this group.

Sense of Community in a Polish American Nursing Home

Royal Nursing Centre is a skilled- and intermediate-care facility located in a northwestern suburb in the Polish community that begins in the inner city and extends into the suburbs. New immigrants are clustered at the southeastern end of the Polish community, named Jackowo after the local Catholic parish church (Saint Hyacinth, or Swieta Jacek). As they and later their children became more prosperous, they tended to move out to the northwestern part of the city and the northwestern suburbs. Royal Nursing Centre was part of an ethnographic study of ethnic nursing homes conducted by Berdes (forthcoming).

The facility is privately owned, consisting of five patient-care floors of sixty beds each, or three hundred beds in total. The highest-functioning residents live on the first floor, and each higher floor houses successively more impaired residents; on the fifth floor there is a special-care unit for those who have Alzheimer's disease. The nursing home was built in 1972 and has been under the present ownership (a for-profit corporation) since 1976. It is nearly always full. In its most recent state inspections, the facility had only "level C" violations of regulations, indicating good quality of care. The typical resident of Royal Nursing Centre is a woman in her eighties, of working- or lower-middle-class origin. The resident population is completely white, and as might be expected in a heavily Polish facility, most residents are Catholics. About half the residents pay for their own care, and the other half are paid for by the Medicare or Medicaid programs.

Royal Nursing Centre was a good place to study community in nursing homes because, unlike most such institutional facilities, both residents and staff are ethnically homogeneous. Eighty percent of the residents and 80 percent of the staff are Polish-speaking or Polish- and English-speaking. Most nursing homes have resident populations that are economically homogeneous but ethnically heterogeneous. Moreover, few nursing homes have Royal Nursing Centre's level of ethnic congruence between residents and staff.

The resident population at Royal Nursing Centre consists largely of elderly immigrant Poles and first-generation Americans of Polish descent; its staff consists largely of younger immigrant Poles. This is possible because Poland is one of the few countries that has had multiple waves of migration to the United States, extending from before the turn of the twentieth century to the present. Thus, today's nursing home residents (people in their eighties) either immigrated before 1925 as children or young people; immigrated as adults between 1925 and 1950; immigrated as old people in the last twenty years; or are the children of immigrants of the first wave. The staff members are people who have immigrated in the last twenty years. The cultural homogeneity of residents and cultural congruity between residents and staff led me to believe I might find Polish community at Royal Nursing Centre.

There was some evidence of Polish community at the home but even greater evidence of factors that result in cleavages in that community (see Berdes, forthcoming). Polishness within Royal Nursing Centre took the following forms:

- Polish food. Food comes up again and again as the main evidence of Polishness, unsurprising in light of research that shows that common food preferences are a major index of ethnicity. Residents repeatedly express their desire for Polish food. However, Polish food is not really available in the Royal Nursing Centre. Staff explained that the Polish diet is unhealthy and cannot be given to people with dietary restrictions.

- Religious practice. Similarly, residents expend great efforts to attend advertised religious services. However, what was advertised as a Catholic mass turned out only to be a short blessing service.
- Forms of address. Polish and English forms of address are used in interesting ways to denote status in this setting. Top staff are addressed by residents as "Pani" (Mrs.), the Polish formal term. Polish immigrant staff are addressed by residents as Pani (First Name), a formal but intimate wording. Although in Polish usage residents should also be addressed in the same way, residents are called by their first names alone.
- Ethnic identity-checking. Residents and staff comment on their own ethnic identity or check on the ethnic identity of others. They want to determine whether others are Polish.
- Preference for Polish staff. Polish staff was believed to be preferable to other ethnic groups. As one staff member said (with some irony), "Poles know how to take care of old people because when I was in Poland I never saw a nursing home."

On the other hand, Polish community at Royal Nursing Centre was fragmented in the following ways:

- By language. The top staff community is separated from the other communities in the nursing home by its lack of Polish. The management team of the facility operates in English, and Poles have access to middle-management jobs only when they can speak English. There is a group of midlevel staff that speaks both English and Polish, using that skill to bridge the upper- and lower-level staff communities as well as staff and resident populations. The top staff uses midlevel staff as informal translators to communicate with lower staff and Polish-speaking residents. Beyond that, midlevel staff seem to have an important mediating role.
- By length of time in the United States. Not uncommonly in immigrant communities, long-term immigrants have greater status than recent ones and take on a "big brother" role, helping the latter to find work and teaching them the ropes of life in America. Here too, long-term immigrants occupy a different social space from recent immigrants. These distinctions are made more complex by the different characteristics of these waves of immigration. In the Polish community, social distinctions are drawn between the post-1980 immigrants, who included large numbers of urban, educated people coming here mainly for political reasons, and earlier waves of immigrants, consisting largely of rural, uneducated people who came here for economic reasons. This distinction is recognized by people at Royal Nursing Centre: according to the social services director, they have had people

take jobs as nursing assistants who were doctors, nurses, and teachers in Poland, as well as those who previously worked on farms. For the former, nursing home work represents a social demotion; for the latter, a promotion. So earlier immigrants had higher status by virtue of their longer experience in the United States but lower status by virtue of their demotion in professional position.

- By generation, or rather, by experience of war. As in many other countries, there may be less of a generation gap in the Polish community than a deep divide between people who have had personal experiences of war and those who have not. One staff member likened the behavior of residents in the context of nursing home life to their survival strategies during World War II: they "did what they had to to survive."

Polishness thus serves as a basis for community at Royal Nursing Centre, but it is a quasi community, one that is both ersatz and dysfunctional: despite its claims to be a Polish community, the nursing home only imitates real Polish culture and functions poorly even at that. Indeed, the major symbols of Polish life— Polish food and the Polish Catholic mass—are poor imitations of the real thing.

The imitative and dysfunctional nature of community in this predominantly Polish nursing home may be attributable, in part, to the fact that placing an elder in a nursing home produces much shame and guilt in Polish families, often inhibiting later contact between the generations. Without a strong link to the broader Polish community through residents' families, the non-Polish management staff has difficulty building a true Polish environment. Thus, though these residents may have reaped the benefits of immigration through an improved standard of living, they have done so at a high price. Their American children are willing to place them in nursing homes, an action that would have been unlikely in Poland. At the same time, many of the Polish staff members have left behind their own parents in Poland, who may themselves need to seek nursing homes there because their children are working in the United States. Thus as Americans hire immigrants to care for our elderly in institutions, we doom the immigrants' parents to the same fate.

Polish Immigrants as Home Health Care Workers for the Elderly

The steady growth of the home health care industry has been complicated by the instability of its labor force. Agencies and clients find it increasingly difficult to recruit and retain workers. Undesirable market conditions (e.g., low wages and few benefits) either keep workers away or drive them out of this sector. The gap created by an expanding industry and an unstable work force provides an occupational niche for illegal immigrants.

I interviewed thirty-five Polish immigrants working as home health care workers for the elderly in Chicago during 1992 (Erdmans 1996a; Erdmans 1996b). Since most of them had had more than one home care position during their time in the United States, I collected data on their total positions, which amounted to 110. The sample was predominantly female (77 percent), and the mean age of the workers was forty (their ages ranged from twenty-four to fifty-nine). Over 90 percent had postsecondary education, and 63 percent had graduate degrees. In addition, many of them had significant education and experience in the health professions: five were doctors, two had completed medical school, three were registered nurses, and three were medical technicians. There were also a midwife, a physical therapist, a pharmacist, a dentist, and a chemist among them. Three-fourths of the workers spoke English well enough to communicate, and the others spoke the language poorly but said they could understand it.

The families for whom they worked were white, middle-class, and not of Polish background. The workers were hired because they were white (their particular ethnicity was irrelevant) and because they were willing to work as live-in caretakers at below-market wages and without benefits. They averaged $300 to $400 a week (usually six days and nights), or roughly $60 a day. Most of the families who hired these illegal immigrants paid them with their own funds, bypassing agencies, insurance companies, and Medicare. The clients were between the ages of forty-two and one hundred; 58 percent of them were eighty years old or older, and another 38 percent were between sixty and seventy-nine. The workers were usually hired to provide long-term care.

Temporary illegal immigrants are willing to take secondary-labor-market positions such as home-care work because they plan to return home, where the actual value of their U.S. wages is higher and where they will receive health care and other benefits from the home country. Moreover, their status is determined in the home country and not by their previous occupations in the United States. Compared to other opportunities available to these illegal immigrants, such elder-care positions are desirable because they offer higher wages, free room and board (often in pleasant settings), less physical exertion than child care, and fewer chances of getting caught by immigration officials. Despite the illegal nature of the work, a formal structure is in place (employment agencies that operate legally and visibly in the community) to help elderly clients and illegal immigrants find each other and form what appears to be mutually beneficial relationships.

Conclusion and Policy Implications

Polish American elderly have several unique characteristics as well as some that they share with other immigrant-ethnic groups. For one, they have a centuries-long history of immigration to the United States that extends to the present day, resulting in multiple cohorts of both immigrants and Polish American ethnics, with important differences of culture, education, and social class among them. They also are highly concentrated in certain regions of the United States and have well-established institutional communities based on the Roman Catholic Church. Because of their Polish culture, there is a deep commitment to the family and strong norms of reciprocity between the generations. In fact, the responsibility of the family for its elderly supersedes that of the state. Yet, immigration has, to a large extent, weakened these generational ties and obligations. Finally, Poles are represented not only among the elderly in need of care but also among paid caregivers.

As a priest caring for the Polish elderly in 1940 aptly put it: "My people do not live in America, they live underneath America. America goes on over their heads" (Haremski, 1940: 64). To some extent this is still true today and typifies the dilemma of the immigrant and American ethnic aged and those who care for them. Polish immigrant elderly tend to adhere to a culture in which the old person is valued within the family, yet they may not have family members in the United States to provide the assistance they need. At the same time, they cannot access the formal care system because of ignorance of its availability, lack of funds, or concerns about their undocumented status. Many of them are reluctant to use formal services because they believe such services represent a shameful failure of the family system of care.

Polish American elderly, on the other hand, may be more knowledgeable about and able to access the formal care system. Yet, many of their children, who view themselves primarily as Americans, lack the Polish cultural norm that values old age and mandates care for parents. These older people also feel shamed by their lack of informal family assistance. Consequently, neither immigrant nor Polish American elderly receive the care—formal or informal—to which they are surely entitled.

16

Irish American Care of the Aged

Patricia J. Fanning

In a recent survey, 80 percent of the seventy-six Irish Americans polled said that the government should bear some of the responsibility for elder care in the United States. They noted that times and families have changed. With people living longer and families scattered across the country, the accepted paradigm of adult children caring for elderly parents can no longer suffice. They look to creative options in living arrangements, professional caregivers, and government assistance to bridge the gap left by absent or unavailable families (Fanning, 2000). How did we get to this point? What dimensions of Irish American life and experience are reflected in these attitudes? Are they really new? The history of the Irish in America may be a familiar one to many, but the aspects of that history relating to the elderly and elder care have received little serious attention. An examination of the experiences, attitudes, and behavior of the Irish in their homeland, their migration to America, and their circumstances here will help us to understand their attitudes.

Immigration to the United States

Historically, the family system in Ireland was patrilinear, tracing its descent through the father. It also was bilateral, with marriage uniting two families instead of absorbing one into the other. Legally, throughout most of the eighteenth century, British-imposed Penal Laws mandated that land, whether owned or, more likely, rented, had to be divided among all sons equally. This prevented the accumulated acquisition of large tracts of land by Catholics. When these laws were rescinded, the Irish farmer reverted to a stem-family system in which one son or, if there were no sons, one of the daughters inherited the land. This allowed for the evolution of a patriarchal system in which the father was the unquestioned head of the family and his sons remained "boys" until the father retired or died. At that point, his designated heir would become head of the family (Arensberg and Kimball, 1968; Greeley, 1972; Horgan, 1998).

This practice resulted in enforced celibacy and delayed marriage of the designated heir, the migration of unmarried, noninheriting siblings, and familism, which placed the family's welfare above any one individual (Schrier, 1958). Familism, in turn, fostered a strong sense of sibling loyalty among the Irish, characterized by emigrant siblings sending money home to help support the members they had left behind. There was not necessarily an emotional closeness among siblings, as will be discussed later, but rather a loyalty and responsibility to the family as a whole.

Since Arensberg and Kimball, in *Family and Community in Ireland,* make no mention of the Irish matriarch, instead focusing on the dominance of the rural father, Andrew Greeley (1972) postulates that the power of the Irish mother emerged in urban areas. When the family shifted to an urban environment in Ireland, and later to the United States, the wife was frequently more employable than her husband. This fact diminished the husband's role as provider and leader and increased the importance and power of the Irish mother. Greeley (1972) also cites the research of Herbert Gutman, who contended that the number of absent fathers was higher among Irish immigrants than among other ethnic groups. Thus the mother-supported, matriarchal family system was more likely to exist among the Irish here in America.

In addition, the subordinate status of women within the patriarchal system, combined with the family's inability to provide for more than one dowry, resulted in single women who were more autonomous than their counterparts among other ethnic groups (Diner, 1983). This made it possible for unmarried female children to leave home, find employment, or emigrate independently. This migration brought to America a substantial number of strong, self-sufficient women who would be reluctant to take on a subservient role once married. An examination of the migration of the Irish to America provides ample evidence of this phenomenon.

The first significant influx of Irish immigrants to America began around 1717, when Scottish settlers in Ulster lost their leases because of a combination of rising rents and crop failures. For the remainder of the eighteenth century, this Ulster migration of mainly Scottish Presbyterians continued at the steady rate of 3,000 to 5,000 per year. Emigration from other parts of Ireland rose following a serious potato crop failure in 1740–1741. These eighteenth-century immigrants, mostly men, included small farmers, indentured servants, and convict transportees. After 1815, emigration from Ireland increased substantially, topping a total of 400,000 by 1845. These immigrants were tradesmen, fishermen, shopkeepers, domestic servants, and small farmers, spurred on by partial potato failures throughout the 1830s. Also by the mid-1830s, a larger proportion of immigrants were women, Irish-speaking, and poor (Adams, 1932; Shannon, 1963; Handlin, 1979; Miller, 1985; Fanning, 1997; Horgan, 1998).

It was, of course, the Great Hunger of the late 1840s that changed everything, beginning with the ruination of the potato crop over one-third of Ireland in 1845. Failures continued each year through the final universal blight of 1848 in which virtually the entire potato harvest was lost. The Great Famine that followed, the result of natural, cultural, and political forces, drove close to 1.5 million primarily poverty-stricken Catholic Irish to America between the years 1846 and 1855. For the remainder of the nineteenth century, the incredible migration continued at the rate of over 500,000 people every decade (Schrier, 1958; Fanning, 1997; Horgan, 1998).

What is more, it was a migration not only of the poor but also of the young. During the third quarter of the nineteenth century, over 60 percent of emigrants were between the ages of fifteen and thirty-five; for the rest of the century, the proportion in that age bracket was never less than 80 percent (Schrier, 1958; Horgan, 1998). In addition, between 1846 and 1875, nearly half the people fleeing Ireland were women, a pattern vastly different from other ethnic migrations (Diner, 1983; Nolan, 1989; Horgan, 1998). The results were devastating for Ireland. Prior to 1845, the population had been nearly 9 million. By the time the first immigration restriction laws were enacted in the United States in 1921, more than 4.6 million had come to America, leaving Ireland with an unprecedented net decrease in population, a pattern that was not reversed until the mid-twentieth century (Sarbaugh, 1991).

After permanent immigration restriction legislation was enacted in the 1920s, Irish immigration declined steadily to an average of only 2,500 a year between 1960 and 1980 (Sarbaugh, 1991). During the 1980s, however, a new influx of Irish immigrants arrived, driven out of their homeland by a debt-ridden economy, high unemployment, and oppressive taxation. Some studies claim that as many as 250,000 Irish immigrants, both legal and illegal, made the journey during that decade (Sarbaugh, 1991). Unlike the 1840s, however, most of these immigrants were educated and middle-class (Sarbaugh, 1991). A recent economic recovery in Ireland, coupled with progress on the contentious political front, may spell the end of significant Irish immigration to the United States. But, with more than 40 million Americans claiming Irish descent, the impact of American Irish attitudes and behaviors will continue to have considerable influence on the shape of policy and politics in America.

The Irish American Family

It is the social context of the American Irish we are most interested in as a predictor of behavior and attitudes related to health, illness, family, and care of the elderly. As many researchers have pointed out, the Irish are full of contradictions (Greeley, 1972; McGoldrick, 1996; Horgan, 1998). Nowhere is this demonstrated more clearly than in the structure and relationships of the Irish American family. Traditionally, the American Irish family has been depicted as more authoritarian and less affectionate than other ethnic groups, with the mother playing a subsidiary and somewhat subservient role to the male head of the household (Greeley, 1981). Yet, realities are more complicated than that.

In most Irish American families, the mother is a very important figure, providing stability, strength, and service to her children and spouse. She is often seen as the pragmatic, morally superior partner, who tolerates the childish delusions of her husband. She is a religious, loving, and loyal mother. The father, on the other hand, remains a shadowy, indistinct figure. Often literally absent, at work or elsewhere, even when he is at home, he seems to be one step removed from the center of family activity. A silent presence, he leaves the majority of the discipline and planning to the mother (Greeley, 1972; McGoldrick, 1996; Horgan, 1998). In old age, these roles change very little. The mother remains the emotional center of the family network and glides effortlessly into the role of matriarch over a burgeoning number of grandchildren. The father, if still present, remains somewhat solitary but is seen as gentle, mild mannered, and good humored, known for his reminiscing and storytelling. The mother–son bond is particularly intense, with the Irish mother doting on her sons and expecting her daughters to do the same (Greeley, 1972; McGoldrick, 1996). Yet, the Irish matriarch transmits to her daughters the will, courage, and spirit to strike out on their own.

As noted earlier, in sharp contrast to other ethnic groups, the rate of emigration of single women from Ireland was quite high. During some time periods, it was even higher than that of men (Kennedy, 1973; Diner, 1983; Nolan, 1989; McGoldrick, 1996). This independence and self-sufficiency were carried over to America, where delayed marriage and singlehood continued to be common. A large proportion of Irish American women seemingly were unwilling to give up their economic and emotional self-reliance for marriage and partnership (Greeley, 1972; Diner, 1983; Nolan, 1989; McGoldrick, 1996). As McGoldrick (1996: 557–58) comments: "Irish women have generally had little expectation of or interest in being taken care of by a man. Their hopes have been articulated much less in romantic terms than in aspirations for self-sufficiency." Family life seems to support these goals, with Irish families often encouraging the education of daughters as well as sons (Greeley, 1972), although daughters "knew that the resources of the family would go first to their brothers" (Horgan, 1998: 55). And, as a further acknowledgment of their importance within the Irish family, the unmarried daughter, sibling, or aunt makes significant contributions as a role model for young girls: she often serves as the nucleus of the extended family and/or caregiver to aging parents (Kane, 1968; McGoldrick, 1996; Horgan, 1998).

The American Irish woman's tendency to stand alone is also reflective of a culture that has a less articulated cult of romance than does the United States in general. For some time, Ireland had the highest age for marriages and the lowest rate of any nation in the world (Kennedy, 1973). Charlotte Ikels (1988: 102) notes, "Historically, singlehood has been, and to a lesser extent remains, an honorable state in Ireland." In addition, the Irish place less emphasis than Americans on romance as the foundation for marriage (Miller, 1985; McGoldrick, 1996). This unsentimental attitude has been traced into the second generation of Irish here in

America (Heer, 1961), although in other respects there was considerable assimilation by that time (Greeley, 1972; Horgan, 1998).

Once married, the American Irish remain paradoxical. They are superficially talkative, hospitable, and good humored but do not encourage intimacy. Reticent about their emotions, they tend to avoid effusive demonstrations of tenderness, often relying on humor, teasing, and ridicule as an expression of affection (Barrabee and von Mering, 1953; Spiegel, 1971; Greeley, 1972). Family ties are seemingly weak, with relationships between husband and wife, parents and children, and among siblings loose and apparently indifferent (Zborowski, 1969; Greeley, 1972). Withdrawal and distancing from intense interactions are seen as solutions to interpersonal problems (McGoldrick, 1996). Couples, children, and siblings drift away from one another, usually without causing trauma or distress, in what Mark Zborowski (1969: 227) has called "the centrifugal tendency of the Irish family."

Herein lies yet another paradox. There is evidence to support the contention that sibling loyalty is extraordinarily high among the Irish American population (Greeley, 1972), as it was in Ireland itself. For example, author Ruth-Ann M. Harris (1989) found that 63 percent of all those Irish looking for relatives were siblings seeking siblings. However, that loyalty appears to be more dutiful than emotional. As Greeley (1972: 115) points out, "In many second- and third-generation Irish American families, it seems clear that the siblings are not friends . . . that is to say, often they do not have common interests, [and] they are not especially eager to spend time with one another." Yet, their sense of obligatory familism requires that they show up on holidays, special occasions, and in times of trouble and conflict (Greeley, 1972; Horgan, 1998). This behavior is a significant characteristic of extended family relationships as well, with cousins, aunts, and uncles seeing one another only on holidays or, most notably, at wakes and weddings (Kane, 1968; Greeley, 1972; McGoldrick, 1996). As McGoldrick (1996: 559) explains it, "The Irish have a tremendous respect for personal boundaries, are enormously sensitive to each other's right to privacy, and will make strong efforts not to impose or intrude on one another."

It is not only a sense of privacy but also pride that causes the reluctance. Horgan (1998: 56) recollects that "household members were ambivalent about giving and seeking help, however, for household self-sufficiency was a matter of great pride." McGoldrick (1996: 558) goes a step further and asserts that "family members tend not to rely on one another as a source of support, and when they have a problem, they may even see it as an added burden and embarrassment for the family to find out." Elaine McGivern (1979: 111), in her examination of ethnic Irish in metropolitan Pittsburgh, agrees that Irish American families are reluctant to seek assistance. She found: "The reason is a matter of preserving the family's pride. What was indicated by some in the interviews was that it was very important for the family not to be made to feel that they were accepting a form of charity." McGivern's interviewees acknowledged that "it's easier to give aid than to receive it." Thus, partners, parents, siblings, and children seem to derive and expect little emotional support from one another. While this attitude may develop feelings of independence and self-reliance, it may also result in isolation and loneliness (Zborowski, 1969; McGoldrick, 1996). This aspect of the Irish American family is of particular significance in the consideration of their attitudes toward health, illness, aging, and the utilization of family and outside social supports.

Attitudes toward Illness

Many of their views toward health and illness are predictable within the given structure of the family. The profile of an Irish American patient that emerges from the sociological and medical data is of a stoic, passive person who presents specific symptoms and/or dysfunction, minimizes pain and accepts it without complaint, and is compliant but skeptical (Suchman, 1964; Zola, 1966, 1973; Zborowski, 1969; Greeley, 1972; Lipton and Marbach, 1984). As a group, Irish Americans fear physical disability and internal disease, especially as they relate to their ability to work (Zborowski, 1969). It is this capacity to perform physical labor that dictates whether they are in good health or not.

Even as they grow older, the Irish are more concerned with achievement, independence, and activity than the elderly of some other ethnic backgrounds (Cohler and Lieberman, 1979; McGoldrick, 1998). Thus, as they age, their self-esteem remains tied more to physical activity and ability and, in essence, self-sufficiency, than for other groups. With regard to psychosis and psychopathology, the Irish tolerate mental deviance including delusion, hallucination, fantasy, and dreaming, far more readily than they tolerate emotional expressiveness such as screaming, crying, and hostile action (Opler and Singer, 1956; Singer and Opler, 1956; Wylan and Mintz, 1976; McGoldrick, 1996).

Irving Zola (1966: 627) attributes much of this pattern to the restrictive life of the Irish: "Life was black and long-suffering, and the less said the better." He sees their understatement, restraint, and resignation as the defense mechanism "singularly most appropriate for their psychological and physical survival." Similarly, their reliance on dreams and fantasy may have been crucial to survival during difficult times. Zola (1966) and others also link these behaviors to the unique religious perspective of the Irish, a perspective dominated by sin, guilt, and fear of punishment. When illness or disability strikes, there is a tendency to believe it is punishment from God and must be accepted and endured alone, without complaint. The Irish are therefore more likely to see sickness as a private matter, something to be kept to themselves (Zola, 1966; Zborowski, 1969; McGoldrick, 1996). Consequently, they delay seeking treatment, even when it is obvious they need it, and they have difficulty communicating with one another about their ailments (Zborowski, 1969; Zola, 1973, Fitzpatrick and Barry, 1990).

The withdrawal and distancing of Irish spouses and siblings are mirrored in the reticence of Irish patients. While there is evidence that the American Irish are moving away from this pattern by utilizing community and institutional resources (Cleary and Demone, 1988), this may merely demonstrate their preference for seeking aid through formal rather than familial sources. This would not be surprising, as the Irish in America have always maintained and utilized organizational social support systems as a viable, and often attractive, alternative to familial networks.

Care of the Aged

From their arrival in America, the Irish have created cultural, political, social, and medical institutions that paralleled the institutions of the dominant community. Within that structure, formal caregiving and institutional arrangements to care for the elderly have always been acceptable. The research of Alfred Kutzik (1979) demonstrates that since Colonial times the aged members of ethnic mutual aid societies received benefits along with widows, orphans, and the sick. Initially, Irish Americans tried to take care of their own elderly in this fashion. Through fraternal or religious emigrant aid societies, the Irish offered financial assistance to the functionally independent aged. Another common practice was to board an elderly parent in a private third-party home for a fixed fee. This rather formal arrangement is consistent with the recognized Irish tendencies toward emotional and physical distance. As Seamus Metress (1985: 19) points out: "Treatment rendered on a contract basis by a third party could be less stressful to the family, as well as the elderly parent, whose status and self-image might be transformed as a result of their dependent state."

Issues of privacy, emotional reticence, and the perception of independence are thus successfully avoided. It is far easier for the Irish to give and receive aid through a third party than it is to articulate a direct expression of need and a reciprocal acknowledgment of love and support. Even recent data demonstrate that third- or fourth-generation Irish Americans consistently indicate that it is a bad idea for older people to live with their grown children. In fact, the older they are, the less support Irish Americans indicate for that particular living arrangement (Vosburgh and Juliani, 1990).

As the nineteenth century progressed and Irish immigration increased, there were calls for immigrant groups to care for themselves; poverty and aging, which previously had not been stigmatized conditions, now were labeled as symptomatic of intemperance and unworthiness. However, Irish immigrants, while poor, were overwhelmingly young. Consequently, for a time, there were relatively few elderly Irish immigrants and even fewer who lived long enough to become aged (Shannon, 1963; Woodham-Smith, 1963; Handlin, 1979; Kutzik, 1979). Still, as Kutzik (1979: 48–49) points out, it is likely that a high percentage of the Irish aged were provided for in community poorhouses around the United States. In addition, Irish political machines in many U.S. cities developed their own system of public welfare, offering food, housing, and fuel assistance to the poor and aged without the risk of humiliation (Metress, 1985).

In both these options, it is the self-esteem and perception of independence that are significant to the Irish aged. They had migrated from rural Ireland, where the older generation maintained control of the family and its resources until death or voluntary retirement. This afforded the aged a certain status: "Irish culture is well-known for both its emphasis on familialism and for the honor, power and privilege that it afforded to its elderly" (Dickerson-Putman, 1997: 366). In America, however, all that changed. The older generation, as well as the younger, often arrived destitute; they had no control over the family's assets and suffered a disturbing further decline in status when they could no longer perform physical labor. Seeking refuge in a poorhouse or accepting other aid from the political system was preferable to becoming a burden to family or extended family in old age (Metress, 1985).

By the late nineteenth century, a third alternative for care had emerged as the American Catholic Church strengthened and became more involved in assistance to the needy of all ages, operating their own asylums, orphanages, hospitals, and homes for the aged. Although care of the aged continued to be secured chiefly by a combination of ethnic organizations, public poorhouses, assistance programs of big-city machines, and families, institutions designed especially for the aged opened for operation. While most of these formal homes for the aged were affiliated with the Catholic Church and were technically not ethnic, they were overwhelmingly staffed by Irish nuns and run by Irish priests. In essence, at the outset, they were primarily homes providing care for the Irish by the Irish (Kutzik, 1979; Metress, 1985).

It is well known that the Catholic Church was a significant institution in the day-to-day life of the American Irish. As Ellen Somers Horgan (1998: 49) puts it, for the Catholic Irish, "the quasi-ghetto neighborhoods in the cities . . . were replaced by the parish as the unit of community living." The parish provided a structure to family life through its religious, educational, social, cultural, and sometimes political activities, all of which bound individuals to the family and the family to the community at large (Skerrett, 1997; Horgan, 1998). Eventually, individual local parishes also saw to the needs of their aged parishioners, especially those without family support. The parish hierarchy provided financial allowances that enabled the elderly to remain independent. In addition, pastors made referrals to Catholic hospitals when illness struck or to Catholic homes for the aged when the need arose (Kutzik, 1979; Metress, 1985; Horgan, 1998). For the aged with families, Horgan (1998: 55) recalls, "All cared for elderly parents but in different ways, depending on their resources—paying bills, shopping, visiting, and having the parents live in their homes." Certainly this is the paradigm most often seen in Irish American literature, with the novels of James T. Farrell providing notable examples of Irish families keeping their aged parents and relatives at home (Loughman, 1985).

But, as Judith Witt (1994: 68) notes, in the United States in general, "a noticeable shift in responsibility for the growing aged population from the family to the community" took place in the early twentieth century. In response to the growing elderly population and emerging cultural beliefs in personal growth and individualism, placing aging parents or relatives in nursing homes became more acceptable. Subsequently, the Great Depression and the Social Security Act of 1935 transformed the delivery of formal public assistance to the aged. Mutual aid societies and ethnic charities, including homes for the aged, disappeared when new government programs took over these functions (Kutzik, 1979; Metress, 1985). The government's willingness to take responsibility for the aged coalesced with the family's newfound individualism. The result was lower expectations of kin support. By the mid-twentieth century, families of all types were relying more on government and institutional supports to care for the aged (Witt, 1994; Sokolovsky, 1997).

While appealing to the Irish, who already had a history of third-party and non-familial assistance, this shift led to another dilemma. Studies of the interactions between the aged and their kin, especially when the health of the elderly weakens, confirm the awkwardness of role reversals between the generations and the reluctance on the part of children to acknowledge the growing dependency of a parent (Hill, 1970; Kutzik, 1979; Gordon, Vaughan and Whelan, 1981; Metress, 1985). There is also evidence that, in some instances, this reluctance can lead to avoidance (Hill, 1970). The ambivalence this creates within the Irish family is particularly acute. Certain aspects of the American Irish family—loose attachments, lack of emotional support, and self-sufficiency for young and old—are compromised by the ever present guilt over familial obligations. In families where physical prowess and self-sufficiency are highly valued, the increasing dependency and frailty of a parent are difficult to confront. Moreover, since intimate interactions are to be avoided, the illness and even impending death of a parent are extraordinarily difficult to manage.

The provision of care to the aged in Ireland today is a complex matter. Singlehood remains a respected, unquestioned lifestyle choice, and, because of this, the widowed are not pressured to remarry. In fact, the most common housing arrangement for the elderly in Ireland remains independent living (Gordon, Vaughan and Whelan, 1981). Overall, this is seen as a positive time of life, satisfying and characterized by self-reliance and freedom from responsibility. Not surprisingly, because of what we know of the Irish, it is illness or disability, rather than old age itself, that causes anxiety among the aged (Fahey and Murray, 1994).

Most believe the best way to maintain their preferred lifestyle is to combine aspects of state assistance, family support, and community-based informal sources of care (Gordon, Vaughan and Whelan, 1981; Larragy, 1993; Dickerson-Putman, 1997). State-supported pension benefits will cover visits by a district nurse if needed and will help the aged maintain their self-sufficiency. Daily or weekly contact with, but not necessarily live-in care by, family members provides confirmation of familial support while maintaining comfortable boundaries of privacy and status. Children, or siblings if there are no children, provide assistance through occasional visits, calls, and crucial services in times of crisis

(Gordan, Vaughan and Whelan, 1981). It is the family's availability when needed that is important, not their continual presence. And, finally, access to activities for the aged assists in the continued integration into, and interaction with, the community at large.

There are similar patterns within the American Irish community. Older Irish American men and women, perhaps as a result of their distinctive solo migration pattern, are reluctant to lose their self-sufficiency to become a dependent part of a relative's household. More than other ethnic groups, the Irish indicate an increased concern with achievement, physical health, and self-reliance as they age (Cohler and Lieberman, 1979). They continue to consider independence and living alone the most desirable alternative. Again and again respondents in a recent study report self-sufficiency and independence as their primary goals. They consider housing for the elderly and assisted-living facilities as options preferable to living with the family of an adult child. It is vital for them to maintain their independence for as long as possible (Fanning, 2000). When the elderly become too frail or too ill to be left alone, however, Irish Americans are ambivalent about the delivery of care (Fanning, 2000). Horgan (1998: 63) confirms that there is no blueprint for satisfaction: "Today, some middle-aged children prefer expanding families to include older adults, others prefer care within a long-term care residence managed by Catholic orders, and still others prefer use of public or private long-term care settings."

While it is difficult to generalize about a group as large and diverse as the Irish in America today, it seems that in times of need they believe it is primarily the family's responsibility to care for the aged (Larragy, 1993, Horgan, 1998; Fanning, 2000). Although in rural nineteenth-century Ireland the wife of the inheriting son was expected to look after her parents-in-law (Shannon, 1963; Arensberg and Kimball, 1968; Kane, 1968; Horgan, 1998), that is not the case for the Irish in America. Here, gender, marital status, and proximity are all predictors of an individual's likelihood of becoming a caregiver (Ikels, 1983b; Fanning, 2000). American Irish daughters are more likely to live near their parents and provide physical care to them. Thus, the Irish aged look first to their own daughters to take on the primary caregiving role and to their sons for more financial and instrumental assistance (Horgan, 1998; Fanning, 2000). There is also evidence that marital status affects caretaker selection. An unmarried child is seen by both parents and siblings as the person most likely to assume the caregiving role (Ikels, 1983b; Fanning, 2000). Geographical distance is another important factor in the selection of a caretaker for the American Irish.

Studies have demonstrated that "the frequency of primary kin contacts is to a large extent determined by proximity" (Gordon, Vaughan and Whelan, 1981: 504). Even when variables such as affection, financial capabilities, and occupational commitments are examined, location is seen as a salient factor in determining the caregiving function (Fanning, 2000). As Charlotte Ikels (1983b: 494–95) summarizes: "Leaving town is one of the most acceptable ways of avoiding a caretaking future. . . . Proximity exerts tremendous influence on these decisions. If there is only one child in the area at the time of the crisis, that child has no choice but to step forward. . . . When several children of the appropriate sex are more or less equally proximate, other practical considerations arise." Those who are married, and especially those with children, have competing obligations that are seen as lessening their ability to provide continual care.

There is evidence to suggest that the Irish expect long-term assistance to be provided by family members, with a division of the caregiver roles (Fanning, 2000). Still, they remain ambivalent, and a sizable number believe that institutional resources should alleviate the financial, emotional, and physical burdens of elder care. Over 80 percent in a recent study indicated that the government should bear some of the responsibility for such assistance (Fanning, 2000). This expectation of institutional support is consistent with Irish Americans' historical pattern of using third-party providers, homes for the aged, and formal resources in the care of the elderly. Today's health care system, however, structurally limits these formal options through financial cost controls, economic-need assessments, and numerical restrictions on home-care visits. Likewise, an individual caretaker's or family's emotional ability to cope with the stress of elder care is rarely given serious consideration. This can become particularly difficult within the Irish family, where issues surrounding personal boundaries and emotionally charged communication remain problematic.

Also, within the Irish family network, siblings are an important source of support for the childless, never-married, or widowed aged, reflective of the importance placed on obligations and loyalty among siblings, both in Ireland and here in America. Unmarried or widowed siblings often live together, providing support to one another as they age. These arrangements are found most often in sister–sister relationships, with sister–brother households seen less frequently. Brother–brother households are the least likely to occur (Ikels, 1983b, 1988; Horgan, 1998). Ikel's (1983b, 1988) research has also revealed the informal reciprocity of caregiving within the Irish family. In exchange for helping an aged parent, the caregiver is provided care by siblings, nieces, or nephews in tacit acknowledgment of familism and sibling loyalty. For those without family, social supports are more difficult to obtain, especially with the gradual loss of informal social networks through retirement and the death of friends. Need can also be exacerbated by the Irish Americans' characteristic reticence and reluctance to share problems with others.

Although data indicate that ethnic heritage is of at least sentimental importance and that a majority of their friends are of Irish descent (McGivern, 1979; Fanning, 2000), most Irish Americans have emerged from the parish enclave community described by Horgan (1998). In fact, as Lawrence McCaffrey (1997: ix) points out, "A majority of people in the United States who now define themselves as Irish or partly Irish are not Catholic." Still, those Irish who remain in the parish setting may be more likely to avail themselves of the services of a parish nurse. This recently rejuvenated position offers medical assistance and also bridges the gap between the medical and religious communities. Parish nursing

programs provide education, advocacy, counseling, screening, and referral services. Of particular importance to the Irish, these nurses focus on health promotion and disease prevention and encourage control, independence, and self-care
techniques (Boland, 1998).

Conclusion and Policy Implications

In summary, the attitudes of the Irish in America toward elder care demonstrate a
certain degree of consistency. Among Irish American families, sibling loyalty and
familism persist; education, self-sufficiency, and independence are highly valued;
singlehood continues to be an acceptable alternative to marriage; and the aged remain resistant to dependence on the younger generation. The American Irish are
aware of available formal resources and are likely to utilize social services, including hospice, visiting nurses, and support groups (Cleary and Demone, 1988;
Levkoff, 1997; McGoldrick, 1998). This seems to confirm McGoldrick's (1998:
548) contention that while the Irish are "the least likely to report problems, they
are the most likely to seek help for problems they do acknowledge, especially if
there is a formal, nonfamilial solution available." Thus, Irish Americans quite naturally look for paradigms of care that include institutional alternatives so as to
maintain their independence from family and secure the receipt of aid, support,
and financial relief. Community living, housing for the elderly, and assisted-living facilities are all seen as positive possibilities that ensure and enhance their
self-reliance and independence as long as possible (Fanning, 2000). Although
Irish Americans still view the family as the primary providers of care, when need
arises, they look for institutional assistance to ease the burden. Especially when a
long-term care situation arises, be it an acute medical condition or daily living assistance, they expect to supplement family support with home visits by nursing,
rehabilitation, or care services (Fanning, 2000).

In a recent study, nearly 40 percent of respondents proposed that the government pay the family for care delivered to an older member (Fanning, 2000). Others suggest tax credits for providing elder care (Fanning, 2000). As with most
Americans, nursing homes are seen as the institutional solution of last resort
(Fanning, 2000). As the debate over the responsibilities of family and the appropriate place for government assistance continues, the American Irish may well
contribute to the creation of, and support for, new institutional paradigms of care.

17

The Status of Older People
in the Italian American Family

Colleen L. Johnson

In a collection on ethnicity and caregiving of older people, Italian Americans are most suitable examples to illustrate ethnic contrasts with the dominant American family type. In this chapter, I will illustrate how Italian Americans view their responsibilities to their elders by assessing the relevant norms and values of their subculture. As these cultural dimensions are translated into day-to-day behavior, I will analyze those family processes and allegiances that are activated to meet the needs of older people.

This chapter uses illustrations from research on Italian American families that was conducted in the mid-1970s in an upstate New York city (Johnson, 1982, 1985). Over 400 individuals were interviewed, including 100 Italian American men and women married to other Italians; 121 intermarried families with one spouse being non-Italian; 66 Italian Americans sixty-five years and older, many of whom were immigrants; and a control group of 56 Protestants of Western and Northern European origin. Although I assume that there have been some transformations in the Italian family over the intervening years, the evidence suggests that the role of elders, especially their high status, has not changed measurably. The findings reported below indicate that this is an area of Italian family life that is most resistant to change.

Most respondents, selected through public records of marriages occurring from 1948 to 1960, were middle-aged at the time of the research. This age group was chosen because at that stage in the family cycle, parents must deal with issues of dependence, independence, and interdependence among family members. The general question guiding the research was, "How do these middle-aged parents deal with the increasing independence of their teen-age children and the increasing dependence of elderly parents?" Instead of instilling independence from family, the second-generation parents attempted to prolong the period of dependency of teenage children to keep them under their protection.

As a corollary, they accept the dependence of their own parents as they become disabled in old age.

Consequently, values favoring independence are either rejected or deemphasized. This acceptance of a more dependent status of parents as they age stands in marked contrast to dominant American values. A dominant American value orientation extols independence, individualism, and self-reliance, while most forms of dependency after childhood are considered deviant from the norm. Schneider and Smith (1973), in their study of American kinship, quote a string of clichés that are repeatedly expressed as truisms: "Stand on your own two feet," "Be independent," and "Make your own way in life." Thus, the onset of dependency with age-related disabilities potentially entails a demotion to an undesirable status.

Most likely as a reflection of these values, theories of successful aging currently rest upon the initiative of individuals as they age to maintain their own good health, well-being, and productivity. In the past, activity theory mandated that to be contented in later life, one must be active and engaged, implying that a middle-aged life style should continue (Cavan, Burgess and Havighurst, 1949). At the same time, the theory of disengagement (Cumming and Henry, 1961) has been rejected by gerontologists who tend to favor the much endorsed idea of continuity rather than change in transitions from middle age into old age. More recently, successful aging has been conceptualized as having a sense of control (Ryff and Essex, 1991) or using a process of selection, optimization, and compensation (Baltes and Baltes, 1990). The Balteses (1990: 1) describe these components as depending upon "the specific personal and societal circumstances individuals may face and produce in old age." In other words, older people are viewed as creating their own problems rather than being confronted with social and physical forces that may be beyond their capacity to control.

In studies of dependent elderly, most researchers focus upon the stresses and burdens of caregiving that the family must bear (Barer and Johnson, 1990). Instead of studying the processes of social supports from multiple sources, researchers refer to caregiving as a social role, usually enacted by one overburdened individual. Such an emphasis neglects cultural diversity in family processes where multiple family members initiate a joint effort to meet the needs of older members. In ethnic groups such as Italian Americans that elevate the status of older relatives, caregiving is not invariably viewed as stressful. Instead, it is likely to be viewed as a predictable and accepted phase of one's life course.

Theoretical Framework for Studying Ethnic Families

Over the years, students of ethnicity have usually endorsed one of three points of view about Catholics of European origin, who are often referred to as the "white ethnics." First, in the 1970s Greeley (1974) and Novak (1972) maintained that the importance of ethnicity was being overlooked because of false assumptions about the inevitability of assimilation. A second view has persisted, particularly among sociologists who conclude that these white ethnics are merging into their respective social-class position, typically identified as a working-class status (Duncan and Duncan, 1968; Yancey, Ericsen and Juliani, 1976). Third, still others argue that ethnic groups persist but in a new social form that is unlike their country of origin or the dominant American group (Glazer and Moynihan, 1963).

In light of the spirited "rise of the unmeltable ethnics" in the 1970s, it is surprising to find that in the ensuing years there has been a marked decline in research on this subject. In 1988, a third edition of *Ethnic Families in America* appeared with a chapter on Italian Americans by Squier and Quadagno. In the fourth edition in 1999, they again coauthored a chapter on this subject that, with a few exceptions, was printed verbatim from the 1988 chapter. Over the twelve years, moreover, they added only four new references, a book by Habra (1994) and three census reports in 1973, 1974, and 1993. Questions arise about the dearth of interest in the subject. Does it mean that the assimilationists are correct in their contention that ethnic groups are melding into a nonethnic working class?

This chapter takes the view that ethnicity continues to be relevant among groups like the Italian Americans and is particularly observable in both the social and the cultural dimensions of the family. These ethnic dimensions usually center on two competing forces: the younger generation responding to pressures for assimilation, on one hand, and their parents and grandparents attempting to preserve Italian ways on the other. Two processes usually operate that influence the pace of assimilation and ultimate changes in the family. First, structural variables such as intermarriage bring in-laws into the family who are not members of the ethnic group, while social and geographic mobility diminishes the influence of insular ethnic communities. Second, the cultural dimensions can provide insights into either the persistence of norms and values that extol the traditional Italian family or the change in these beliefs that leads to ambivalence about or a rejection of a shared ethnic past.

Structural Determinants of Family Solidarity

Most immigrants came from Southern Italy's peasant culture, and they initially resisted education, a stance that persisted among some members of the second generation (Covello, 1967; Squier and Quadagno, 1999). Not only were children expected to work at a young age, but parents also feared that education would undermine family solidarity. Consequently, social mobility among them was slower than among similar immigrant groups. National surveys indicate that by 1973 only 16.5 percent of the Italian Americans ages twenty-five to thirty-four had four years of college and 6 percent who were thirty-five and older had a college degree (Squier and Qaudagno. 1999), figures that are similar to the upstate New York sample described here (Johnson, 1985). Even by the 1990 census report, that percentage only reached 20.9 percent for those twenty-five and older. In the upstate

New York sample of middle-aged Italians, only 23 percent of the men had some college education or a college degree.

In occupational status in 1973, 27 percent of Italian men were in professional or managerial occupations, a proportion that only increased to 30 percent by 1990 (Squier and Quadagno, 1999). In the upstate New York sample, only 13 percent of the Italian men were in the professional or managerial status but as many as 39 percent were in other white-collar positions. This slow movement into higher socioeconomic brackets was most likely associated with low rates of geographic mobility, a trend that reinforced family solidarity. Most respondents in upstate New York remained near their parents either in the old immigrant neighborhood or in adjacent neighborhoods (Johnson, 1985). In agreement, Greeley (1974) noted that more than other ethnic groups, Italian Americans were likely to live near their parents and relatives, a factor that has encouraged a retention of ethnic characteristics.

Probably more than social and geographic stability, intermarriage has resulted in changes in family life. A number of studies report that Italian Americans were less likely to marry outside their group than were other European Catholic groups (Abramson, 1973). In going through public marriage records from 1948 to 1960, we noticed so many intermarriages that we drew a sample of these families to study the effects (Johnson, 1985). In these families, the non-Italian spouse was usually accepted. Either parents had no strong objections to intermarriage or they were resigned to this inevitable process of blending with other groups.

Nevertheless, intermarried families in upstate New York differed from the in-married families in almost every area of family life except for the strong filial behaviors in both samples. Statistical comparisons found that intermarried families had less-traditional, more-companionate marriages; less-traditional child-rearing practices; and lower kinship solidarity (Johnson, 1985: 122). Consequently, intermarried Italians were less connected to their extended family network than were the in-married families, a unit that usually reinforced ethnic identity. Instead, networks of the intermarried families had more heterogeneous members, who potentially introduced new family values. Despite this influence, the filial behaviors toward parents in intermarried families did not differ from those in in-married families. Consequently, it is likely that the relationship between parent and adult child is the most resistant to change, as other areas of family life are affected by assimilation.

Cultural Determinants of Family Solidarity

The Italian immigrants who came to the United States early in the twentieth century brought strong values endorsing the traditional family system, values their children referred to as the "old-fashioned way" (Barzini, 1964; Cronin, 1970; Lopreato, 1970; Moss and Thompson, 1959; McLaughlin, 1971). As an ideal type, the elderly in the traditional family had high status and were to be treated with both respect and affection. The hierarchical family was organized by the dominance of old over young, who were expected to conform to family ways, and men's dominance over women. For men, hard work, frugality, and home ownership defined status, while women were expected to provide a clean home, good food, love, and nurturance (Gambino, 1974). Even though members of the later generation modified aspects of the traditional family, these values are still discernible, particularly those that endorse a high status for elderly family members (Johnson, 1985).

Traditional ways were instilled in a lifelong socialization process that emphasized respect and conformity to family goals. These were achieved by dispensing love and affection as well as social control. Continuity of these values was observed in our study. When middle-aged children were asked about their relationship with older parents, respondents described their filial bonds as a unilateral mandate. "It's a special feeling that has been absorbed throughout life." "We're programmed for it." "It's an unwritten law." "That's the way it's supposed to be." "It's a tie that can't be broken."

The motives were varied. Some expressed a need to repay parents for raising them or for the parental gift of life itself. Others maintained that they helped their parent out of love, so they disliked the notion of obligation. In fact, some respondents objected to our using the latter term in our questioning. In-married spouses tended to take different views of the bond: "Parents won't let go. They want to bury their child." "Love and gratefulness have become burdensome obligations." As will be described below, these cultural directives in Italian American families stem from values and beliefs that are translated into extensive supports for older parents.

Socialization to Family Attachments

When asked about the sources of strong family bonds, respondents often said it was so basic in their life that they rarely thought about it. In open-ended interviews, they emphasized that values were instilled early in life and continued as a lifelong process. Three child-rearing themes emerged in interviews. These mothers focused upon the realm of emotions such as love and affection; the use of social control to instill respect through strict disciplinary techniques; and the encouragement of interdependence among family members.

In agreement with qualitative data, statistical tests indicate that Italian American parents differ from the Protestant control group in three dimensions of child rearing. First, Italian American mothers have significantly higher nurturing behaviors. The concept of maternal unconditional love was repeatedly discussed. A mother should remember no wrongs, avoid being too demanding, be forgiving and self-sacrificing, and strive for her children's happiness. In some cases, mothers treated these serious goals with a sense of humor: "I try to find an appropriate balance between a mother's love and being a martyr."

Second, Italian parents differ significantly from non-Italians in their attempts to delay the independence of their children. Teenagers are supervised closely in their choice of friends, their activities outside the home, and adherence to strict curfews. As teenagers become young adults and economically independent, they may want to move to an apartment. Parents view such a change as distasteful for a son and unthinkable for a daughter. In any case, a mother's love can moderate the effects of traditional strict parenting, compelling children to meet parental demands, often with resignation.

Third, social control over children is significantly higher among Italian parents. The idea expressed is, "Any mother who doesn't discipline is not showing love." Some mothers are familiar with widely used child-rearing manuals but reject their more permissive views as being unworkable in Italian families. As one mother commented, "Dr. Spock didn't have an Italian mother." Another mother avoided these advice givers because, she concluded, "They make children feel guilty."

When asked, "What are the most desirable personality characteristics you would like to see in your children?" Italian parents differ significantly from Protestants. Protestants are more likely to choose personality traits related to self-direction, while Italians emphasize those related to behavioral conformity, such as respect for elders and the priority of family interests over individual interests.

In terms of achievement goals, Italian Americans do not differ from non-Italians of similar social class. In working-class families, if money is available, those with ability are expected to go to college. If resources are limited, a son takes precedence over a daughter. In contrast, middle-class parents view a college education as the best way to get ahead, but most prefer that their children attend a local Catholic college rather than the large heterogeneous university in their hometown. If children insist upon going elsewhere, some parents confine them to colleges within a one-to-two-hour drive from home. Most parents are uneasy about advanced education undermining their children's family values. Nevertheless, education is encouraged as long as it is compatible with family goals (Gambino, 1974).

Respondents commonly describe their child-rearing approach as using "lots of love and the back of the hand." These findings are in agreement with Pearlin's (1970: 45) interpretation of family processes in his research in Northern Italy. He found that "Italian parents want love and affection between their children and themselves. But while love might be enjoyed for its own sake, it is employed as a means to manage and control the behavior of children. Parental control, in turn, serves to discourage independence and autonomy, in turn, serves to cement family solidarity."

Kinship and the Connectedness of Networks

In addition to the values that shape the socialization of children, a further mechanism enhancing family solidarity is the close-knit nature of the kinship network. Two network theories clarify this process. Fredrik Barth (1969) conceptualized the ethnic group as a unit of self-ascription and ascription by others. Such an ascription leads to common agreement on the norms and strategies of interaction that form the boundary around the group. In other words, the ethnic boundary rests upon a mutual agreement on ethnic norms, particularly those that offer directives about family life.

For practical purposes, according to Bott (1971), this ethnic boundary of the network consists of normative directives about family life that are potentially reinforced by one's network members of family and friends. When these individuals are Italians from similar social settings, members of the network tend to agree on the norms that regulate family life. A consensus is then reached on the norms of family solidarity, the high status of older people, and family priorities over individual interests. As a result, with the acceptance of these norms, the ethnic family is reinforced and those attitudes at odds with family goals are rejected.

Most family activities take place in a group larger than merely parents, children, and grandparents. For example, on a weekday afternoon, we arrived for an interview to find the respondent hosting a spontaneous lunch that included ten people: her father, her sister, four nieces, and three of her sister's grandchildren. The gathering resulted from the gloomy weather. The respondent and her sister decided to cheer up their father by inviting him to lunch. Her sister's daughters heard about it and wanted to join them, bringing their children.

Kinship relationships dominate the social life of most Italians in the study. The expansive nature of the kinship system can be traced to the solidarity of siblings, who maintain continuous patterns of mutual aid and sociability. When siblings are in frequent contact, their children also visit and communicate regularly. Consequently, they form close relationships that continue over the life cycle. When these collateral relationships among siblings, cousins, and nieces and nephews are added to generational bonds, a larger kinship network emerges that provides extra resources for the dependent older members.

A series of correlations supports the proposition that the high status older family members enjoy can be traced not only to a conformity to family norms but also to the influence of Italian-dominated networks. Membership in these close-knit networks is significantly associated with having higher filial behaviors. Likewise, ethnically dominated networks are significantly associated with those child-rearing practices that tend to reinforce key elements of the traditional family system. Consequently, the mechanisms used to enforce conformity to family interests and the elevated status of older people are reinforced by some insularity from the outside community. When family connections are given the highest priority and alternatives to the family are limited, there are fewer adjustments to be made when an aging family member needs assistance.

Escape Valves to Family Encirclement

Certainly most people growing up in our society spend large blocks of time outside the family. They usually cannot ignore the differences between their ethnic

norms and values and those of mainstream America. Most middle-aged parents
and their children in this study are no exception; they tend to view the old-fashioned way with some ambivalence. They know that if they are to get ahead in life,
their parents' idealized conceptions of the family are not always expedient.

While most respondents feel that they cannot escape family demands, they
usually find some means to deal with the pressures. One means to moderate the
effects is through the expression of emotions. Venting feelings of anger and resentment as well as love and affection is usually acceptable to family members.
Also, in their ideology, most immigrants and many second-generation Italians
tend to view basic human nature as innate. Thus, personal actions are beyond the
capacity of any one individual to control. When an individual behaves at odds
with family expectations, the fault can be assigned to forces beyond the person's
control rather than to a personal deficiency. Even though expectations are high in
Italian families, penalties for failure to meet them are not rigidly enforced.

Conclusion and Policy Implications

This chapter has described how a lifelong socialization process creates strong
family solidarity that secures a high status for older family members. One major
feature of the socialization of children is a complex blend of emotional and social
controlling elements. The expression of emotions potentially creates close bonds
at the same time that it satisfies a child's dependency needs. In turn, the controlling features in the hierarchy of family roles serve to enforce conformity to family interests. As a consequence, Italian American families are not as child centered as most American families, for adults are very much in charge (Gans, 1962).
In this sense, these factors work together instrumentally to further family goals at
the expense of individual ones.

Children grow up in a secure family environment where their needs are well
met. When they stray from parental expectations, the system of social control is
set into motion with few reservations. Errant young people may also face the
many relatives who can step into a parent role and remind them of their family responsibilities. The techniques of social control appear to impel individuals back
into the family rather than into alternative relationships, most likely because of
the impressive affectual component.

How these same processes operate at later stages in the family life cycle is
more difficult to interpret, because developmental theories of family processes are
only now being extended to later stages in the family cycle. From an analysis of
the interviews, it is difficult to see how high filial devotion can exist without both
affection and social control, those important components in childhood socialization. Unlike earlier stages, however, the affectual and nurturing behaviors after
childhood are at odds with societal values. In our country, one is expected to be
independent and free from parental control in adulthood. Consequently, when situations arise that demand a choice between personal interests and family inter-

ests, the common cultural directive is to place priority on individual interests, a decision that is alien to most Italian Americans.

When families combine control over their children with security and affection, they can instill a strong sense of filial attachment to, and obligation for, parents. However, as adult children move into middle age, they tend to reach a stage of maturity that allows them to reverse roles and care for a parent. When offspring are dispensers of both affection and control to their parents, they have reached a stage of filial maturity (Blenkner, 1965). The large resources in Italian American extended families and the tradition of frequent family gatherings, combined with the psychological and social processes described here, appear to serve the elderly well.

Note

This chapter and my other publications cited here stem from research funded by the National Institute of Mental Health grants MH26417 and MH31907. The analysis of Italian American family processes is adapted from my book, *Growing Up and Growing Old in Italian American Families,* so it reflects that status of the family in the mid to late 1970s.

18

The Interplay of Aging and Ethnicity: Filial Responsibility and Greek Americans

Chrysie M. Constantakos

All societies for which we have records have had some concept of the nature of old age. Biologically, the stages of development over the life span, from birth to death, are similar for past and present generations. Yet, the way in which the life cycle has been articulated, both culturally and institutionally, has differed significantly among different groups and in different periods of history. "Certainly, there are biological imperatives, but what is truly remarkable," writes Bengston (1979: 12), "is that these imperatives are handled in quite different ways by various cultural, socioeconomic, and ethnic groups. There appear to be wide variations in attitudes, values, and practices concerning aging which are social, not biological in nature." To better understand the process of aging and related attitudinal and behavioral variations, it is important to focus on the sociocultural context in which aging occurs. The interplay of aging and ethnicity allows us to look intensively at the basic elements that bind families together, the culturally sanctioned dependency of older people on the family institution, and the types of assistance and relationships between generations that are most important in family continuity.

The family has always played an important role in determining the status and security of older people. With all the structural and functional changes of the family in the past few decades, however, the impact on the aged has been extensively addressed in the context of family decline. Proponents of the family decline thesis (Cowill, 1972; Dinkel, 1944; Macklin, 1987; Martin, 1990; Wake and Sporakowski, 1972) argue that modernization, urbanization, mass education, and suburban exodus have created residential mobility and status inversion (children acquiring higher status than their parents), resulting in a decrease in family-based assistance to the aged and greater reliance on formal institutions of elder care. According to this view, a number of trends point to a reluctance on the part of young adults to support aged parents and to a change in the norm of filial responsibility, a "life for the young" attitude, and a shifting away from familism as a cultural value. These include demographic increases in the elderly population, both in absolute numbers and in proportions of the very old; socioeconomic shifts relating to the entry of women into the labor force; higher divorce rates; and a decrease in fertility, diminishing the pool of filial providers.

The issue of family decline, however, is far from settled and continues to be debated. The prevailing position among family researchers appears to be one that considers the theme of family decline as a "myth" and takes the position that the family today is strong but changing. Data suggest that familial responsibility still holds and encompasses duty both to older parents and to other family members (Piercy, 1998). Adherents of this position (Brody et al., 1983; Brody, 1985, 1990; Cicirelli, 1983; Coontz, 1992; Day, 1985; Dornbusch and Strober, 1988; Skolnick, 1991; Zill and Rogers, 1988) report that the family continues to be a viable social institution, manifesting itself in a "modified extended family" form, or what has been labeled an "intimacy at a distance." Although families are less likely to live together, they maintain regular contact, remain in substantial proximity to each other, exhibit positive concern for the welfare of members, and provide considerable aid and services (money, shopping, assistance in times of illness, child care, emotional support, rituals, and social activities), often with a degree of reciprocity. Filial obligation is reported by some studies as more intensified, and the aged as more integrated in modern society, than previously thought. Others maintain that insufficient attention has been given to the emotional interplay and "feeling tone" of relationships between aging parents and adult children and how this affects the delivery of care (Pyke, 1999). Such a position looks at filial responsibility as behaving sensitively to one's older parents' needs for safety, comfort, autonomy, attention, and companionship. It emphasizes a conception of filial responsibility that goes beyond instrumental assistance and incorporates noninstrumental, or what is referred to as "socioemotional," aid (Walker, Pratt and Eddy, 1995).

The debate over the changing role of families, however, has not focused on ethnicity as such, and relatively little is known about the composition, needs, and potential resources of ethnic elderly. The state of knowledge relating to aging, ethnicity, and family is thus rather limited, especially as it pertains to support systems in these families (Dillworth-Anderson, Burton and Turner,1993; Rosenthal, 1986). Because ethnic minorities are rarely included in family investigations, the ability to use comparative methodologies to understand differences both within and between groups is somewhat restricted (Brubaker and Roberto, 1993; Butler, 1984; Woehrer, 1978). This is true to an even greater degree with specific ethnic groups such as Greek Americans.

Greek American Families

It is difficult to provide the exact number of Greek Americans nationwide: estimates vary from a high of 3 million (according to the Greek Orthodox Archdiocese), to 2 million (according to the Greek embassy), to slightly over 1 million (reported in census documents). There are approximately 250,000 first-, 400,000 second-, 250,000 third-, and 100,000 fourth-generation Greek Americans (Moskos, 1989). Approximately 11 percent of the Greek American population is sixty-five or older.

Greek America is overwhelmingly urban. New York City is home to the largest such community in North America. Though Greek ethnic agencies claim that approximately 250,000 to 300,000 Americans of Greek ancestry live in New York City, census data indicate that there are 76,328 people, 33,800 of whom are foreign born (29,878 from Greece, 1,471 from Cyprus, and 637 from Turkey).

The literature is scanty with regard to aging and Greek ethnicity. A review of existing research reveals writings focusing on the Greek family and intergenerational relations (Constantinou, 1989; Costantakos, 1980, 1993; Kourvetaris, 1988; Moskos, 1989; Saloutos, 1964; Scourby, 1984). Several of these works have reflected on the traditional value of filial obligation as it has been emerging among the younger generations. The point has been made that, as with the case of the immigrant generation, second-generation Greek American families have stressed respect for parents in general and the elderly in particular. Grandparents *(papou and yiayia)* are important figures in the Greek American family (Kourvetaris, 1988). Moskos (1989) speaks of a generalized respect for the elderly ingrained in both Greek and Greek American norms and suggests that filial loyalties are strongly observed. It is commonly held among Greek Americans, Moskos writes, that second-generation children are much more likely to look after their aged parents, including having elderly parents move in with them, than is the practice in American society overall. In an early intergenerational study of the Greek American family and mobility, Tavuchis (1972) underscored the persistence of cultural norms related to filial piety and respect for parents and the elderly.

In another early study, Safilios-Rothschild and Georgiopoulos (1970) researched parental and filial role definitions testing concepts developed by Parsons and Duvall, respectively, along instrumental-expressive and traditional-developmental components. The study compared couples in Detroit with those in Athens, Greece. One distinction was quite clear: Greek parents much more than the American ones stressed "financial help in case of need." Thus, it seemed that the traditional notion of children as a form of financial security persisted among the former. A more recent study, specifically focusing on the aged, was conducted in Chicago by Kathryn Kozaitis (1987), who examined the influence that a common heritage, shared history, collective identity, traditional customs and rituals, common language, and similar lifestyles has on how elderly Greeks perceive and experience aging, what expectations they have from the community, and what strategies they employ to resolve problems intrinsic to aging. Kozaitis segmented her sample into three groups: the Americanized Greeks, those who either were born in the United States or immigrated at the turn of the century as youths; Greek Americans, individuals who immigrated before World War II; and recent migrants, individuals who immigrated in the late 1950s, 1960s, or 1970s to join their children in America. A segmented acculturation continuum of these groups strongly correlated with how aging is perceived and how problems of life and aging are confronted, with the acculturated group exhibiting the most security, satisfaction with life, and comfort with American mainstream values. Among other recommendations, Kozaitis advised teaching Greek American elderly adaptive skills conducive to "bi-functionalism" (e.g., facility in English) so that they can function comfortably within both the ethnic subcommunity and the larger society.

In view of the above, the discussion that follows examines attitudes of filial obligation or responsibility in three generations of Greek Americans. It focuses on possible changes in value orientation and the implications they might hold for the future care of elderly Greek Americans. It is hypothesized that the norm of filial responsibility, though it might be decreasing in nonimmigrant generations, continues with considerable strength, at least at the attitudinal level, lagging behind demographic and sociocultural changes in this group. In qualitative terms, any perceived decline in filial duty appears to be one of change rather than disappearance of the value.

This study draws from a concept of filial obligation that implies obligations on the part of adult offspring to meet the needs of aging parents. It emphasizes duties associated with notions of economic support, protection, and care for aging parents (Lee, Netzer and Raymond, 1994; Schorr, 1960). Filial obligation is central in societies of familistic orientation, such as traditional Greek society. It encompasses the belief "in a strong sense of family identification and loyalty, mutual assistance among family members, a concern for the perpetuation of the family unit, and the subordination of the interests and personality of individual family members to the interests and welfare of the family group" (Popenoe, 1993: 537–38). Regardless of personal motivation, cultural prescriptions of obligations and sanctions for noncompliance encouraged the development of family responsibility and a concept of piety, promoting both mutual support and cooperation among generations.

Greek Culture and the Life Cycle

This chapter assumes that ethnicity is an important dimension of differentiation among older people and may be expected to have an impact on their family relationships and supports (Rosenthal, 1986: 19). The underpinnings of ethnicity, however, are affected by changing social, economic, and political conditions. Ethnicity thus emerges as a complex, dynamic variable that alters in response to changes in the individual's or the group's life.

A discussion of ethnic families in the context of aging and ethnicity would not be complete without a consideration of the ways ethnic families have changed and are changing and their effects on elderly members and intergenerational relations. Immigrant families frequently attempted to recreate in this country the value systems of their homeland. Many froze the ethnic culture in their memory, attempting to pass it intact to younger generations. Despite these efforts, however, the value systems have transformed, especially as one moves along the continuum of successive generations, and have progressively emerged as new, distinctive entities in our pluralistic society, more homegrown than imported. Simultaneously, significant changes have occurred and are occurring in the country of origin. Thus, it is important to recognize the heterogeneity of the Greek American subcommunity, including those who are native born as well as immigrant groups of varying degrees of acculturation.

Within the framework of definitional considerations related to ethnicity, aging is addressed as a process of human development, with the underlying notion that health in old age includes all aspects of well-being: the physical, emotional/psychological, spiritual, and cultural. The nature of the aging experience is shaped by the cultural and social context at the time at which aging occurs. Parents and children are connected throughout their lives, and each generation experiences life-course transitions that influence the lives of the other generation. Early family experiences have an effect on the quality of adult–parent relationships and on the extent of instrumental and emotional support provided to elderly parents.

In my view, a life-course perspective provides the means of "tracking the development of the person through his or her lifetime to determine the quality of life at different stages" (Barresi, 1987: 19). It includes biological, psychological, and sociological influences, with ethnicity intertwining throughout the various stages. Such a perspective allows us to understand role transitions and differences in role adjustment during the aging process. Moreover, attitudes about aging itself have changed over time, including ideas about the time periods at which certain roles are assumed and relinquished, income status, health, and self-definitions of well-being.

Within this framework, ethnic group membership is seen as a major shaping force throughout the life cycle. However, the ethnic group also is influenced by the cultural norms of the host society, the measure of influence depending on factors such as early socialization, opportunities for ethnic contact, and the strength of adherence to traditional values and norms (Barresi, 1987). Age, stage in the family life cycle, generational status, education, social class, recency of immigration, experiences in the host country, gender, and position in the kin network all have an impact on cultural norms as well.

An individual is born into, shaped by, and nurtured in his/her family, peer groups, community, and other particular environments, such as religion, that inculcate cultural values, traditions, practices, and worldviews. For traditional Greek culture, with its strong familistic, collectivistic orientation, the family provided the introductory vehicle for relationships, and through it the individual was socially located in the kinship system, the community, and the church. It was within the context of the family that young Greek children developed their sense of self. Their identity was intimately tied to kin: the individual was known and knew himself/herself as a member of a particular family. The traditional Greek family was viewed as a lifelong system of emotional support and, if need be, of economic assistance. A strong cultural value inherent in this orientation was that of mutual aid within the family (Pyke and Bengston, 1996). Greek culture has been characterized, at least on the ideal level, by familism, intergenerational cohesion, collectivism, subcultural continuity, and high levels of support for older parents, especially in their later years. Moreover, adults, and especially the elderly, were always to be respected. To a large extent, this is related to an age hierarchy, with status associated with older ages, but it is also due to the continuing functional roles that elders played in the extended family (Costantakos, 1980, 1993).

Demographic Characteristics

This study looks at filial obligations to elderly parents using three generations of Greek Americans in New York City. It seeks to explore the extent to which the traditional Greek values of respect for, and assistance to, elderly family members remain intact, despite changing socioeconomic conditions. The sample consists of 119 people of Greek descent who were drawn from a variety of sources, including student organizations, chiefly from the campuses of the City University of New York, community organizations, and church groups. No distinction was made between older (before World War I) and more recent immigrants (following World War II), as the former cohort is greatly diminished and difficult to reach. With regard to the intergenerational mix, the group includes 34 percent first-generation, 41 percent second-generation, and 25 percent third-generation Greek Americans.

Respondents ranged from twelve to eighty-seven years of age: 38 percent were between the ages of twelve and twenty-nine; 36 percent between the ages of thirty and forty-nine; and 26 percent over the age of fifty. Thirty-six per cent were males and 64 percent females. Most of them were born in the United States (67 percent) and the rest in Greece (30 percent) or other areas previously under Greek control (3 percent). A large majority were educated solely in the United States (78 per cent), with only 5 percent schooled in Greece and 17 percent in both countries. Interestingly, the self-evaluated Greek-language proficiency of the group is quite high, with almost 54 percent reporting fluency in, and 22 percent good knowledge of, Greek. Approximately 86 percent were fluent in English, and another 13 percent reported good or fair knowledge of the language. The group is high on the occupational scale: 40 percent were professionals and 16 percent students. Approximately 62 percent are single, separated, divorced, or widowed, while 38 percent are married, all to Greek American spouses. Significantly, there is a low percentage of multigenerational households (approximately 10 percent). Overall, the group is highly active in church-related and community organizations.

Methodological limitations are acknowledged in view of the inherent weaknesses of the data-collection instruments and the difficulties encountered in gaining access to the group for research purposes. However, the results allow us to make tentative interpretations and inferences about some basic elements that bind families together, the importance of intergenerational relationships, and the strength of filial responsibility among Greek Americans.

Attitudes toward Elder Care

Respondents were asked whether they agreed, disagreed, or had no opinion on five statements related to elder-care obligations. They were also given a number of open-ended questions.

In answer to the statement "A family should be willing to sacrifice some of the things they want for their children in order to help support their aged parents," designed to measure the extent of their willingness to help aged parents, a full 83 percent of the respondents agreed, 10 percent had no opinion, and only 6 percent disagreed. This positive attitude toward elders cuts across the generations.

The strongest agreement is shown by the second generation (91 percent), followed by the first (83 percent). One possibility accounting for the small difference is the distinction between norms and expectations: that is, a person brings shame on himself/herself by expecting support in old age from children; yet one could be accused of shameful behavior in failing to care for aged parents (Ogawa and Retherford, 1993: 585). The lower positive reaction (71 percent) of the third generation and their greater ambivalence (18 percent) indicates a slightly lesser willingness to sacrifice children's needs for those of elderly parents. However, it also could reflect the fact that many of them are the offspring whose wants would be surrendered.

There was a reversal in the response to the statement that "Parents are entitled to some return for all the sacrifices they have made for their children," with the second generation responding somewhat less positively (75 percent) than either the first (88 percent) or third (90 percent) generations. The latter seem a bit more comfortable with the idea of having some debt to their elderly parents. Moreover, they tended to express reciprocity, and in ideal forms. Overall, however, generational differences were not very significant; the responses represented a consistent acknowledgment of obligation and responsibility toward parents, as well as strength in the parent–child bond.

In an open-ended question, typical statements include:

> It is the obligation of children to take care of their parents in their old age. Respect, love, consideration, any kind of help possible.

> It is an honor and duty for children to take care of their parents who in turn had sacrificed to bring up their children, gave them support and education. Their twilight years should be lived with dignity and love.

> Greek parents take excellent care of their young children. Later the children must

take equally good care of parents. Give back to the parents and support them. Give back love and support.

The children must respect their parents. To respect and help them the way they invested in us.

Respondents also were asked "What in your opinion are the obligations of children toward aged parents?" and "Are those obligations seen differently by Greek Americans vis-à-vis Americans in general?" The answers to these open-ended questions reinforce the sense of support for filial responsibility but also point to some emerging shifts and transformations regarding the maintenance of this norm.

Nearly half of the respondents indicated that children should take care of their parents' physical, emotional, and financial needs, and many mentioned a willingness to sacrifice. However, there was a shift toward the affectional aspects of the norm of filial responsibility, rather than the obligatory ones. Moreover, one-third felt that parents deserve assistance with some needs, but with conditions placed on such duties (for example, "if children can afford it," "to the best of their ability," "to a point") and not at the expense of one's own spouse and children. Respondents tended to emphasize compassion, respect, companionship, love, and dignity. To the extent that these were perceived as more voluntary than required, any potential feelings of guilt or resentment would be minimized.

In terms of the difference between Greek Americans and the larger society, 58 percent contended that there were much greater obligations for elder care among the former. Typical responses included:

Yes! Differently!! Amongst Greek Americans, there is the belief that children are responsible for elderly and sick parents, regardless of the child's own personal obligations. Non-Greeks have a greater sense of independence from the family than Greek American families.

Yes!! Greek Americans for the most part do see those obligations differently because of the Greek morals and value system. Absolutely, we see it differently. We have a higher regard for the dignity and respect for our parents.

In general, Greek Americans believe that the sense of obligation toward parents is stronger among Greek Americans.

Another question explores attitudes toward old-age homes. The responses to the statement "Aging parents who are incapacitated are best placed in a nursing home" reveal an interesting breakdown, with the least agreement (15 percent) from the first generation; fully one-third of them expressed ambivalence. The highest degree of disagreement is indicated by the second generation, the group that was also the most willing to sacrifice for their elderly parents. The third generation shows the greatest uncertainty (41 percent) and the least disagreement (35 percent), possibly the consequence of acculturation influences and a shift to patterns more in congruence with those of the larger society, including a greater acceptance of formal systems of assistance.

Respondents were split between those agreeing with the statement "It is considered a stigma for American children of Greek descent to place their parents in a home for the aged. Parents belong with their children" and those disagreeing or projecting uncertainty. For example, one respondent noted: "[It is] better to be cared for in an old age home by professionals. I might consider the alternative." On the other hand, another explained:

> Greek young people do those things (burial customs, rituals surrounding death) because they want to please the family and because it is expected of them by the community. I cannot see, with my parents' position in the community, how we really can avoid it. . . . The community has that strong of a hold. I cannot shirk my duty to my parents, even if it is not easy. If I do, I will have to contend with exclamations "What a pity! What did they do? They dumped their parents in an institution." This would bother me and my brother so much. It would be like selling the name of the family.

In general, it is apparent that the idea of placing parents in a nursing home is not entirely acceptable to Greek Americans of any of the three generations. In answer to open-ended questions, most respondents expressed a reluctance to put parents in an old-age home, barring serious illness or a situation that left no alternative.

The data point to a strong sense of obligation toward aged parents, an obligation that is only beginning to erode among third-generation respondents. The second generation upholds the value in considerable strength, close to, if not surpassing, the first generation, thus indicating that responsibility toward one's elders has been deeply internalized among the immediate descendants of immigrants.

Assistance does not necessarily include coresidence. In fact, there is a decline in multigenerational households. In the small percentage of extended families living together, only grandparents are included—there are no other relatives. Respondents also indicated high intergenerational agreement (88 to 90 percent) on the importance of helping aging parents maintain their independence. In answer to the statement, "For the sake of the family happiness, one should help aging parents who are physically able to maintain themselves independently if this is financially possible," both those who might be recipients of assistance and those who would be the caregivers if the need arose left little doubt about the desirability of independent living for aged parents.

Economic affluence provides the freedom for independent living desired by both the elderly and their adult children. It seems that there is an emerging "intimacy at a distance," rendering filial obligations easier. There also is a growing mutuality of services, with some help flowing from the older generation to the young, especially where adult children have dual-career households. Moreover, changes in Greece itself have had an impact. For example, according to one respondent, since the adoption of a retirement pension system in that nation, many parents have separated from their children and one may currently find parents in homes for the aged.

Conclusion and Policy Implications

This study reveals the predominance of the family as a source of support for aged parents. There also was a consistent theme of filial obligation toward them that cut across the three generations of Greek Americans, with only a slight erosion over time, despite significant demographic and socioeconomic changes within the group and society at large. It shows the ongoing strength of what has been one of the tenets of traditional Greek morality, namely, that adult children who have benefited from responsible parents feel obligated to care for them as they grow old.

Cultural prescriptions and sanctions for noncompliance are strong forces within Greek American society. Even those no longer involved in the ethnic community seem to carry on the tradition of respect for, and assistance to, their elders. Such values seem to be strongly internalized and resistant to change. One could argue that the enduring strength of filial obligations may very well be due, in part, to the impact of ethnicity renewal, the recent shift from a negative to a positive view of ethnicity "from curse to pride and from host group to ethnic identity" (Tabachnik, 1985: 68). In addition, many Greek Americans may view themselves as carrying the burden of preserving their cultural identity.

The survey underscored the emotive function of the family unit, as most respondents interpreted their filial role as including a great deal of emotional support. There also is evidence that interdependence among the generations and the growth of independent living can occur simultaneously. A "family at a distance" orientation is taking hold, with a desire for geographic proximity, frequent contact, and affectional intergenerational bonds. The emotional aspects of assistance were emphasized, with stress on love, honor, respect, and dignity. The extremely positive response to economic assistance for parental independence may well be related to the upward mobility and status of the group overall, and thus its ability to provide such help. Moreover, many of the elderly have achieved financial security of their own, rendering family aid less necessary.

Yet, a decreasing pool of caregivers, faced with increased longevity, and with it more older people with chronic illnesses, may sorely test the ability of Greek Americans to act on their expressed support of filial obligations. The Greek American community and the Greek Orthodox Archdiocese in particular have not addressed this issue sufficiently. There are presently 58 senior residences in the United States for elderly Greek Americans, consisting of apartments, and only one nursing home (Hellenic Nursing Home for the Aged in Canton, Massachusetts). Forty-six of the apartment complexes represent the efforts of AHEPA (American Hellenic Educational Progressive Association), while the rest have resulted from various Greek American communities, churches, and other organizations. New

York City claims two such housing complexes, one (St. Michael's Home) under the auspices of the Greek Orthodox Archdiocese and serving fifty-six elderly; and another, a nonsectarian facility (Archbishop Iakovos Senior Citizens Residence) sponsored by HANAC (Hellenic American Neighborhood Action Committee), a social services agency (Greek Orthodox Archdiocese 1999).

There is an obvious lack of nursing homes and other facilities and services to meet the specific needs of the Greek American elderly, thus leaving significant burdens on their families now and in the future. The Greek American community would do well to help adult children, who feel strongly about their filial responsibility, provide a quality life for their frail elders.

19

Caring for Gay and Lesbian Elderly

Jacalyn A. Claes and Wayne R. Moore

During the past two decades the number of people over the age of sixty-five in the United States has been increasing twice as fast as the rest of the population. Within this diverse group, gerontologists are increasingly aware that there also exists a large and growing population of older lesbians, gay men, and bisexuals. Available data show that their number over the age of sixty ranges from 1.75 million to 3.5 million (Jacobson and Grossman, 1996). Richard Bannin, executive director of the New York City–based Senior Action in a Gay Environment (SAGE), notes that every year an estimated 400,000 lesbians and gay men in America turn fifty. With more people living with AIDS through new drugs and other treatments, an even more dramatic increase in the senior gay population will occur over the next several decades (Mann, 1999). The need for medical care and community- and home-based services will increase concomitantly.

Health and service providers must acknowledge and work with older lesbians and gay men as they become more prevalent and visible in society. In particular, physicians, nurses, social workers, administrators, nurse's aides, and others in the field have to learn about the special challenges and needs of this diverse group as well as the negative impacts of homophobia and heterosexism on their well-being. If they are to receive professional, quality services by knowledgeable and compassionate personnel, we must examine and overcome the current barriers to adequate and sensitive care.

Lesbians', Gay Men's, and Bisexuals' Concerns about Aging

Much of the research concerning older lesbians and gay men is limited. The models and theories that have been constructed are based on a heterosexual view of society, individuals, and their proper roles. Gerontologists note that most older

Americans are concerned about their health, financial situation, loss of family members and friends, any alterations in their living arrangements, personal safety, and their functional ability. Aging homosexuals, of course, have similar problems, but they may be experienced differently. Many, for instance, suffer loneliness, having lost numerous friends and their life partner to AIDS. A large percentage of lesbians and gay men worry about becoming seriously ill themselves and losing their independence. Money is another issue for most seniors, including homosexuals, many of whom don't have sufficient retirement income and savings to sustain themselves adequately or provide a decent quality of life (Quam and Whitford, 1992).

Institutionalization is a particularly dreaded prospect for those who become functionally disabled. In addition to losing their independence, lesbians and gay men also fear an environment that is insensitive, antagonistic, and discriminatory towards them and their needs (Taylor and Robertson, 1994). Many of the services for older adults are heterosexist, and older homosexuals are placed in a position either of denying their sexual identity or of being shunned. When examining problems with growing old, Quam (1993) points out, the tendency has been to look at issues affecting the heterosexual population as representative of the concerns and needs of older lesbians and gay men. Yet, as the following examples show, this is not always the case:

> An older lesbian's life partner is in the intensive care unit and now the staff has hinted about disconnecting her life-support system. They have asked about the patient's legal next of kin, even though at admission the hospital was informed of the patient's power of attorney for health care. Should her partner again have to talk about their thirty-year relationship? Will the hospital recognize her right to make decisions for the patient?

> A sixty-five-year-old gay man continues the responsibility for his seventy-year-old life partner, whose Alzheimer's disease is progressing. He has joined a support group but hasn't told them that he is gay. He also has decided to put his partner in an adult day-care program. Should he reveal more to the support group members? What about the day-care program? Will he be turned down again, as they were when they applied to the retirement village two years ago?

> The estranged daughter of a seventy-year-old lesbian suddenly appears at the in-patient hospice unit where her mother has been admitted to die. She demands that the nursing unit not allow her mother's partner to visit. She further demands that the physician order another series of chemotherapy, a treatment that the couple does not want.

> A seventy-eight-year-old gay man has been in the local skilled nursing facility after another stroke but, with rehabilitation, uses a quad cane. He needs more help than can be provided at home. His eighty-year-old life partner spends a great deal of time at the nursing home, helping feed, support, and care for the resident. After inquiring about admission and expressing his plan to share a small apartment on the

grounds of the retirement village, the partner receives a call on Wednesday informing him that "his friend" is being discharged Friday.

Clearly, one must be very cautious in assuming that the aging of heterosexual and homosexual populations is the same. Hospitals, long-term care institutions, and community-based services will confront many issues related to sexual identity, sexuality, and even the health care practices of older homosexuals (Quam and Whitford, 1992; Jacobson and Grossman, 1996; Weeks, 1981; Wojciechowski, 1998).

Homophobia and Heterosexism

Lesbians and gay men are made invisible to health care providers through heterosexist and homophobic practices. Heterosexism is "a world view, a value system that prizes heterosexuality, assumes it is the only appropriate manifestation of love and sexuality, and devalues homosexuality and all that is not heterosexual" (Herek, 1986: 925). Providers who unconsciously see through a heterosexist lens when caring for patients or clients ask questions reflecting this bias.

Hospital and nursing home admission procedures, medical history and intake forms, and routine questions asked by providers generally assume that patients or clients are heterosexual. According to Stevens and Hall (1988), these practices do not provide a safe or comfortable means to let health or service staff know that certain heterosexual assumptions are not applicable to them. Providers should use language inclusive of both homosexuals and heterosexuals.

For example, instead of asking "Are you married?" the provider could recast the question as "Are you partnered?" The latter would allow homosexuals in a long-term relationship to share a fundamental piece of their lives, information that could prove vital in planning for their care. In addition, it would allow them to be seen and known for who they are.

In working with frail elders, it is also essential to be aware of the intergenerational support system that is in place. For older people, children and grandchildren are not only important sources of assistance but also can provide pleasure, warmth, and comfort. Many of today's older lesbians and gay men have not been parents, although they may have had the desire to do so: artificial insemination, surrogate parenting, and adoption were not options for this generation. However, most of them have young people who are significant in their lives, children and young adults who share holidays and birthdays with them, send letters, visit, or call and who have built memories with their treasured "aunts" and "uncles." These surrogate family members may be nieces or nephews, a partner's children from a heterosexual marriage, or those of longtime friends. The standard question "Do you have children?" makes these connections invisible. On the other hand, "Who are the significant children in your life?" raises the visibility of these attachments and invites patients or clients to share important stories in their lives.

In addition to heterosexist practices that promote the invisibility of lesbians and gay men, homophobia is also prevalent in health care and social service institutions. Homophobia is "the prejudice, discrimination, and hostility directed at gay men and lesbian women because of their sexual orientation. . . . In its most overt form homophobia results in violence ranging from verbal harassment to murder" (Murphy, 1992: 230). Older homosexuals have dealt with the consequences of homophobia all of their lives. If they claim or reveal their sexual identity, they are at risk of joining the 92 percent of their fellow homosexuals who report being the targets of antigay verbal abuse and the 24 percent who report physical attacks because of their sexual identity (Herek, 1984).

In health care institutions and social service settings, homophobia may be conveyed through nonverbal communication, such as avoiding eye contact, maintaining distance, or refraining from touching a patient or client who is lesbian, gay, or bisexual. The message is conveyed that the provider is uncomfortable with, or disapproving of, that person. Even though the words "We don't treat your kind here" may not be said, the point can be made nevertheless. In a study of hospital nurses, Jay and Young (1992) found that the majority of them believed that "homosexuality is a sickness that should be cured or abolished." Since society prefers to see older people as sexless, and since lesbians and gay men are identified primarily through their sexuality, it is not surprising that they experience even greater homophobia than their younger counterparts. As Brower (1995) concludes, heterosexism and ageism are mutually reinforcing.

Sexual Identity of Older Lesbians and Gay Men

It is important to understand the historical context in which older homosexuals formed their sexual identity. "Coming out," or acknowledging one's sexual orientation, has only recently been brought into public discourse by younger people as a part of their need to assert their true selves. The gay rights movement or post–"Stonewall Period" is not a part of the life experience of today's older lesbians and gay men. As young adults, these elders tended to admit their sexual orientation only to themselves—if at all. Hiding it was often a survival strategy in a homophobic society whose laws and policies labeled homosexuality as immoral, pathological, and even illegal. Churches forbade membership to homosexuals who were open and honest about their identity. Most states had laws that criminalized romantic sexual expression by two consenting adults of the same gender. If lesbians and gay men were brave enough to acknowledge their sexual identity to a family physician or psychiatrist, they could be viewed as mentally ill and could be institutionalized. During the McCarthy era, the hunt for Communists in government, the armed forces, and the entertainment world linked homosexuality to such subversive activity. It was not possible to be both a good citizen of the United States and a homosexual. This age cohort was so bound by social pressures and fear of disclosure, immediate discharge from employment, and humiliation that they were forced to create a hidden life (Fassinger, 1991).

Consequently, many older lesbians and gay men have never disclosed their homosexuality. It has been quite acceptable for older single females living together to be "roommates," sharing housing for economic reasons. Their cohabitation generally was dismissed with little suspicion, and they were labeled "just two old spinsters" or "old, retired school teachers" living together. Gay men in later life were labeled "confirmed bachelors" or considered just not to have found the right person to marry. Some gays found safety in marriage while having sexual relationships with men. Lesbians often married and had children while living their emotional life with a significant woman friend. Some moved in with a significant female other later in life.

In working with women and men of this age cohort, health care and other providers must listen for subtle messages to learn more about their sexual identity, and therefore their needs. Some indicators are: (1) having the same roommate for a long time; (2) having a roommate as the emergency contact, although the patient or client has a child; or (3) making statements about being different, such as "women like us" or "men like me" (Wojciechowski, 1998).

Strengths of Lesbian and Gay Elders

Gays' and lesbians' experience of "feeling different" throughout their lives allows many of them to see and hear in divergent ways, thus encouraging them to challenge conventional wisdom on many issues. Lacking clear rules as to how to be lesbian, gay, or bisexual in the world, these women and men have had to be creative in making up their own directives in life as they went along. This can broaden one's worldview and encourage flexibility (Brown, 1989).

For example, the adaptability of gender roles within lesbian and gay couples is an asset in the aging process (Friend, 1991). In addition, anxiety among lesbians about the outward signs of aging is low, since they tend to feel less need than other women to live up to societal expectations of physical appearance. Having never fit the stereotype of traditional womanhood, they appear to enjoy many aspects of the aging process. Gay men, unlike their lesbian sisters, live in a community that extols youth, physical fitness, and sexual prowess. Those who have measured themselves by these standards sometimes struggle with self-esteem as they age and are forced to redefine their assets and strengths. Overall, however, older homosexuals can have a strong sense of self, developed through painful circumstances and the constant fears and tensions stemming from lifelong confrontations with homophobia.

Even though they may have fewer biological family members to assist them, lesbians and gay men often compensate by creating a large support system of friends in addition to their significant other, if they have one (Dorfman et al., 1995). This chosen family can be counted on for support; celebrating birthdays, holidays, and other meaningful events; and sharing the trials and tribulations of life in general (Wojciechowski, 1998). Lipman (1986) notes that homosexuals tend to have more friends on whom they can depend than do heterosexuals of the same age. Such a support system can provide a strong sense of security, since they know that they will be aging with others who care about them and with whom they can be genuine and honest (Quam and Whitford, 1992).

Similar to the aging population as a whole, lesbians and gay men have a desire for immortality; to pass on some legacy provides them with a sense of continuity. Accordingly, older lesbians and gay men often mentor young people. They may become their surrogate parents or grandparents, or mentors for their professional, personal, or political aspirations. If the younger individuals are also lesbian or gay, the elders can help them deal with discrimination, homophobia, and any struggles they may have in claiming their identity. Since most parents of lesbians and gays are heterosexual, it is especially important for these elders to serve as role models. Such connections with the younger generation also prevent stagnation of ideas and beliefs among older homosexuals and expand their self-contained world of peers (Kimmel, 1992).

Attitudes of Health Care Professionals

Good medical care is predicated upon the establishment of a positive relationship between the patient and his or her primary health care professional, mainly the physician. Unfortunately, studies of older persons and their experiences with medical personnel are limited and do not represent the full range of problems faced by homosexuals. However, the available research on attitudes of physicians and other providers in caring for this sector of society does provide some insight into how they respond to nonheterosexuals. Researchers have found that although older lesbians and gay men do well on all measures of psychological adaptation, life satisfaction, and acceptance of the aging process, they have numerous problems and fears as a result of discrimination in the health care delivery system (Deevey, 1990; Eliason, 1996; Harrison, 1996; Kehoe, 1986; Quam and Whitford, 1992).

Physicians in both medicine and psychiatry express discomfort when providing care and services to homosexuals; studies continue to show the ambivalence of medical providers in responding to their needs. In 1986, Matthes et al. surveyed members of a California county medical society and found that 40 percent of the respondents were "sometimes" or "often" uncomfortable in treating homosexual patients. In a 1989 survey of general medical practitioners, only 32 percent felt comfortable with treating gay men. In a national survey of 1,121 primary care physicians, 35 percent of the respondents indicated that they felt nervous when they were with homosexuals, and 33 percent agreed that homosexuality was a threat to the basic social institutions of society (Gerbert, Maguire and Bleecker, 1991).

In a survey by Schatz and O'Hanlan (1994), members of the American Association of Physicians for Human Rights found that physicians' attitudes may compromise the medical care and support provided to homosexual patients. Their research revealed that over 67 percent of the association's members knew of lesbian and gay clients who had received substandard medical care or had been denied care because of their sexual orientation. Fifty-two percent of the respondents had direct knowledge of or had observed professionals who had provided poor care or who had denied care entirely. Eighty-eight percent reported overhearing their peers make disparaging remarks about such patients. Just as alarming, two-thirds of the 711 respondents felt that many of their fellow physicians would seek to jeopardize the medical practices of homosexual physicians through discrimination, harassment, or ostracism. These data are supported by a survey conducted by the Gay and Lesbian Medical Association (Robb, 1996). It found that 88 percent of its membership had heard colleagues disparage homosexual patients, and 67 percent knew of associates who denied or reduced care to lesbians and gay men.

Physicians learn medicine and how to care for patients in medical schools, hospitals, and clinic environments that assume heterosexuality and in an environment that may be hostile or negative to homosexuals. They receive scant formal education about sexual orientation. In a study of how homosexuality is taught, Wallick, Cambre, and Townsend (1992) found that, on average, medical schools devote a total of less than one hour a year to this subject. Reviews of medical texts yield very little information about lesbians; issues pertaining to gay men were found only in the context of human immune deficiency virus (HIV), acquired immune deficiency syndrome (AIDS), and other sexually transmitted diseases.

Attitudes about lesbians and gay men held by psychiatrists reflect those of their medical peers. In Chaimowitz's (1991) study of the psychiatric faculty of a medical school, it was found that 25 percent of the respondents admitted that they were prejudiced against gay men and lesbians. And this is despite the fact that in 1973 the American Psychiatric Association officially removed homosexuality as a category of mental disorder and in 1986 removed the diagnosis of egodystonic homosexuality, or excessive concern about one's homosexuality (Stein, 1993). Moreover, as late as 1991, one in seven family practice and internal medicine residents still considered homosexuality a mental disorder (Hayward and Weissfeld, 1993; Harrison, 1996).

Concern has been raised that nurses, too, may have negative attitudes towards their homosexual patients; they may have cognitively accepted them, but many continue to have homophobic feelings while providing health services. One of the earliest studies found that nurses were less willing to care for homosexuals than heterosexual patients with the same illness (Kelly et al., 1988). Nursing curricula and textbooks have been found to have little or no content regarding sexual orientation (Garnets and D'Augelli, 1994; Misene et al., 1997).

Schwanberg's (1990) review of fifty-nine articles on homosexuality in the health care literature found that over 61 percent of the studies expressed negative attitudes towards lesbians and gay men, especially those with AIDS. In fact, Schwanberg observed an alarming shift from neutral to negative attitudes over time. Such a change, including increased stereotyping of homosexual behaviors, may induce even lower quality of care for these patients in health and human service settings. Smith (1992) provides evidence that this indeed has occurred.

It is rare for homosexuals to be asked directly about their sexual identity. In a study of almost two thousand lesbians who were questioned about whether their health care provider ever raised this issue, only 9 percent responded in the affirmative. Moreover, over a third of these women were fearful that bringing it up on their own would put them at risk for compromised health care (Smith, Johnson and Guenther, 1985). Most older lesbians and gay men can and do withhold their sexual identity from their health care providers because they are fearful of being judged negatively or receiving inferior care.

People who are forced to hide pieces of their true selves may experience many emotional difficulties. It takes a great deal of energy to monitor oneself constantly for spontaneous remarks that might reveal one's sexual identity. When individuals must conceal certain aspects of themselves to avoid mistreatment, they may internalize a sense of shame: there must be something wrong with them (Eliason, 1996).

Given the sensitive nature and the continuing societal stigmatization of homosexuality, medical education should prepare physicians, psychologists, psychiatrists, and nurses to respond more appropriately to this population. It is also crucial for social workers, nurse's aides, and other providers to become better educated about the needs and concerns of such clients. To do this, they must begin by acknowledging their own views and assumptions about homosexuality and sexual identity. They should be aware that some of their coworkers in health care institutions and human service organizations are themselves lesbian, gay, or bisexual. Consequently, negative comments or derogatory remarks about patients or clients also create a hostile work environment for many staff members.

Therefore, agencies and organizations should offer training programs that include issues related to sexual orientation and identity. Special programs, workshops, and seminars focusing on the needs, concerns, and anxieties of older homosexuals should be a regular part of the continuing education program for all providers working in human service organizations and institutions.

Given the perceived and actual hostility of the health care environment, it is not surprising that the number one health risk for lesbians and gay men is the fear of seeking medical care: many are concerned that their sexual orientation will be discovered (Davison and Friedman, 1981; Robb, 1996; Robertson and Schacter, 1981). According to Harrison (1996), even routine care is avoided for this reason. This concern is undoubtedly compounded for older homosexuals, since most of them have been closeted for much of their lives. The results may be devastating if they seek care only at later stages of an illness, when treatment is more invasive and intensive and the risk of disability or death is greater.

Moreover, older gay men may be at a higher risk for developing lung cancer, colon cancer, heart disease, and stroke. Although studies focusing specifically on those who are elderly are not available, the data on young gay men suggest that they are more likely than heterosexuals to abuse alcohol and to smoke and less likely to utilize screening exams (Harrison, 1996). Zeidenstein (1990) found that older lesbians, including those with university degrees and business or professional careers, rarely or never sought routine gynecological care or a regular breast examination. Without such care, they are at risk for a host of diseases, including endometrial and breast cancer. Even if they have access to health care, lesbians and gay men, both young and old, often choose not to seek routine preventive health care because of negative experiences with providers (Eliason, 1996; O'Neill and Shalit, 1992; Robertson and Schachter, 1981; Stevens and Hall, 1988; Trippet and Bain, 1990). The quality of life and potential for independent living as one ages are dependent upon early diagnosis and consistent primary care. Without a supportive and nondiscriminatory system, older homosexuals suffer compromised health care as they age.

According to Harrison (1996), it is imperative that all health and human service providers discuss directly with older lesbians and gay men any documentation of their sexual orientation in their records. Some individuals and couples may be reluctant to have such information written down for fear of disclosure. Even though medical offices, hospitals, and service agencies may stress that their charts are "confidential," a large number of people have access to them. These include office workers, other staff, insurers, or the employing company if it is self-insured (Harrison, 1996). Patients and clients should be informed about who may read their records and how they could be used.

On the other hand, it can be pointed out to the patient that a health provider's awareness of his or her sexual orientation may, in fact, be relevant to any discussion of health risks, care options, and potential social or community support services. If the client is reluctant to have such information in writing, an oral discussion could suffice.

Life Partners

In situations where clients are unable to speak for themselves, life partners should be drawn into health care decisions and long-term care planning. However, the existence of significant others often is not officially recognized even though lesbian and gay couples may have lived together and established a stable and supportive relationship for many years. Physicians, hospitals, and home-care services need to consider these relationships when making medical decisions about life-sustaining or maintenance treatment. It is imperative that physicians be aware of whom a lesbian or gay patient has designated as their surrogate decision maker. Because of shorter hospital stays under Medicare, the Council on Scientific Affairs of the American Medical Association (1996) has encouraged physicians to explore surrogate decision making with their older homosexual patients even before the need arises. Moreover, even though all hospitals, hospice programs, and home-care agencies have enacted various versions of end-of-life decision programs or initiatives for establishing health care power of attorney, many institutions and professionals are hesitant when such designated persons are not immediate or even indirect family members. State and local laws must be clearly explained to, and understood by, all concerned.

According to Eliason (1996), some critical-care settings continue to enforce policies that restrict visitors to the immediate family or legal spouse. Significantly, where the life partner is not explicitly designated as the person in charge, or where such declarations are ignored, the partner can be excluded from all aspects of the decision making process. In these instances, blood relatives, who may have direct knowledge of a life partner but who are opposed to the relationship, can control treatment options, visitation, finances, transfers to other institutions, and discharge planning.

Hospitals, nursing facilities, in-patient hospice programs, retirement homes, assisted living facilities, and adult day-care programs may directly or indirectly seek to create barriers between life partners, thus adding greater stress and anxiety to a person's already overwhelmed psychological and emotional state. Holding hands or hugging may be comforting gestures of reassurance during times of distress; yet staff workers often discourage or obstruct outward signs of affection through their comments, indirect communications, or "policies."

Even though hospitals may readily make arrangements for husbands or wives to spend the night in the patient's room, lesbians and gay men may encounter indifference or downright hostility from the hospital staff when they ask if such accommodations can be arranged for them. Reid (1995) underscores the fact that administrators of hospitals, nursing homes, senior programs, and agencies that provide home-based support services should have specific policy statements granting rights to life partners.

Isolation

In a 1992 study, Quam and Whitford found that, among other factors, the adjustment of lesbians and gay men to later life is dependent upon their acceptance of aging, maintenance of high levels of life satisfaction, and active participation in the lesbian and gay community. However, elders often feel ignored or dismissed by their younger counterparts. According to Reid (1995), this generational division within the homosexual community reflects changes brought about by the gay rights movement. In the past, younger people were introduced by older homosexuals into safe social circles, where they learned about supportive individuals and professionals. Beginning in the late 1960s, the young began to form their own social, political, and economic organizations, especially in large and midsize metropolitan areas, as well as in college and university towns. By the 1980s, these groups began focusing on the AIDS crisis, many of them providing case management and home services to people suffering from the disease. While these efforts are commendable, they often ignore or fail to examine the issues and needs of older lesbians and gay men who may need different or additional services to remain independent in their homes. This has exacerbated the isolation and separation within homosexual communities between the young and old (Bell and Weinberg, 1978; Gross, 1999; Grube, 1991; Reid, 1995; Slusher, Mayer and Dunkle, 1996; Westefeld and Winkelpeck, 1983).

In examining the unique challenges facing aging lesbians and gay men today, Richard Bannin, executive director of SAGE, notes that isolation is the biggest threat to their well-being. According to Bannin, "Many of today's seniors did not have the benefit of spending their adult lives as out gay men or lesbians. . . . Many only came out later in life and so do not feel connected [with the gay community]" (Mann, 1999: 3).

Housing and Long-Term Care

With aging and the potential loss of income, concern over independent and supportive living arrangements heightens. For older homosexuals, such anxieties can be exacerbated by the early loss of a life partner to AIDS or seeing one's supportive friendship network diminish because of disability, chronic illness, or death. The lack of marriage rights and spousal benefits, protections that heterosexual couples enjoy, can create serious financial hardships, especially if one partner dies. A few corporations, institutions, agencies, and municipalities now provide domestic partners with health and retirement benefits. However, the vast majority of today's older lesbian and gay couples did not have such options available during their working years—and most younger people will not have them in the near future unless greater progress is made. Without careful financial and estate planning, the surviving partner may be forced out of his or her home or face other income-related housing problems.

Even those lesbian and gay couples who are financially secure and have planned ahead by investigating housing options, such as life-care communities or assisted living facilities, may find that they are not allowed to live together or that their application is suddenly withdrawn if their relationship is disclosed. Certainly, as Mann (1999: 5) notes, "People who have been out their whole lives are not going to go back into the closet in a nursing home or in a retirement community."

In some larger metropolitan areas, informal housing networks have evolved, primarily composed of middle-class lesbians and gay men; however, development of retirement, assisted living, and life-care facilities elsewhere has not expanded to meet the growing need of this elderly population overall. Significantly, despite the potential market for these housing options, there have been no large-scale corporate initiatives to develop them. Such efforts would, in fact, be quite timely given the large number of aging lesbian and gay baby boomers today.

These opportunities have not gone completely unnoticed, however. For example, Rainbow Gardens (1999) of Durango, Colorado is seeking to build retirement and assisted living centers throughout the United States that are friendly to homosexuals. Recently the New York Community Trust, a city grants organization, awarded SAGE money to study the feasibility of building a lesbian- and-gay-oriented retirement home (Mann, 1999).

Conclusion and Policy Implications

Only a few programs or services are aimed specifically at older lesbians and gay men, and the majority of them are found in larger metropolitan areas. SAGE, established in 1977, has twelve chapters in the United States and Canada. Gay and Lesbian Outreach to Elderly (GLOE), founded in San Francisco, has been used as a model to develop services to elderly homosexuals in other areas. The types of assistance provided by these programs include a full range of social services such as information and referral, transportation, care management, support groups, and social events (Berger and Kelley, 1992; Slusher, Mayer and Dunkle, 1996).

Loss, whether physical or psychological, is an integral part of the aging process. Little notice has been given to the problems or issues facing lesbians and gay men who have experienced the death of a partner (Taylor and Robertson 1994). Yet the loss of a longtime partner can be especially difficult for older homosexuals. Even though many of them have constructed extensive social support systems, they often have to conceal their grief in the outside world of family, church, and neighbors. There may even be friction with the biological family regarding the partner's right to make funeral arrangements.

While bereavement services and counseling are readily available to the heterosexual community, programs and support for older lesbians and gay men may not be so accessible. Community programs serving AIDS/HIV patients and families, along with collateral ones established by hospices, may be possible avenues for offering sensitive, supportive grief counseling.

Moreover, violence, abuse, and exploitation in homes or institutions tend to go unreported for older people overall; this is an even greater problem for homosexuals. It is imperative for adult protective service workers to realize that gays and lesbians are especially reluctant to report abuse, sometimes owing to past negative experiences with physicians and other health care professionals, law enforcement personnel, and community agencies. They may also be afraid that their sexual orientation will be exposed. Thus, they become open to victimization by society's agents who may directly or indirectly ridicule, dismiss, and negate or minimize their fears, needs, privacy, independence, and choices.

Abuse and neglect of the elderly in nursing homes are prevalent, regardless of sexual orientation. For example, one survey found that 36 percent of nursing home aides had observed other staff psychologically and/or physically abusing residents (Pilemer and Moore, 1989). Such abuse included using excessive restraints; grabbing, kicking, pushing, or shoving patients; throwing things; yelling and swearing at residents; and denying them food and privileges. These problems are compounded for older homosexuals, who may encounter discrimination, prejudice, or violence based upon their sexual identity as well. Negligence by care providers may be direct or subtle. Some accounts report nursing home aides who refuse to bathe or even touch residents who are identified as gay or lesbian. Others may threaten to reveal the patient's sexual orientation if their abusive behavior or negligent care is reported.

In addition, lesbians and gay men, both young and old, face the same range of violence in their relationships and from informal care providers as do heterosexuals: physical abuse, economic exploitation, property destruction or misuse, isolation, and threats of harm or intimidation (Gentry, 1992; Hanson, 1996). Unfortunately, few studies focus specifically on older homosexuals. Within the larger context of elder abuse, it has been found that more than 1.5 million older people are victims each year, with physical and mental abuse or neglect affecting one in twenty persons over the age of sixty-five (Rosenblatt, 1990).

Medical and human service professionals should be alert for indications that an individual or couple is at risk for abuse or neglect. Minimizing physical injuries, reluctance to discuss their home life or care provided by a life partner or paid staff, fear of care providers, and even suggestions of "giving up" or suicide are all indicators of possible abuse; older lesbians and gay men are especially vulnerable.

It is the responsibility of every professional, from executive director to direct service provider, to examine his or her biases and seek to eliminate attitudes, values, or stereotypical thinking and assumptions that interfere with the delivery of quality and compassionate care and services. It should be the mission of every health and human service organization to offer competent health care and community-based services sensitive to their patients' ethnicity, religion, race, social class, and sexual orientation. Certainly, as Quam (1993: 5) notes, "As today's gay men and lesbians become a more openly recognized part of the group referred to as 'older adults,' they will become more assertive about having their needs met by traditional social service agencies and programs." Institutional or agency policies, both formal and informal, that demean, denigrate, or erode the social and psychological support of lesbian and gay elders must be abolished. Physicians, nurses, social workers, nurse's aides, and community service providers must learn about the special challenges and needs of this diverse group.

20

Gender and Long-Term Care: Women as Family Caregivers, Workers, and Recipients

Laura Katz Olson

It has become increasingly clear that feminists and gerontologists have given short shrift to the issues of older women. Recently, a number of progressive scholars have begun to fill the void, with keen analyses and insights (see, e.g., Browne, 1998). This new recognition of the relevance of gender to the aging process reveals how sex and age are defined, constructed, and perpetuated by our patriarchal social structures and power relationships. Just as important, research is starting to address how they are shaped by multiple and interlocking oppressions as well, especially those related to race and socioeconomic class.

This chapter will look at aging and long-term care through a feminist age lens, rendering women central to the inquiry. As Browne (1998) points out, gender-neutral approaches often mask the marginality, special circumstances, and impoverishment of women. I will look at the actual experiences of females as they pertain to elder care and focus on how these realities are affected by American culture, social constructs, and policies.

A number of feminist writers suggest that women's oppression can be found in four major places: the domestic sphere; the public domain; control over one's body; and vulnerability to violence. Their studies, however, tend to center on younger females, emphasizing such critical issues as reproductive responsibilities, employment discrimination, day care, poverty, abortion rights, domestic abuse, sexual harassment, and rape. In this chapter, I will broaden this analytic framework to illuminate the encumbrances of old age. The chapter also explores the interconnections among these spheres as well as intergenerational concerns.

This inquiry begins with the problems encountered by family caregivers. I then examine issues faced by formal caretakers, followed by those experienced by the frail elderly themselves. The investigation takes a life-cycle perspective, asserting that current approaches to long-term care adversely affect women as family caregivers, workers and recipients. These impacts are compounded by the complex dynamics of race/ethnicity and class.

The Domestic Sphere: Family Caretakers

During the nineteenth century, social and economic life was increasingly fragmented into private and public spheres, with reproductive labor relegated to women. For white middle- and upper-class families, it was assumed that female nurturing within individual households would allow men to compete and achieve successfully in the external world (Coontz, 1992). Women's role thus was socially constructed to mean unpaid work in the home, especially the bearing and raising of children, but it also included kin keeping and support for other dependent people (Fineman, 1995). Since few parents reached old age, most women did not have to take care of frail elders.

With growing longevity, elder care had become more common by the mid-twentieth century. In particular, the eighty-five-and-over age group, which experiences a high level of chronic illness and dependency, began expanding rapidly—by 154 percent between 1940 and 1960, and 142 percent from 1960 to 1980 (Abel, 1991).

Today, this age group is the fastest-growing sector of our population, representing over 3.9 million people, or 11.5 percent of the aged (U.S. Census, 1999). As a result, about 25 percent of American households are responsible for some form of elder care (Gould, 1999). A significant number of women now spend more years caring for aging parents than they do raising children; the evidence suggests that this responsibility will become even more a part of the lives of middle-aged and older women in the future (Abel, 1991; Gannon, 1999). Thus, unlike men, who can choose to retire at some point in their lives, women have caring roles that tend to be ongoing throughout their life span (Ray, 1996).

Policies and programs grounded on government retrenchment, decentralization, individualism, familism, residualism, and privatization ignore the centrality of gender. As Hooyman and Gonyea (1995: 20) explain, "In most instances, family care giving is a euphemism for one primary care giver, typically female." For older couples, the spouse—ordinarily the wife—is the primary provider of care. Single, frail elders usually are assisted by their adult children, mostly daughters; sons, and sometimes daughters-in-law, tend to take on such responsibilities only when there is no daughter available (Abel, 1991; Hooyman, 1992). Since the vast majority of elder care is provided by women, current social, economic, and political trends portend even greater burdens for them in the coming decades.

In fact, as Fineman (1995) astutely observes, since families in American society are expected to look after their dependents, including elders, without seeking any public aid, full-time care actually necessitates a two-adult household unit with differentiated gender roles. Therefore, in privatizing dependency, we generate derivative dependencies: female caretakers who require a spouse for financial support. These caretakers, of course, cannot meet our idealistic notions of individualism, independence, and autonomy.

Nor are families themselves self-sufficient. According to Coontz (1992: 67), we fiercely retain the myth that the gendered division of labor within traditional families created a unit that worked coactively and succeeded on its own. She points out that "the self-reliant family is the moral centerpiece of both liberal capitalism and the ideology of separate spheres for men and women." However, despite the political jargon, families have always relied on others, especially government, for their well-being. The American political system continues to support and advantage middle- and upper-class traditional family units through tax legislation, inheritance laws, health care rules, retirement benefits, and other private and public measures (Fineman, 1995).

Moreover, the functions assigned to traditional families are clearly incompatible with social realities today. Despite the renewed emphasis on "natural" families by the New Right and others, over the last several decades American society increasingly has spawned new, nonpatriarchal family types. Single parenthood, divorce, and early widowhood are common, leaving growing numbers of adult daughters to care for their parents alone.

The number of dependent elderly per carer also is increasing steadily owing to declining family size and greater life spans. In one study, Brody (1995) reports that about one-fifth of her respondents were caring for more than one older person at the same time, a situation that is likely to become more prevalent over the next thirty years.

Because of the private wall surrounding family work, women's care of frail older people is invisible, undervalued, and lonely. At the same time, in the name of family values, current political discourse depicts informal care as preferable to paid, outside assistance. While celebrating spousal/filial domesticity and commitment, such rhetoric translates into a social disregard for the substantial financial, physical, social, and psychological costs experienced by those providing elder care. The not-so-hidden agenda is to save public costs on the backs of women caretakers.

For most females, whether single or married, public and private roles have blurred. Despite the persistence of unpaid caregiving as their special task, the vast majority of women today work, and their income often is essential for supporting themselves and their families. In fact, about half of unpaid caregivers are employed full- or part-time, and this is expected to rise. Yet, as several researchers have reported, employment status is not a major factor in the amount of time or type of help provided; even women with paid jobs provide substantial aid to their functionally impaired parents (Hooyman, 1992). And many of these females are disadvantaged at work as they struggle to balance their occupations with elder care; some are forced to quit (Abel, 1991).

The economic consequences for those who are either unemployed or shift into part-time jobs can be considerable: they often face financial hardship, compromise their retirement security, and encounter difficulties reentering the labor force (Hooyman and Gonyea, 1995). One study shows that adult children lose nearly $5 billion in earnings annually because they are caring for a disabled parent (Spalter-Roth and Hartman, 1988). In addition, despite some positive benefits of care work, depression, social isolation, guilt, and deteriorating health and well-being are common among caregivers.

Nor do women seem to have a meaningful choice about whether or when to provide hands-on assistance to their spouses or parents; it generally is unpredictable, unplanned, and expected of them. The paucity of publicly funded services limits women's options even further (Abel, 1991). Browne (1998), for one, insists that this lack of government support is a form of gender discrimination. Other feminists warn that providing potential female carers with limited but woefully insufficient supplementary aid could actually reinforce their hands-on familial obligations (Hooyman, 1992).

There is considerable debate about compensating families for home care through cash grants and vouchers. American policy is based on the assumption that such payments would not only increase government involvement in private matters and raise public costs but also would undermine familial obligations. Consequently, current rules are quite restrictive: though about thirty-five states allow personal-care funding under Medicaid and/or state programs, the majority exclude spouses, many disallow adult children, about one-fourth force family carers to leave their jobs, most wait until institutionalization is imminent, and all are insufficiently funded and provide low reimbursement levels (Linsk and Keigher, 1995; Barusch, 1995). Moreover, any available remuneration is limited to those elders poor enough to qualify for Medicaid, Supplemental Security Income, or state income supplements. Linsk and Keigher (1995: 146) put it well: "Concern for community care appears to be focused on government providing only what it cannot get families to do for free."

Some feminists argue that society will recognize the importance of caring for dependent kin only if women are paid—and adequately so—for these services (Abel, 1991; Hooyman and Gonyea, 1995). On the other hand, while concurring that rewarding women financially "could be a gender responsive policy," Browne (1998: 244), for one, cautions that it also "reaffirms gender-role stereotypes and prevents long term structural change." She and others conclude that a better approach would be to provide universal coverage for a wide range of supportive services.

Similarly, many existing programs, such as respite care, educational projects, counseling, and support groups, help women cope with their elder-care duties while reinforcing the inevitability of their situation (Abel, 1991). According to Abel (1991: 66), "The overriding issue is not how to relieve stress but how to organize society to make care for the dependent population more just and humane." In other words, while these types of services can help individual women adjust to their situation, the focus on personal responsibility diverts attention from our collective obligation for dependent older people.

It is essential that we place greater emphasis on the emotional aspects of at-home care as well. As many feminist researchers recognize, spouses and adult children can care about, without physically caring for, their frail kin. Emotional closeness among family members does not necessitate hands-on assistance (Baines, Evans and Neysmith, 1998).

Despite its gendered subtext, the current push toward home- and community-based care is not necessarily detrimental to women. The real issue is the lack of social responsibility for dependent elders as well as the shortage of affordable housing alternatives and available, publicly funded programs to help with personal care, day-to-day living, and household chores.

Public Domain of Work: Paid Caregivers

The devaluation and invisibility of family caregiving clearly spill over into the public sector: hired-care work, which mirrors that in the private domain, is merely gendered social reproduction commodified (Hooyman and Gonyea, 1995; Glenn, 1992). Women, especially Latinos, African Americans, and increasingly immigrants of color, make up the vast majority of institutional and home-based personal-care attendants (Diamond, 1992). In most urban areas, such workers predominate, and the evidence indicates that long-term care will depend even more on imported labor in the coming years.

Racial and class stratifications are also evident within institutional facilities themselves: white males hold positions of power at the top; white women are lower-level professionals, responsible mostly for the day-to-day supervision and paperwork; and minority/immigrant women are situated at the bottom, delivering the actual care (Diamond, 1992; Glenn, 1992). Analysts have noted that members of the last group often are subject to arbitrary rules and regulations from above (Glenn, 1992), have few rights and privileges, and are expected to behave deferentially toward their supervisors (Foner, 1994).

Clearly, the experiences and conditions of personal-care workers and middle-class white America are worlds apart (Tellis-Nayek and Tellis-Nayek, 1989). Overall, the American public, nursing facilities, home health care agencies, and government regulators are little concerned with the problems experienced by women providing formal services or with their rights.

Nurse's aides and home-care assistants make up a large and growing segment of the generally low-wage female labor force. They are also the most poorly paid, with many attendants earning the minimum wage. Inadequate salaries and an absence of benefits leave most full-time personal-care workers in dire economic circumstances, most often hovering at or below the official poverty level. In the main, they are in dead-end positions, with the potential for only meager, incremental raises (Diamond, 1992).

To maintain themselves and their families, a significant percentage of nurse's aides are forced to hold two jobs or work double shifts (Diamond, 1992). Since they tend to be single parents, they must also provide hands-on care for their children, as well as arrange for their care, often at difficult hours such as early mornings or late at night. Many aides must depend on limited available public transportation, face family illness without either health care coverage or adequate time off from work, and deal with other stressful situations stemming from responsibilities for their own kin and inflexible, difficult working conditions (Foner, 1994).

Compared to medical care, the long-term care industry does not consist of highly trained technical or professional personnel (Kane, 1994). In nursing homes, these low-paid aides are the primary caregivers, accounting for about 80 to 90 percent of direct patient services (Glenn, 1992). Since the introduction of prospective reimbursements based on Diagnostically Related Groups in the 1980s, hospitals have discharged patients to institutions and their homes both "quicker and sicker." Thus, while nursing assistants tend to have limited expertise, they are increasingly required to take care of severely ill and disabled patients, frequently with overwhelmingly large patient-to-staff ratios and inadequate medical backup, as reported in a 1996 study for the Institute of Medicine (Wunderlich, Sloan and Davis, 1996).

The same study found that nursing homes also are an especially hazardous place to work. Although injury and illness among workers in the private sector have decreased since 1980, the rate for nurse's aides has actually increased by 62 percent. Much of the labor is physically demanding—lifting, turning, dressing, and cleaning heavy, sometimes immobile patients—and back ailments are common. It is also exhausting work: aides are responsible for emptying bedpans, toileting, changing sheets, wiping up incontinent patients, and maintaining a strict routine and time schedule for residents' eating, showering, waking, and sleeping. To save on labor costs, the pace in nursing homes has quickened in recent years (Diamond, 1992), sapping even further the strength of already overworked aides. These frontline laborers also are subject to resistant patients, some of whom inflict abuse on them, including racial slurs and physical violence (Foner, 1994). Diamond (1992: 117) sums it up incisively: nursing home work "is both back-breaking physically and emotionally heart-breaking."

Home health agencies, also caring for increasingly complex cases, often require their aides to act on their own, despite low levels of education and technical skill (Wunderlich, Sloan and Davis, 1996). To cut costs, they too are subject to more rigid schedules and greater productivity goals, allowing for less time per patient. Aronson and Neysmith (1996) found that these aides are highly vulnerable to exploitation. Since they have few marketable skills and occupational choices, paid homemakers are susceptible to demands by their clients and clients' families to put in additional, unpaid hours to satisfy any unmet needs. And, given that they are alone in the older person's home and often are a last resort for patients, they can feel a moral pressure to do so as well.

According to Kane and Penrod (1995), employed baby boomers seem more inclined than previous generations to rely on privately paid help to care for their frail elders. Obviously, a willingness to use formal services to substitute for, or more likely supplement, informal caregiving tends to be directly related to one's ability to pay (Browne, 1998). Similar to nursing homes and home health agencies, privately purchased care under current conditions depends on exploiting the nurturing labor of others.

The Frail Elderly: Loss of Autonomy and Violence

Feminists argue that since control over one's body and vulnerability to violence are two primary sites of women's oppression, females must fight for abortion rights and freedom from poverty, domestic abuse, rape, and sexual harassment. However, for the frail elderly, these areas of oppression engender additional problems that adversely affect their lives and well-being.

The experiences of people at advanced ages are clearly at odds with the dominant individualistic norms of self-reliance and independence. A majority of the elderly over eighty-five require ongoing help with at least some activities and will never become entirely self-sufficient (Baines, Evans and Neysmith, 1995). Most of them are single women whose poverty is compounded by functional impairments and dependency, leaving them open to new forces of exploitation and violence as well as to deprivation of their rights, liberty, power, and choices. Increased privatization, individualism, government retrenchment, and familism have put even more older females at the mercy of others.

Among elderly women, alternative household forms are as common as, and at the oldest ages more common than, the conventional patriarchal types. In the United States, 72 percent of the eighty-five-and-older population is female (Hooyman, 1997). Fully one-third of all older people, primarily widows, divorcées, and never-married females, live alone. A significant number of women also live with their adult children, generally daughters. At more advanced ages, however, their chances of nursing home placement rise dramatically. Though only 5 percent of the elderly overall are institutionalized, this percentage increases to about 23 percent for the eighty-five-and-over age group (Birenbaum, 1995).

Though older women's living arrangements are not labeled as deviant, nor are the women blamed for their unmarried status as younger women are, they are penalized by the state nonetheless. Since the Social Security program and private retirement systems are based on a traditional patriarchal family structure, adequate benefits accrue primarily to two-adult households. Upon the death of, or divorce from, their spouse, many elderly females—similar to young mothers without husbands—tend to be relegated to lives of poverty.

The evidence suggests that single older women suffer from a higher incidence than men of chronic diseases and disabilities, conditions that are associated with their low socioeconomic status (Kane, Kane and Ladd, 1998; Gannon, 1999). There are cumulative negative health effects as well, since females have higher rates of poverty than men at younger ages and are less likely to be covered under medical insurance (Gannon, 1999; Hooyman, 1999).

Despite a lifetime of providing care to others, women also are more at risk than men of lacking any care for themselves (Hooyman, 1999). Chronically ill older men generally receive hands-on assistance from their wives. When low-income, single women become frail and dependent, they have difficulty remaining in the community unless they can rely on their adult children (i.e., daughters) for support. They cannot afford to purchase help privately, nor do they have legitimate claims on the resources of society. Yet, nearly one-fifth of dependent widows, divorcées, or never-married females do not have children to assist them, and about 10 percent lack any kin (Abel, 1991; Brody, 1995). Many have sons and daughters who are geographically distant or old and incapacitated themselves.

Though home ownership is common among the elderly and many live mortgage free, single women often cannot afford to repair or modify their houses to make them suitable for a person with disabilities (Liebig, 1998). Moreover, the number of rental units for low-income older people is steadily declining and is now at a crisis level (OAR, 1999), also threatening the ability of unmarried elderly women to stay in their own dwellings.

A number of factors, then, converge to push economically disadvantaged frail widows, divorcées, and never-married women into nursing homes. Their precarious situation is exacerbated by the fact that Medicaid primarily funds institutional rather than home- and community-based care. In 1999, there were 1.5 million disabled older people, of whom over 80 percent were female, in 17,039 nursing homes in the United States (OAR, 1999).

The primary goal in private, for-profit long-term care is cost effectiveness, efficiency, and productivity rather than concern for the patient's well-being, service needs, or the quality of care. For the most part, nursing homes have become big business, primarily accountable to individual owners and/or stockholders. As such, they are driven by balance sheets, bottom lines, and short-term return on investments. Consequently, as Foner (1994) indicates, there are significant structural forces that work against compassionate, supportive care. They also promote seriously abusive practices.

Within institutional facilities, both older people and their assistants "are made into commodities and cost-accountable units" (Diamond, 1992: 172). The social structure strips residents of any semblance of control over their daily lives. They must eat, sleep, and bathe on rigid schedules, allowing for little individuality in needs and preferences. Even their leisure activities are limited and strictly managed. For the most part, they become passive recipients of services that are organized for the private profit of others.

Since nurse's aides are rated by what is quantifiable and therefore reimbursable, their ability to perform emotional tasks is seriously curtailed (Foner, 1994). Diamond (1992: 137), who was a participant-observer in four nursing homes, noticed that much of the aides' caring work, including listening to the residents' stories and concerns, building relationships, and maintaining their sense of dignity, is not recorded on official charts and, for administrators, regulators, and policymakers, "if it wasn't charted, it didn't happen." According to Foner (1994: 59), aides in many nursing homes "are castigated for spending too much time on 'emotional work' with residents. Those who take the initiative in trying to improve patient care and respond to patients' special needs can find themselves punished rather than rewarded." In addition, since staff turnover is inordinately high, with a large number of nursing homes experiencing a rate of 100 percent annually, residents have little continuity in their lives (Tellis-Nayek and Tellis-Nayek, 1989).

For many institutionalized older people, these frontline workers play a major, and sometimes sole, role in day-to-day existence: about 75 percent do not have anyone visiting them regularly (U.S. Senate, 1995). Studies show that it is the human qualities in staff that patients value most—compassion, listening, chatting, gentleness, and responsiveness to their problems and needs (Foner, 1994; Tellis-Nayek and Tellis-Nayek, 1989). The accelerating pace of institutional life allows even less time for emotional and relational labor; it also engenders harsh, often inhumane conditions.

As Diamond (1992: 206) puts it, the industry's cost-cutting measures do not allow staff to concern themselves with "hunger in the night, or [the fact] that stale, urine-drenched air might have accumulated all through the day, or that tomorrow the showers might be cold or the pancakes soggy or . . . [to] puzzle about why this barren care cost[s] so much." He noticed that the food served is neither palatable nor tasty and that some facilities deny even basic amenities, such as lotions and aspirin, if they are not directly reimbursable by the government.

Since nearly 70 percent of nursing home expenditures are on wages, to maintain high profits, proprietors purposely keep staffing levels low. Exploitive labor practices also have led to shortages of both aides and nurses, directly affecting the health and well-being of residents. At a 1997 Senate hearing on malnutrition, a condition that kills or severely injures thousands of residents annually, analysts asserted that a major cause of the problem was insufficient staffing. One observer noted that sometimes aides, who are under severe time pressures, would force-feed patients (U.S. Senate, 1997). Overmedication, especially the use of psychoactive drugs; reliance on restraints; and a host of other problems experienced by frail elders in institutions can be attributed to a paucity of aides as well as to other profiteering approaches to care (Diamond, 1992).

Shortages also lead to lax hiring practices, including failure to screen current or potential workers for prior criminal activity and abuse. Neglect and mistreatment by nurse's aides, overall, is prevalent (Wunderlich, Sloan and Davis, 1996). Mercer, Heacock and Beck (1994) found that most of these assistants enjoyed helping people but were burdened by their own economic situation and shoddy treatment by management. During her experience working in a nursing home, Foner (1994), too, discovered that most aides are decent and considerate people. However, because of their frustration with harsh, restrictive working conditions and personal financial matters, they sometimes vent their anger by abusing residents and disregarding their needs. She views the relationship between these frontline workers and their charges as a "complex tangle of attachments, obligations and antagonisms" (Foner, 1994: 52).

The Tellis-Nayeks (1989) also hold that both nurse's aides and their patients target each other. They conclude: "And that completes the vicious cycle. Two parties, both powerless, little respected, and hardly recognized by society are made to face each other in a difficult setting not of their own making. . . . Neither party controls the institutional environment in which they exist, neither can break the negative cycle, and so the problem feeds on itself" (312).

National studies continue to document the mistreatment of nursing home residents. A General Accounting Office (GAO) investigation of California's facilities in 1998 found that nearly one-third had serious violations that caused death, significantly harmed patients, or immediately jeopardized their health and safety. Its report alleged that the problems are most likely even worse, since many threatening care problems were not even identified or documented by regulators. Medicaid and Medicare paid about $2 billion to California nursing homes in 1997 (GAO, 1998).

A 1999 GAO study of Pennsylvania, Michigan, Texas, and California, which account for 23 percent of the nation's nursing homes, revealed that more than one-fourth of these institutions "had serious deficiencies that caused actual harm to residents or placed them at risk of death or serious harm" (23).

Not surprisingly, an overwhelming majority of older people dread the prospect of entering an institutional facility. In a survey of three thousand seriously ill hospitalized patients, 26 percent said they were unwilling and 30 percent said they would rather die than live in a nursing home; only 7 percent said they would do so voluntarily (Kane, Kane and Ladd, 1998).

Both the national government and states do relatively little to force nursing homes to provide decent, quality care. New federal regulations, standards, and enforcement procedures, enacted under the Omnibus Budget Reconciliation Act of 1987 and later, have not meaningfully improved institutions, nor have they prevented most ongoing abusive practices (GAO, 1998). As Diamond (1992: 231) asserts, policymakers continue to favor solutions that impose more stringent rules and regulations on aides, "the people who have the very least to do with the source of the problems in the first place."

The GAO (1999) and others recommend even stricter federal guidelines, oversight, sanctions, and monetary penalties; more aggressive termination of noncompliant homes from Medicare and Medicaid; an improved national data system; and strengthened monitoring, surveys, and complaint procedures at the state level. While such proposals could ameliorate some of the conditions that endanger residents, they do not address the root causes of the pervasive problems and abuses experienced by frail elders in nursing homes, including the commodification of long-term care; business ethics that depersonalize and dehumanize services; the growth of large, for-profit chains; sorely inadequate wage structures; and other exploitive practices.

Clearly, single older women at advanced ages often have only limited control over their bodies, well-being, and lives. Their real needs depend on notions of reciprocity, interdependence, and mutuality, goals that are achievable only through improving their financial situation and promoting public responsibility for their care.

Conclusion and Policy Implications

In the United States, there has never been a comprehensive long-term care system. Older people have been mostly left to their own devices, with formal services available only to those who can afford to pay. The vast majority of care is done informally by women, mostly wives and adult daughters. The new emphasis on home- and community-based care, with few public resources for any meaningful implementation, translates into even more hands-on assistance by females, especially adult daughters. For many of these women, who must work full-time to support themselves and their families, their private and public roles have become increasingly indistinct. And, as suggested above, most experience significant financial, physical, social, or psychological costs.

We must be careful, however, not to universalize women's caretaking experiences in our country since there are critical cleavages based on class, race, and ethnicity. Significantly, for many who are not white middle- or upper-class, there has never been a sharp demarcation between their private familial duties and financial responsibilities; they have always had to combine paid employment with informal caring labor (Glenn, 1992).

Despite a greater incidence of functional and chronic impairments, primarily because of disadvantaged economic conditions throughout their lives, elderly African American women use fewer formal long-term care services than whites (Hooyman and Gonyea, 1995; Gannon, 1999). They have always been more likely than other groups to be taken care of within extended family structures (Coontz, 1992). Gannon (1999) and others hold that older women of color have larger and more complex support networks. It is unclear, however, whether this is due to tighter kin ties or a paucity of choices. Financial inability to purchase services privately, lack of available nursing home beds for Medicaid-eligible elderly, and other factors related to low income and racial discrimination prevent any consideration of alternative modes of care.

Moreover, American families and long-term care institutions and agencies are increasingly relying on the low-paid labor of minority women, especially immigrants, for their formal service needs. Indeed, as Coontz (1992) suggests, the advantages of certain economic classes have always depended on minorities and lower-income individuals. Thus, under current conditions, any expansion of private services will benefit middle- and upper-class women at the expense of their less-well-off counterparts. Critically, in her study of adult daughters who had hired private domestic workers, Abel (1991: 143) observes that "although many women complained about the financial burden on their parents, only one questioned whether the wages were sufficient to permit aides and attendants to maintain a decent standard of living."

As suggested earlier, poverty contributes substantially to a decreased sense of agency among disabled female elders overall. After a lifetime of caring for others, a large percentage of functionally impaired single older women—many of whom are or had been middle class—end up in nursing homes where they lose all control over their personal existence. They also become vulnerable to countless forms of violence, including malnutrition, physical and emotional abuse, neglect, and even rape. Moreover, even those individuals with some assets are forced to impoverish themselves to finance such care.

Nursing facilities should be a viable option for those who cannot be cared for at home. In a recent study, Abel (1991) observes that many exhausted caregivers refuse to consider institutional placement for their severely disabled relatives primarily because of their fear of maltreatment. Others are deterred because of long waiting lists for the relatively desirable nursing homes, especially if the elder is Medicaid eligible. The underlying issue is not institutional care, per se, but rather its prohibitive cost, short supply, and low quality, often abusive, conditions.

We must begin to seek long-term care solutions that empower frail older women, policies that do not rob them of their dignity, choices, and sense of self or deprive them of any control over their own bodies, safety, and physical health. For the vast majority of disabled older people and their families, resources available for paid services are limited. With private responsibility for financing care, most cannot afford to pay significantly higher wages for the services they require. The obvious conclusion, as Glenn and others point out, is to provide universal coverage for a broad range of continuous, quality services at decent salaries for the frontline workers who supply them (Glenn, 1992).

21

Long-Term Care:
The Case of the Rural Elderly

Jean Pearson Scott

This chapter considers diversity of older adults from the perspective of rural environments, contexts that create unique challenges for the planning, delivery, and quality of long-term care and that also shape many characteristics of its residents. Rural older adults are disadvantaged relative to their metropolitan or urban counterparts by being on average poorer, more functionally impaired, and less educated and having less access to, and a more limited range of, health care services. As health care costs increase and older adults live to advanced ages, access to, and use of, long-term care will be of considerable importance to rural older adults and their families, the major providers of long-term care assistance. This chapter describes characteristics of rural elderly that have implications for long-term care services; examines factors affecting availability, use, and quality of services in rural areas; and discusses issues essential for the improvement of long-term care for rural elders.

Who Are Rural Older Adults?

Identifying the characteristics and needs of rural elders is complicated by the diversity represented by rurality. Rurality refers to a continuum of characteristics (e.g., population size, density, degree of urbanization, distance from urban centers) associated with rural environments (Coward et al., 1994). Because of more common usage, the U.S. Bureau of the Census's dichotomous definitions of rural versus urban and metropolitan/nonmetropolitan (metro/nonmetro) are cited in this chapter as well as more descriptive definitions when they are available. Rural residents are defined as those persons living outside urbanized areas in places with populations of less than 2,500 (U.S. Census, 1992a). Approximately 24 percent of adults age sixty-five and over live in places designated as rural (farm and nonfarm). Rural farm residents are those who live on farms—residences with at least $1,000 in agricultural sales in 1989 (McLaughlin and Jensen, 1998: 17). Few older adults live on farms (2.0 percent). Even within a rural or urban designation, a wide range of population sizes and densities exist. A rural area could be a small town or a large, sparsely populated area many miles from a town. An urban area may include small towns of over 2,500 population to cities of several million—a wide range.

According to U.S. Bureau of the Census definitions, "rural" and "nonmetropolitan" are not synonymous terms. A metropolitan area is a county that contains one or more places that have a population of at least 50,000 or a U.S. Census urbanized area with a total population of at least 100,000 persons. Nonmetropolitan areas are those *counties* that do *not* meet the metropolitan designation. An urbanized area is one or more places along with the adjacent densely settled surrounding territory that together have a population of at least 50,000. By definition, metropolitan counties include surrounding counties that are socially and economically tied to a central one. The nonmetropolitan designation is based on counties, whereas the rural designation is based on urbanization and places within counties (Angel et al., 1995; McLaughlin and Jensen, 1998).

An area defined as rural, therefore, could be part of an area designated as metropolitan or an area designated as nonmetropolitan. The metro/nonmetro dichotomy also lumps quite diverse counties together. A metropolitan county may include open country and farmland not far from a city with a population of 50,000. A nonmetropolitan county may include a heavily populated area with a population approaching 100,000. Approximately a fourth (26 percent) of all elderly reside in nonmetropolitan counties, a disproportionate number compared to 22 percent of the population as a whole. Elders appear only slightly more urban when rural/urban comparisons are used; 23.5 percent are rural, compared to 24.3 percent of all Americans who live in rural areas.

More recently, continuums for identifying residence have been proposed (Coward et al., 1994). The Beale codes, for example, use a ten-category scale ranging from central counties in large metropolitan areas to completely rural counties not adjacent to metropolitan areas. While these models may better reflect the diversity across areas, the underlying dimensions on which to base distinctions along the continuum have been difficult to identify. These attempts to more accurately capture the residential setting are welcomed by researchers and will no doubt become more widely used. Presently, however, most of the literature on rural aging uses one or both U.S. Census definitions (rural/urban, metro/nonmetro). Despite the rather arbitrary nature of these dichotomies, the designations for residence have important implications for research and social policies.

Over the last two decades, the percentage rate of growth of the older population has been greater in metro counties than in nonmetro counties despite the higher proportion of elders in the latter. This trend reflects the larger cohorts of the population growing older in metro areas in comparison to nonmetro areas (McLaughlin and Jensen, 1998). An important factor to consider in service provision is the concentration of older adults. The Northeast region and Mid-Atlantic Division have the highest proportions of older adults (14 percent). The states with the highest percentage of nonmetro elders are Florida (18.3 percent), Pennsylvania (15.4 percent), and Iowa (17.8 percent). Interestingly, Iowa was one of the slowest-growing states in terms of percentage growth of all elderly (21.6 percent) and nonmetro elderly (14.9 percent) between 1970 and 1990. Florida and Arizona, popular retirement states, experienced high percentage increases in growth of elderly persons between 1970 and 1990. Census data reflect a pattern of slow growth in states where older adults are "aging in place" and the fastest growth in those states that attract retirees or states with previously very small elderly populations (West Region and Mountain Division). States with fast-growing percentages of elders include, for example, Alaska (194 percent) and Nevada (313 percent), states with low base populations of older adults. These trends have implications for service needs in rural areas, particularly for those states that have not had a great need for long-term care services in the past (McLaughlin and Jensen, 1998: 27–28).

The availability, quality, and use of long-term care services by older rural adults are affected by the poverty rate, employment and economic structure, family composition, educational attainment, migration, population densities, and the pool of human resources. For example, McLaughlin and Jensen (1998) note that smaller rural communities are more likely to have experienced increasing concentrations of older adults due to outmigration of youth, aging-in-place of elders, or immigration of older people. The age dependency ratio, which is a crude indicator of the number of persons who must be supported by one working person, bears this out. The age dependency ratio, calculated as the number of elderly and children divided by the number of working individuals (age nineteen to sixty-four), is largest for nonmetropolitan areas. Thus, smaller rural communities may be least capable of providing the social and economic resources to sustain an aging population. In turn, personal characteristics such as the financial and health status of older adults will affect needs and resources of rural communities.

A related concern for rural areas is that despite a high proportion of elderly in some areas, their actual numbers may not be sufficient to justify specialized services. An important implication of nonmetro/metro labeling is that many social and health care policies stipulate variations according to residence (Angel et al., 1995). Medicare, for example, has a different schedule for reimbursement to hospitals in metropolitan and nonmetropolitan areas. Nonmetropolitan hospitals may be financially vulnerable because of a lower reimbursement rate in comparison to those designated as metro.

Rural elderly have well-documented disadvantages in comparison to their urban counterparts with respect to education, income, health, housing, and access to services such as transportation (Krout, 1997). Recent reviews of the literature show that rural elders have more functional limitations, a greater incidence of many chronic health conditions, more falls, a higher proportion of heavy drinkers, and poorer perceived health than metro/urban groups. Older people from small towns and rural nonfarm areas have a higher Medicare hospital discharge rate per one thousand persons than those living in metropolitan areas. Nonmetropolitan/ rural elderly are more reliant on Medicaid as a primary source of payment and cite cost of care as a barrier to service use more than their metropolitan/urban counterparts (Blazer et al., 1995). The combination of disadvantaging conditions in rural environments suggests that needs are prevalent in rural areas.

Although these needs are well substantiated in rural communities via statistics, need is also a perceptual phenomenon. Rural communities place especially strong value on independence and being able to do for others. Asking for help or admitting to need may be embarrassing or even stigmatizing to rural elders and create barriers to seeing a problem as correctable with outside help. The social milieu and values held by rural elderly and their families are often ignored, resulting in a long-term care system that misinterprets their needs and impedes their use of services. Trust, for example, rather than expertise, is the basis for accepting the authority of health professionals in rural communities (Vissing, Salloway and Siress, 1994).

Availability, Use, and Quality of Community Long-Term Care

A consistent theme in the literature on rural areas is their general lack of a range of institutional and noninstitutional long-term care services. A pervasive stereotype is that rural elderly have stronger and more extensive extended family ties than their urban counterparts. Though research on family relations generally shows more similarities than differences between rural and urban families, the differences that are observed often reveal rural vulnerability with respect to availability of familial support to older members. Some consistent differences emerge, however, along the rural–urban continuum, such as the greater percentage of married elderly, the lower divorce rate, and greater difficulties for widowed elderly in rural as opposed to urban areas. Percentages of elderly who are married range from 70 percent in rural farm areas to 48 percent in urban inner cities. Among farm laborers, however, a high percentage are lifelong singles. The greater proportion of married elderly reflects a slightly younger elderly population in rural areas than in urban areas, more traditional values that weigh against divorce, and the joint nature of farm activity. Much of the marital difference is eliminated when age is controlled. Even when age is not controlled, the marital status difference disappears at age eighty-five and above. Rural elderly of advanced ages are no more likely to have a spouse than are those who are urban.

Regardless of age or residential status, more women than men live alone. For women of advanced age (eighty-five and over), 45 percent of rural nonfarm women and 57 percent of small-town women live alone, as compared to 25 percent and 30 percent, respectively, of men. For those who live alone and need long-term care, rural environments pose added challenges owing to the likelihood that there will be few nearby family caregivers and limited access to formal long-term care services.

In general, rural elderly have more children and are less likely to be childless than urban elderly. (This finding varies according to region, as no differences were found in the Southwest between rural and urban elderly with respect to number of children [Scott and Roberto, 1987]). Rural elderly are no more likely to live with family members than are urban elderly, and, in fact, the proportion of elders coresiding with an adult child is highest in central cities (Coward, Lee and Dwyer, 1993). Only rural farm elderly are more likely than urban elderly to have a nearby adult child. Rural nonfarm and small-town elderly are disadvantaged with respect to availability of, and face-to-face contact with, adult children. Some research suggests that out-migration of young people accounts for this situation (Lorenz et al., 1993). Proximity to adult children is one of the most important factors, if not the most important, influencing the exchange of aid between the generations. Expectations of giving and receiving assistance appear to be greater for people living in rural than in urban areas. In one study, when proximity of children, marital status, and gender were controlled, differences in help received from children favored rural elderly over their urban counterparts, particularly when an elderly parent was ill (Scott and Roberto, 1987). Though few differences were found between rural and urban elderly with respect to the help given to children, rural elderly males gave significantly more financial assistance to proximate adult children, and rural residents gave more aid when an adult child was ill. Actual support between generations in a rural Southwest area reflected a strong reliance on proximate adult children for most assistance (Scott and Roberto, 1985). Greater needs of rural residents may also account for the stronger pattern of reciprocity between them and their adult children.

There is evidence that rural elderly have more salient friendship networks that function as both social and instrumental sources of support. Older rural widows use friendship networks more than other marital status groups, and, for all rural elderly, friends provide a compensatory support when there are few proximate kin (Scott and Roberto, 1987). However, researchers have noted that the voluntary nature of friendships makes them less reliable as a source of support over long periods of time.

With regard to the configuration of informal/formal service use, rural elderly rely almost exclusively on informal support until those resources are exceeded and then add formal services (Freudenberger Jett et al., 1996). Rural elderly generally use fewer long-term care services even in situations where need is greatest. For example, Coward, Cutler and Mullens (1990) found that those rural older adults who were the frailest (those who needed assistance with more than nine activities of daily living) were less likely to be using formal services than similarly situated urban residents.

In summary, rural elderly are more likely to have support from a spouse, but for elderly of advanced ages where need may be greatest, there is little difference across residential groups in the proportion of those married. Rural nonfarm and small-town elderly are less likely than other residential groups to have a nearby child; however, when proximity and other relevant factors are controlled, frequency of interaction and exchanges between older parents and adult children are similar. Patterns of exchange of assistance indicate that rural older adults receive more help from children during times of illness than do urban elderly. Rural older adults, especially elderly widows, rely upon friendship networks for instrumental and social support, whereas in urban areas these networks serve more exclusively social functions.

Formal in-home services straddle the fence between health service and social service delivery systems (Nelson, 1994). These services comprise a broad range of assistance to meet chronic health conditions (such as giving therapy or administering medical regimes) and to satisfy maintenance and social requirements (cooking, cleaning, personal care, bathing, companionship, and respite care). Though the need factors most predictive of in-home service use are disproportionately greater among rural populations, the relationship between need and residence is not linear. That is, the range of predisposing conditions—functional status, poverty, medical conditions, housing, cultural and racial backgrounds, and perceived need for services—is not the same across rural/nonmetropolitan areas, thereby rendering general statements about need in rural areas difficult. Furthermore, the availability of informal and formal care, community structure, local leadership, and community climate all influence perceived need for, and use of, services. Despite the variety of factors that are difficult to compare across residences, a body of research continues to document the lack of in-home services in rural areas, fewer auxiliary aids, and less use of home health care and mental health services (Ganguli et al., 1997; Rabiner, 1995; Rokke and Klenow, 1998).

In studies examining the use of Medicare home health benefits with hospital use variables, Kenney (1991) and Kenney and Dubay (1992) found Medicare beneficiaries were 17 percent less likely to use home health services in rural than in urban areas (Nelson, 1994: 70). In the same series of studies, rural home health agencies offered fewer auxiliary services than urban home health agencies. For example, whereas occupational therapy was offered by 80 percent of urban agencies, it was available only through 35 percent of rural agencies. The comparable percentages for speech therapy were 86 percent and 60 percent, respectively (Nelson, 1994: 71). Recent cuts in Medicare for such services under the 1997 Balanced Budget Act have only exacerbated the problems.

Though research is scant with respect to social in-home services, studies concur that the availability of social services in rural areas is nearly comparable to that in urban areas, but considerable unevenness exists in their provision across rural areas. Krout's (1989) national study of Area Agencies on Aging (AAAs) found no differences between rural and urban areas in their provision of case management, chore services, housekeeping, home-delivered meals, and transportation. Rural AAAs provided significantly less adult day care and respite services (Nelson, 1994: 72). In rural localities more so than urban places, case management may only be available in one or two counties of a service area (Krout, 1997). Urv-Wong and McDowell (1994) observed that even though small rural service agencies reported that they provided case management, in many cases it meant only integration between nutrition and transportation and not the full scope of planning and service coordination.

In a national sample of rural case management providers, the major difficulties cited in the delivery of case management in rural, open country, and/or combinations of rural and small-city locales were lack of transportation, too many regulations, inadequate funds for services and case management, and insufficient community financial support (Krout, 1997: 146–47). Despite difficulties, planning and coordination of services is believed to offer rural constituents a number of advantages including preserving scarce financial resources; preventing unnecessary and costly hospital and nursing home stays; increasing awareness of, and access to, community-based services; containing costs; targeting resources; and coordinating aging services (Krout, 1997: 143). Another consistent finding was that per capita costs were greater for services for AAAs in rural areas than for those in urban places. The small population size, coupled with low population densities, invariably reduce the economy of service delivery (Krout, 1997: 143). Although Older Americans Act programs cost more to deliver in rural areas, less than half of state units on aging use a rural factor in their funding formulas (Nelson, 1994: 72).

Barriers to home care services are a major theme in the home and community care literature. Several structural, organizational, and workforce barriers that affect access to, and use of, home care have been examined (Nelson, 1994: 74). The number of home health agencies in a community is positively associated with use of home health services, particularly when they are provided by the Visiting Nurse Association. Evidence of a substitution effect is apparent, with less Medicare-funded home health use in states with more nursing home beds. There are also fewer home health agencies per enrollee in areas that operate under certificate-of-need regulations (Kenney and Dubay, 1992). Kenney (1991) found that there were fewer home health services in states that had a moratorium on nursing home beds. Another barrier to use was the Medicare reimbursement ceiling differential, which was approximately 10 percent lower for rural areas than urban localities. Another frequently cited concern is the need to allocate more resources to transportation to enhance service delivery in rural regions (Krout, 1997).

A deficiency of health care professionals in rural areas is a long-standing problem, one that will continue to be a barrier to the availability and use of long-term care. Shortages of physicians, nurses, nurse practitioners, physician's assistants, and allied health practitioners in rural communities are projected to remain critical issues. Nelson (1994) noted that the bulk of literature on the supply of professional health care providers has been limited to acute care. There are virtually no data on the impact of the number of home health personnel and medical social workers on the use of home health services. Benjamin (1986) and Hammond (1985) observed that the supply of physicians, who serve as a source of referrals, is a predictor of use of home health services, whereas Kenney and Dubay (1992) found no significant influence of health personnel variables on use.

Despite a number of limitations, community development initiatives in rural areas can be a successful strategy for providing at-home formal assistance. However, careful attention must be paid to political climate, values and attitudes, and community leadership to build communication channels with, and common goals among, rural older people and their families (Nelson, 1994: 78).

Institutional Care

Institutional long-term care settings include nursing homes with skilled nursing facilities (SNFs) as well as intermediate care facilities. Also, hospitals now are settings for "short-term" long-term care in the form of rehabilitation, units with swing beds, hospital-based SNFs, and institutional hospice services for terminally ill persons (Shaughnessy, 1994: 169). The rural hospital swing-bed program, initiated in the 1980s, has been successful in improving near-acute care needs in approximately 1,300 rural hospitals. In rural areas, nursing homes are the major providers of institutional long-term care.

More long-term care is required in rural than in urban locales as evidenced by the former's higher per capita need for services and its greater number of functionally impaired older adults. Need, however, must be juxtaposed against the allowances of the Medicare and Medicaid programs, the cost of services, the supply of health care personnel, and the quality and availability of long-term care services in rural communities. Although the number of hospitals that have remained fiscally sound has declined in recent years, the number of nursing home beds is higher in rural areas. When considering only Medicare/Medicaid-certified facilities, approximately 40 percent of all nursing homes are in rural areas, which translates into a bed-to-elderly ratio of 62 beds per 1,000 elderly for rural areas versus a ratio of 45 per 1,000 for urban localities. Moreover, nursing homes in rural regions have more beds designated for intermediate care than do urban nursing homes, which have a larger number of SNF beds. According to one researcher, the quality of nursing home care in rural settings runs the whole continuum from poor to excellent (Shaughnessy, 1994).

Shaughnessy (1994) notes a number of nursing home issues that must be considered in planning services in rural areas: (1) nursing homes appear to address the needs of chronic-care patients more successfully than those requiring rehabilitation; (2) the supply of health care professionals for rehabilitation services is insufficient; (3) proper assessment and coordination of services is inadequate or lacking; and (4) integration of institutional and noninstitutional care is often inadequate in rural communities.

Conclusion and Policy Implications

Sensitivity to the diversity of rural environments and the people who inhabit them must be an important consideration before implementing new strategies of long-term assistance. Recommendations to improve long-term care in rural and nonmetro communities include:

- Improve coordination and integration of institutional and noninstitutional long-term care services (Foster et al., 1994).
- Place greater emphasis on utilization of case management appropriate for rural contexts (Foster et al., 1994; Kelley and MacLean, 1997).
- Develop leadership and community strategies for underserved rural areas (Nelson, 1994: 83).
- Implement new combinations of noninstitutional and institutional assistance (e.g., provide respite services in assisted living and nursing home settings; combine short- and long-term services such as swing-bed programs).
- Build relationships where trust, not expertise, is the basis for authority. Health professionals also should encourage reciprocal relationships with elders (Craig, 1994).
- Identify ways to train, certify, and increase the use of alternative-care providers in community-based agencies (e.g., nurse practitioners, physician assistants) (Barens, 1997; Nelson, 1994: 82).
- Expand outreach programs, since they have proved successful in identifying elders in need and improving appropriate referrals. Many such programs use gatekeepers (postal service personnel, neighbors, meter readers) who help locate and keep track of high-risk elderly. Others are based on educational models that target, for example, family caregivers or indigenous helpers such as clergy (Bane, 1997).
- Restore Medicare home health care cuts enacted under the 1997 Balanced Budget Act.

The need for long-term care in rural areas will not diminish in the future, and services will remain more costly to deliver than in urban areas. Although strategies to better coordinate and utilize resources will be essential, policies that stem from misconceptions about the realities of rural residence for older adults and their families must be challenged. Similarly, the changing demographic composition of rural areas will require a reexamination of the match between the needs of older persons and the availability of, and options for, long-term care.

References

AARP. 2000. *Bulletin*, May, 5.

Abel, E. K. 1991. *Who Cares for the Elderly? Public Policy and the Experiences of Adult Daughters*. Philadelphia: Temple University Press.

Abramson, H. 1973. *Ethnic Diversity in America*. New York: John Wiley & Sons.

Adams, J. P. 1981. "Service Arrangements Preferred by Minority Elderly: A Cross-Cultural Survey." *Journal of Gerontological Social Work* 3: 39–57.

Adams, William Forbes. 1932. *Ireland and Irish Emigration to the New World from 1815 to the Famine*. New Haven: Yale University Press.

Adelman, M. 1990. "Stigma, Gay Lifestyles, and Adjustment to Aging: A Study of Later-Life Gay Men and Lesbians." *Journal of Homosexuality* 20, nos. 3/4: 7–32.

Albrecht, Stan L., and Marie Cornwall. 1998. "Life Events and Religious Change." Pp. 231–52 in *Latter-day Saint Social Life: Social Research on the LDS Church and Its Membership*, ed. James T. Duke. Provo, Utah: Religious Study Center, Specialized Monograph Service.

Alder, Elaine R. 1987. "Growing Older." *Ensign* 17 (June): 44–46.

Allen, A., and J. Hayes. 1994. "Patient Satisfaction with Telemedicine in a Rural Clinic." *American Journal of Public Health* 84: 1693.

Andersen, R., S. Z. Lewis, A. L. Giachello, L. A. Aday, and G. Chiu. 1981. "Access to Medical Care among the Hispanic Population of the Southwestern United States." *Journal of Health and Social Behavior* 22, no. 1 (March): 78–89.

Angel, J., G. DeJong, G. Cornwell, and J. Wilmoth. 1995. "Diminished Health and Living Arrangements of Rural Elderly Americans." *National Journal of Sociology* 9, no. 1: 31–57.

Angel, R. J., and J. L. Angel. 1997. *Who Will Care for Us? Aging and Long-Term Care in Multicultural America*. New York: New York University Press.

Aranda, M. P., and B. G. Knight. 1997. "The Influence of Ethnicity and Culture on the Caregiver Stress and Coping Process: A Sociocultural Review and Analysis." *Gerontologist* 37, no. 3 (June): 342–54.

Arensberg, Conrad M., and Solon T. Kimball. 1968. *Family and Community in Ireland*. Cambridge: Harvard University Press.

Aronson, J., and S. Neysmith. 1996. "You're Not Just in There to Do the Work: Depersonalizing Policies and the Exploitation of Home Care Workers' Labor." *Gender and Society* 10, no. 1: 59–77.

Arrington, Leonard, Feramorz Y. Fox, and Dean L. May. 1976. "Taking Care of Their

Own: The Mormon Welfare System 1936–1975." Chap. 15 in *Building the City of God: Community and Cooperation among the Mormons.* Salt Lake City: Deseret.

Atchley, Robert. 1997. *Social Forces and Aging: An Introduction to Social Gerontology.* 8th ed. Belmont, Calif.: Wadsworth.

Baines, C., P. Evans, and S. Neysmith. 1998. "Women's Caring: Work Expanding, State Contracting." Pp. 3–22 in *Women's Caring: Feminist Perspectives on Social Welfare,* ed. C. Baines, P. Evans, and S. Neysmith. New York: Oxford University Press.

Baker, F. M. 1994. "Suicide among Ethnic Minority Elderly: A Statistical and Psychosocial Perspective." *Journal of Geriatric Psychiatry* 27: 241–64.

Baltes, P. G., and M. Baltes. 1990. "Psychological Perspectives on Successful Aging." Pp. 1–34 in *Successful Aging: Perspectives from the Behavioral Sciences,* ed. B. Maltes and M. M. Bates. New York: Cambridge University Press.

Bane, S. D. 1997. "Rural Mental Health and Aging: Implications for Case Management." *Journal of Case Management* 6: 158–61.

Barens, N. D. 1997. "Examining the Long-Term Care Needs of Rural Older Women." *Journal of Case Management* 6: 162–65.

Barer, B. M., and C. L. Johnson. 1990. "A Critique of the Caregiving Literature." *Gerontologist* 30: 26–29.

Barrabee, P., and O. von Mering. 1953. "Ethnic Variations in Mental Stress in Families with Psychotic Children." *Social Problems* 1: 48–53.

Barresi, C. M. 1987. "Ethnic Aging and the Life Course." Pp. 18–34 in *Ethnic Dimensions of Aging,* ed. D. E. Garland and C. M. Barresi. New York: Springer.

Barrow, G. 1992. *Aging, the Individual, and Society.* New York: West.

Barth, F. 1969. *Ethnic Groups and Boundaries.* Boston: Little, Brown.

Barusch, A. S. 1995. "Programming for Family Care of Elderly Dependents: Mandates, Incentives, and Service Rationing." *Social Work* 40: 315–22.

Barzini, L. 1964. *The Italians.* New York: Atheneum.

Beauregard, K., P. Cunningham, and L. Cornelius. 1991. *Access to Health Care: Findings from the Survey of American Indians and Alaska Natives.* Rockville, Md.: Public Health Service, Agency for Health Care and Policy Research.

Becker, T. M., C. L. Wiggins, C. R. Key, and J. M. Samet. 1990. "Symptoms, Signs, and Ill-Defined Conditions: A Leading Cause of Death among Minorities." *American Journal of Epidemiology* 131: 664–68.

Belgrave, L. L., M. L. Wykle, and J. M. Choi. 1993. "Health, Double Jeopardy, and Culture: The Use of Institutionalization by African Americans." *Gerontologist* 33: 379–85.

Bell, A., and M. Weinberg. 1978. *Homosexualities: A Study of Diversity among Men and Women.* New York: Simon & Schuster.

Bengtson, V. 1979. "Ethnicity and Aging: Problems and Issues in Current Social Science Inquiry." Pp. 9–31 in *Ethnicity and Aging: Theory, Research, and Policy,* ed. D. E. Gelfand and A. J. Kutzik. New York: Springer.

Bengtson, V., C. Rosenthal, and L. Burton. 1990. "Families and Aging: Diversity and Heterogeneity." Pp. 263–80 in *Handbook of Aging and the Social Sciences,* ed. R. H. Binstock and L. K. George. 3d ed. San Diego: Academic Press.

Benjamin, A. E. 1986. "Determinants of State Variations in Home Health Utilization and Expenditures under Medicare." *Medical Care* 24: 535–47.

Benson, Ezra T. 1989. "To the Elderly in the Church." *Ensign* 19 (November): 4.

Berdes, Celia. 2001. "Sense of Community in Residential Facilities for the Elderly." Ph.D. diss., Northwestern University.

Berdes, Celia, and Adam A. Zych. 1996. "The Quality of Life of Polish Immigrant and Polish American Ethnic Elderly." *Polish American Studies* 53, no. 1: 17–62.

———. Forthcoming. "Subjective Quality of Life of Polish, Polish Immigrant, and Polish American Elderly." *International Journal of Aging and Human Development.*

Berger, R., and J. Kelley.1992. "The Older Gay Man." Pp. 121–29 in *Positively Gay: New Approaches to Gay and Lesbian Life,* ed. B. Berzon. Berkeley, Calif.: Celestial Arts.

Biegel, D., and Z. Harel. 1994. "Diverse Jewish Aged: Challenges for Program Planning and Service Delivery." Pp. 103–22 in *Jewish Aged in the United States and Israel: Diversity, Programs, and Services,* ed. Z. Harel, D. Biegel, and D. Guttmann. New York: Springer.

Billingsley, A. 1999. *Mighty like a River: The Black Church and Social Reform.* New York: Oxford University Press.

Binstock, R. H. 1996. "The Politics of Enacting Long-Term Care Insurance." Pp. 215–38 in *The Future of Long-Term Care: Social and Policy Issues,* ed. R. H. Binstock, L. E. Cluff, and O. von Mering. Baltimore, Md.: Johns Hopkins University Press.

———. 1997. "The 1996 Election: Older Voters and Implications for Policies on Aging." *Gerontologist* 37, no. 1: 15–19.

———. 1998. "Introduction: The Financing and Organization of Long-Term Care." Pp. 1–34 in *Public and Private Responsibilities in Long-Term Care: Finding the Balance,* ed. L. C. Walker, E. H. Bradley, and T. Wetle. Baltimore, Md.: Johns Hopkins University Press.

———. 1999. "Challenges to U.S. Policies on Aging in the New Millennium." *Hallym International Journal of Aging* 1, no. 1: 3–13.

Birenbaum, A. 1995. *Putting Health Care on the National Agenda.* Westport, Conn.: Praeger.

Black, S. A., K. S. Markides, and T. Q. Miller. 1998. "Correlates of Depressive Symptomatology among Older Community-Dwelling Mexican Americans: The Hispanic EPESE." *Journal of Gerontology: Social Sciences* 53, no. 4 (July): 198–208.

Blakemore, K., and M. Boneham. 1994. *Age, Race, and Ethnicity: A Comparative Approach.* Philadelphia: Open University Press.

Blazer, D., L. Landerman, G. Fillenbaum, and R. Horner. 1995. "Health Services Access and Use among Older Adults in North Carolina: Urban and Rural Residents." *American Journal of Public Health* 85: 1384–90.

Blejwas, Stanislaus. 1981. "Old and New Polonias: Tension within an Ethnic Community." *Polish American Studies* 38, no. 2: 55–83.

———. 1995. "The Evolving Polish Parish in the United States: St. Stanislaus Kostka, Bristol, Connecticut." *Analecta Cracoviensia* 27: 383–94.

Blenkner, M. 1965. "Social Work in Family Relationships in Later Life." In *Social Structure and the Family: Intergenerational Relations,* ed. E. Shanas and G. Stribe. Englewood Cliffs, N.J.: Prentice Hall.

Boland, Clara S. 1998. "Parish Nursing." *Journal of Holistic Nursing* 16, no. 3 (September): 355–69.

Bott, E. 1971. *Family and Social Network.* New York: Free Press.

Braun, Kathryn L., and Colette V. Browne. 1998. "Perceptions of Dementia, Caregiving, and Help Seeking among Asian and Pacific Islander Americans." *Health and Social Work* 23, no. 4: 262–74.

Braun, Kathryn L., and R. Nichols. 1997. "Death and Dying in Four Asian American Cultures: A Descriptive Study." *Death Studies* 21: 327–60.

Brody, E. M. 1985. "Parent Care as Normative Stress." *Gerontologist* 25: 1–29.

———. 1990. *Women in the Middle: Their Parent Care Years.* New York: Springer.

———. 1995. "Prospects for Family Caregiving: Response to Change, Continuity and Diversity." In *Family Caregiving in an Aging Society,* ed. R. Kane and J. Penrod. Thousand Oaks, Calif.: Sage.

Brody, E. M, P. T. Johnsen, M. C. Fulcomorend, and A. M. Lang. 1983. "Women's Changing Roles and Help to Elderly Parents: Attitudes of Three Generations of Women." *Journal of Gerontology: Social Sciences* 38: 597–607.

Brooks, C. 2000. "In the Twilight Zone between Black and White: Japanese American Resettlement and Community in Chicago, 1942–1945." *Journal of American History* 86, no. 4: 1655–87.

Broom, L., and J. I. Kitsuse. 1973. *The Managed Casualty: The Japanese-American Family in World War II.* Berkeley and Los Angeles: University of California Press.

Brower, H. T. 1995. "Allowing for Same-Sex Preferences." *Journal of Gerontological Nursing* 21, no. 9: 5–6.

Brown, L. S. 1989. "New Voices, New Visions: Toward a Lesbian/Gay Paradigm for Psychology." *Psychology of Women* 13, no. 4: 445–59.

Browne, Colette V. 1998. *Women, Feminism, and Aging.* New York: Springer.

Browne, Colette, and Alice Broderick. 1994. "Asian and Pacific Island Elders: Issues for Social Work Practice and Education." *Social Work* 39, no. 3: 252–59.

Brozek, Andrzej. 1985. *Polish Americans: 1854–1939.* Trans. Wojciech Worsztynowicz. Warsaw: Interpress.

Brubaker, T. H., and A. K. Roberto. 1993. "Family Life Education for the Later Years." *Family Relations* 42, no. 2: 212–21. .

Bukowczyk, John J. 1987. *And My Children Did Not Know Me: A History of Polish-Americans.* Bloomington: Indiana University Press.

Burr, J. A., and J. E. Mutchler. 1992. "The Living Arrangement of Unmarried Elderly Hispanic Females." *Demography* 29, no. 1: 93–112.

———. 1993. "Nativity, Acculturation, and Economic Status: Explanations of Asian American Living Arrangements in Later Life." *Journal of Gerontology: Social Sciences* 48, no. 2: 55–63.

Burton, L. M., and R. Jayakody. In press. "Rethinking Family Structures and Single Parenthood: Implications for Future Studies of African American Families and Children." In *Family and Child Well-Being: Research and Data Needs,* ed. A. Thornton. Ann Arbor: University of Michigan Press.

Burton, L., J. Kasper, A. Shore, K. Cagney, T. LaVeist, C. Cubbin, and P. German. 1995. "The Structure of Informal Care: Are There Differences by Race?" *Gerontologist* 35: 744–52.

Butler, J. S. 1984. "Social Research and Scholarly Interpretation." *Society* 24: 13–18.

Calasanti, Toni M., and Anna M. Zajicek. 1997. "Gender, the State, and Constructing the Old as Dependent: Lessons from the Economic Transition in Poland." *Gerontologist* 37: 452–61.

Calderón, E. 1984. "Relaciones interpersonales y satisfacción de vida de las viudas enve- jecientes." Ph.D. diss. Graduate School of Social Work, University of Puerto Rico.

Caldwell, C. H., L. M. Chatters, A. Billingsley, and R. J. Taylor. 1995. "Church-Based Support Programs for Elderly Black Adults: Congregational and Clergy Characteris- tics." Pp. 306–24 in *Aging, Spirituality, and Religion: A Handbook*, ed. M. A. Kimble, S. H. McFadden, J. W. Ellor, and J. J. Seeber. Minneapolis: Fortress Press.

Carp, Frances M., and Eunice Kataoka. 1976. "Health Care Problems of the Elderly of San Francisco's Chinatown." *Gerontologist* 16, no. 1: 30–38.

Caserta, M., D. Lund, S. Wright, and P. Redburn. 1987. "Caregiving to Dementia Patients: Use of Community Services." *Gerontologist* 27: 209–13.

Castro, F. G., M. K. Cota, and C. V. Santos. 1998. "Health Promotion in Latino Popula- tions." Pp. 137–68 in *Promoting Health in Multicultural Populations: A Handbook for Practitioners*, ed. R. M. Huff and M. V. Kline. Thousand Oaks, Calif.: Sage.

Cavan, R. S., E. Burgess, and R. J. Havighurst. 1949. *Personal Adjustment in Old Age*. Chicago: Social Research Associated.

Centro de Investigaciones Demográficas. 1998. *Número Especial* 3, no. 2 (October). San Juan: University of Puerto Rico, Graduate School of Public Health.

Chaimowitz, G. 1991. "Homophobia among Psychiatric Residents, Family Practice Resi- dents, and Psychiatric Faculty." *Canadian Journal of Psychiatry* 36: 206–9.

Chan, Kwok B. 1983. "Coping with Aging and Managing Self-Identity: The Social World of Elderly Chinese Women." *Canadian Ethnic Studies* 15, no. 3: 36–50.

Chang, Grace. 2000. *Disposable Domestics: Immigrant Workers in the Global Economy*. Boston: South End Press.

Char, W. F., W. S. Tseng, K. Y. Lum, and J. Hsu. 1980. "The Chinese." Pp. 53–72 in *Peo- ple and Cultures of Hawaii: A Psychocultural Profile*, ed. J. F. McDermott, W. S. Tseng, and T. W. Maretzki. Honolulu: University Press of Hawaii.

Chatters, L. M., R. J. Taylor, and J. S. Jackson. 1986. "Size and Composition of the Infor- mal Helper Network of Elderly Blacks." *Journal of Gerontology: Social Sciences* 40: 605–14.

Chatters, L. M., R. J. Taylor, and R. Jayakody. 1994. "Fictive Kinship Relations in Black Extended Families." *Journal of Comparative Family Studies* 25: 297–312.

Chen, Chiung Hwang, and Ethan Yorganson. 1999. "Those Amazing Mormons: The Media's Construction of Latter-day Saints as a Model Minority." *Dialogue: A Journal of Mormon Thought* 32 (Summer): 107–32.

Chen, Helen. 1984. "Chinese Immigration into the United States: An Analysis of Changes in Immigration Policies." Pp. 44–47 in *The Chinese American Experience: Papers from the Second National Conference on Chinese American Studies*, ed. Genny Lim. San Francisco: Chinese Historical Society of America and the Chinese Culture Foundation of San Francisco.

Chen, Jack. 1980. *The Chinese in America*. San Francisco: Harper & Row.

Chen, Pei Ngor. 1979. "A Study of Chinese-American Elderly Residing in Hotel Rooms." *Social Casework* 60, no. 2: 89–95.

Cheung, Lucia, Eric Yim San, Doman Lum, Tze Yee Tang, and How Boa Yau. 1980. "The Chinese Elderly and Family Structure: Implications for Health Care." *Public Health Reports* 95, no. 5: 491–95.

Cheung, Monit. 1989. "Elderly Chinese Living in the United States: Assimilation or Ad- justment?" *Social Work* 34, no. 5: 457–61.

Chierici, R. M. 1991. *Demele 'Making It.'* New York: AMS Press.

Ching, J. W. J., J. F. McDermott, C. Fukunaga, and E. Yanagida. 1995. "Perception of Family Values and Roles among Japanese Americans: Clinical Considerations." *American Journal of Orthopsychiatry* 65: 216–24.

Chinn, Thomas, H. Mark Lai, and Philip Choy. 1969. *A History of the Chinese in California: A Syllabus.* San Francisco: Chinese Historical Society of America.

Choi, Jae Suck. 1970. "Comparative Study on the Traditional Families in Korea, Japan, and China." In *Families in East and West,* ed. R. Hill and R. Koenig. Paris: Mouton.

Cicirelli, V. G. 1983. "Adult Children's Attachment and Helping Behavior to Elderly Parents: A Path Model." *Journal of Marriage and the Family* 45: 815–24.

Clark, D. O., S. M. Mungai, T. E. Stump, and F. D. Wolinsky. 1997. "Prevalence and Impact of Risk Factors for Lower Body Difficulty among Mexican Americans, African Americans, and Whites." *Journal of Gerontology: Medicine* 52, no. 2 (March): 97–105.

Clark, W. E., and M. Gordon. 1979. "Distance, Closeness, and Recency of Kin Contact in Urban Ireland." *Journal of Comparative Family Studies* 10: 271–75.

Clayton, G., W. Dudley, W. Patterson, L. Lawhorn, L. Poon, M. Johnson, and P. Martin. 1989. "The Influence of Rural/Urban Residence on Health in the Oldest-Old." *International Journal of Aging and Human Development* 36: 65–89.

Cleary, Paul D., and Harold W. Demone Jr. 1988. "Health and Social Service Needs in a Northeastern Metropolitan Area: Ethnic Group Differences." *Journal of Sociology and Social Welfare* 15, no. 4: 63–76.

Cogill, D. 1974. "Aging and Modernization: A Revision of the Theory." In *Late Life Communities and Environmental Policies,* ed. J. Gubrium. Springfield, Ill.: Thomas.

Cohler, Bertram J., and Morton A. Lieberman. 1979. "Personality Change across the Second Half of Life: Findings from a Study of Irish, Italian, and Polish-American Men and Women." Pp. 227–45 in *Ethnicity and Aging: Theory, Research, and Policy,* ed. D. E. Gelfand and A. J. Kutzik. New York: Springer.

Colen, J. L., and R. L. McNeely. 1983. "Minority Aging and Knowledge in the Social Professions: Overview of a Problem." Pp. 15–23 in *Aging in Minority Groups,* ed. R. L. McNeely and J. L. Colen. Beverly Hills, Calif.: Sage.

Comhaire-Sylvain, S. 1975. "Vieillir à Port-au-Prince." *Ethnographie* 69: 61–80; 70: 127–86.

Commonwealth Fund Commission. 1989. *Poverty and Poor Health among Elderly Hispanic Americans.* Baltimore: Commonwealth Fund Commission on Elderly People Living Alone.

Commonwealth of Puerto Rico, Junta de Planificación. 1994. "Informe económico de la población de edad avanzada." *Boletín Social* (San Juan) 2, no. 3.

Constantakos, Chrysie M. 1980. *The American-Greek Subculture: Processes of Continuity.* New York: Arno Press.

———. 1993. "Attitudes of Filial Obligation toward Aging Parents: A Greek American Perspective." *Journal of Modern Hellenism* 10: 1–36.

Constantinou, S. T. 1989. "Dominant Themes in Intergenerational Differences in Ethnicity: The Greek Americans." *Sociological Focus* 22: 99–117.

Cool, Linda Evers. 1987. "The Effects of Social Class and Ethnicity on the Aging Process." Pp. 263–82 in *The Elderly as Modern Pioneers,* ed. Philip Silverman. Bloomington: Indiana University Press.

Coontz, S. 1992. *The Way We Never Were.* New York: Basic Books.

Council on Scientific Affairs. 1996. "Health Care Needs of Gay Men and Lesbians in the United States." *JAMA* 275, no. 17: 1354–59.

Covello, L. 1967. *The Social Background of the Italo-American School Child.* Leiden: E. J. Brill.

Coward, R. T., S. J. Cutler, and R. A. Mullens. 1990. "Residential Differences in the Composition of Helping Networks of Impaired Elders." *Family Relations* 39: 44–50.

Coward, R. T., G. R. Lee, and J. W. Dwyer. 1993. "The Family Relations of Rural Elders." Pp. 216–31 in *Aging in Rural America,* ed. C. N. Bull. Newbury Park, Calif.: Sage.

Coward, R. T., D. K. McLaughlin, R. P. Duncan, and C. N. Bull. 1994. "An Overview of Health and Aging in Rural America." Pp. 1–32 in *Health Services for Rural Elders,* ed. R. T. Coward, C. N. Bull, G. Kukulka, and J. M. Galliher. New York: Springer.

Cowill, D. O. 1972. "A Theory of Aging in Cross-Cultural Perspective." Pp. 1–13 in *Aging and Modernization,* ed. D. O. Cowill and L. D. Holmes. New York: Appleton-Century-Crofts.

Cowill, D. O., and L. D. Holmes, eds. 1972. *Aging and Modernization.* New York: Appleton-Century-Crofts.

Cox, D. 1991. "Social Work Education in the Asia Pacific Region." *Asia Pacific Journal of Social Work* 1: 6–14.

Craig, C. 1994. "Community Determinants of Health for Rural Elderly." *Public Health Nursing* 11, no. 4: 242–46.

Cronin, C. 1970. *The Sting of Change: Sicilians in Sicily and Australia.* Chicago: University of Chicago Press.

Crouch, B. M. 1972. "Age and Institutional Support." 1972. *Journal of Gerontology: Social Sciences* 27: 524–29.

Cruz-López, M., and F. Pearson. 1985. "The Support Needs and Resources of Puerto Rican Elders." *Gerontologist* 25, no. 5: 483–87.

Cubillos, H. L. 1987. *The Hispanic Elderly: A Demographic Profile.* Washington, D.C.: National Council of La Raza.

Cuellar, I., L. C. Harris, and R. Jasso. 1980. "An Acculturation Scale for Mexican-American Normal and Clinical Populations." *Hispanic Journal of Behavioral Sciences* 2: 199–217.

Cuellar, Jose B., and John Weeks. 1980. *Minority Elderly Americans: The Assessment of Needs and Equitable Receipt of Public Benefits as a Prototype in Area Agencies on Aging (Final Report).* San Diego: Allied Home Health Association.

Cumming, E., and W. E. Henry. 1961. *Growing Old: The Process of Disengagement.* New York: Basic Books.

Curb, D. J., N. E. Aluli, B. J. Huang, D. S. Sharp, B. L. Rodriguez, C. M. Burchfiel, and D. Chiu. 1996. "Hypertension in Elderly Japanese Americans and Adult Native Hawaiians." *Public Health Reports* 111 (supp. 2): 53–55.

Curriculum Supplement: Rural Mental Health Training Project. 1995. Tucson: Arizona Center on Aging.

Cu'u, Long Giang, and Anh Toan. 1967. *Nguoi Viet dat Viet* (The people and the land of Vietnam). Saigon: Nam Chi Tung Thu.

Damron-Rodriguez, J., and J. E. Lubben. 2000. "Community Health Care in Aging Societies." Paper presented at the International Meeting on Community Health Care in Ageing Societies, sponsored by the World Health Organization Centre for Health Development, Kobe, Shanghai, China.

Dang, Janet. 1999. "Talkin' about My (Older) Generation: Baby Boomer Jeanette Takamura Leads Agency That Soon Will Impact Her Peers." *Asian Week* 41, no. 4 (September 22): 10.

Dao, Anh Duy. 1961. *Viet Nam van hoa su cuong* (A general history of Vietnamese culture). Saigon: Nha Xuat Ban Bon Phuong.

Dávila, A. L., and M. Sánchez-Ayendez. 1996. "El envejecimiento de la población de Puerto Rico y sus repercusiones en los sistemas informales de apoyo." In *Dinámica demográfica y cambio social,* ed. C. Welti. Mexico City: Ediciones de Buena Tinta.

Davison, G., and S. Friedman. 1981. "Sexual Orientation Stereotype in the Distortion of Clinical Judgment." *Journal of Homosexuality* 6, no. 3: 37–44.

Day, A. T. 1985. "Who Cares? Demographic Trends Challenge Family Norms." *Population Trends and Family Policy* 9: 1–15.

Deevey, S. 1990. "Older Lesbian Women: An Invisible Minority." *Journal of Gerontological Nursing* 16, no. 5: 35–39.

Delgado, M. 1995. "Puerto Rican Elders and Natural Support Systems: Implications for Human Services." *Journal of Gerontological Social Work* 18, no. 2: 192–200.

Delgado, M., and D. Delgado. 1982. "Natural Support Systems: A Source of Strength in Hispanic Communities." *Social Work* 27, no. 1: 83–90.

Delgado, M., and S. Tennstedt. 1997. "Puerto Rican Sons as Primary Caregivers of Elderly Parents." *Social Work* 42, no. 2: 125–34.

Dhoomer, S. S. 1991. "Toward an Effective Response to the Needs of Asian-Americans." *Journal of Multicultural Social Work* 1, no. 2: 65–82.

Diamond, T. 1992. *Making Gold Gray: Narratives of Nursing Home Care.* Chicago: University of Chicago Press.

Dickerson-Putman, Jeanette. 1997. "History, Community Context, and the Perception of Old Age in a Rural Irish Town." Pp. 364–73 in *The Cultural Context of Aging: Worldwide Perspectives,* ed. Jay Sokolovsky. Westport, Conn.: Bergin & Garvey.

Dilworth-Anderson, P. 1996. "Rethinking Family Development: Critical Conceptual Issues in the Study of Diverse Groups." *Journal of Social and Personal Relationships* 13: 325–34.

Dilworth-Anderson, P., and L. M. Burton. 1999. "Critical Issues in Understanding Family Support and Older Minorities." Pp. 93–105 in *Full Color of Aging: Facts, Goals, and Recommendations for America's Diverse Elders,* ed. T. P. Miles. Washington, D.C.: Gerontological Society of America.

Dilworth-Anderson P., L. M. Burton, and W. L. Turner. 1993. "The Importance of Values in the Study of Culturally Diverse Families." *Family Relations* 42, no. 3: 238–48.

Dilworth-Anderson, P., S. Williams, and T. Cooper. 1999. "Family Caregiving to Elderly African Americans: Caregiver Types and Structures." *Journal of Gerontology: Social Sciences* 54: 237–41.

Dilworth-Anderson, P., P. Goodwin, S. Williams, and T. Cooper. In preparation. "The Physical Health Effects of Caregiving among African American Caregivers: A Longitudinal Analysis." University of North Carolina at Greensboro.

Diner, Hasia R. 1983. *Erin's Daughters in America: Irish Immigrant Women in the Nineteenth Century.* Baltimore, Md.: Johns Hopkins University Press.

Dinkel, R. 1944. "Attitudes of Children toward Supporting Aged Parents." *American Sociological Review* 9: 370–79.

Doi, T. 1977. *The Anatomy of Dependence.* Tokyo: Kodansha International.

Dorfman, R., K. Walter, P. Burke, and K. Hardin. 1995. "Issues and Challenges in Working with Lesbian Women and Gay Men." *Counseling Psychologist* 19, no. 2: 157–76.

Dornbusch, S. M., and M. H. Strober, eds. 1988. *Feminism, Children, and the New Families.* New York: Guilford.

Du Bois, B. C., and E. P. C. Stanford. 2000. "Multicultural Managed Care: Focus Group Results."

Duke, James T., and Barry L. Johnson. 1998. "The Religiosity of Mormon Men and Women through the Life Cycle." In *Latter-day Saint Social Life: Social Research on the LDS Church and Its Membership,* ed. James T. Duke. Provo, Utah: Religious Study Center, Specialized Monograph Service.

Duncan, B., and O. Duncan. 1968. "Minorities and the Process of Stratification." *American Sociological Review* 33: 356–64.

Dunkel-Schetter, C., and T. L. Bennett. 1990. "Differentiating the Cognitive and Behavioral Aspects of Social Support." Pp. 267–97 in *Social Support: An Interactional View,* ed. B. R. Sarason, I. G. Sarason, and G. R. Pierce. New York: John Wiley & Sons.

Dunn, Paul H. 1983. "Honour Thy Father and Thy Mother." *Ensign* 13 (November): 25–26.

Durnbaugh, Donald, ed. 1974. *Every Need Supplied: Mutual Aid and Christian Community in the Free Churches, 1525–1675.* Philadelphia: Temple University Press.

Dwyer, Jeffrey W., and R. T. Coward, eds. 1992. *Gender, Families, and Eldercare.* Newbury Park, Calif.: Sage.

Eleazer, G. Paul, Carlton A. Hornung, Carolyn B. Egbert, John R. Egbert, Catherine Eng, Jennifer Hedgepeth, Robert McCann, Harry Strothers, Marc Sapir, Ming Wei, and Malissa Wilson. 1996. "The Relationship between Ethnicity and Advance Directives in a Frail Older Population." *Journal of the American Geriatric Society* 44: 938–43.

Eliason, M. J. 1996. "Caring for the Lesbian, Gay, or Bisexual Patient: Issues for Critical Care Nurses." *Critical Care Nursing Quarterly* 19, no. 1: 65–72.

Elliot, K. S., M. Di Minno, D. Lam, and A. M. Tu. 1996. "Working with Chinese Families in the Context of Dementia." Pp. 89–108 in *Ethnicity and the Dementias,* ed. Gwen Yeo and D. Gallagher-Thompson. Bristol, Pa.: Taylor & Francis.

Elo, I. T. 1997. "Adult Mortality among Asian Americans and Pacific Islanders: A Review of the Evidence." Pp. 41–78 in *Minorities, Aging, and Health,* ed. K. S. Markides and M. R. Miranda. Thousand Oaks, Calif.: Sage.

Enstrom, James E. 1998. "Health Practices and Cancer Mortality among Active California Mormons, 1980–93." In *Latter-day Saint Social Life: Social Research on the LDS Church and Its Membership,* ed. James T. Duke Provo, Utah: Religious Study Center, Specialized Monograph Service.

Erdmans, Mary. 1995. "Immigrants and Ethnics: Conflict and Identity in Polish Chicago." *Sociological Quarterly* 36, no. 1: 175–95.

———. 1996a. "Home Care Workers: Polish Immigrants Caring for American Elderly." *Current Research on Occupations and Professions: A Research Annual* 9: 267–92. Greenwich, Conn.: JAI Press.

———. 1996b. "Illegal Immigrant Home Care Workers: The Non-Market Conditions of Job Satisfaction." *Przeglad Polonijny* (Krakow, Poland: Jagiellonian University) 6.

———. 1998a. *Opposite Poles: Immigrants and Ethnics in Polish Chicago, 1976–1990.* University Park: Pennsylvania State University Press.

———. 1998b. "The Transformation of the Polish National Alliance: From Immigrant to

Ethnic Organization." In *Ethnicity, Culture, City: Polish-Americans in the USA—Cultural Aspects of Urban Life 1870–1950 in Comparative Perspective*, ed. Thomas Gladsky, Adam Walaszek, and Malgorzata M. Wawrykiewicz. Warsaw: Oficyna Akademicka.

Espino, D. V., and D. Maldonado. 1990. "Hypertension and Acculturation in Elderly Mexican Americans: Results from 1982–84 Hispanic HANES." *Journal of Gerontology: Medicine* 45: 209–13.

Fahey, Tony, and Peter Murray. 1994. *Health and Autonomy among the Over-Sixty-fives in Ireland*. Dublin: National Council for the Elderly, report 39.

Fanning, Charles. 1997. *The Exiles of Erin: Nineteenth-Century Irish-American Fiction*. Chester Springs, Pa.: Dufour Editions.

Fanning, Patricia J. 2000. Survey of Irish American attitudes toward elder care.

Farrell, James T. 1940. *Father and Son*. New York: Vanguard.

———. 1953. *The Face of Time*. New York: Vanguard.

Fassinger, Ruth E. "The Hidden Minority: Issues and Challenges in Working with Lesbian Women and Gay Men." *Counseling Psychologist* 19 (April): 27.

Fennell, G., C. Phillipson, and H. Evers. 1988. *The Sociology of Old Age*. Philadelphia: Open University Press.

Ferrara, Peter J. 1993. "Social Security and Taxes." In *The Amish and the State*, ed. Donald B. Kraybill. Baltimore, Md.: Johns Hopkins University Press.

Fineman, M. A. 1995. *The Neutered Mother, the Sexual Family, and Other Twentieth-Century Tragedies*. New York: Routledge.

Fisher, Albert, 1978. "Mormon Welfare Programs: Past and Present." *Social Science Journal* 15 (April): 77–99.

Fitzpatrick, C., and C. Barry. 1990. "Cultural Differences in Family Communication about Duchenne Muscular Dystrophy." *Developmental Medicine and Child Neurology* 32, no. 11: 967–73.

Fitzpatrick, J. 1981. *The Puerto Rican Family*. Pp. 189–215 in *Ethnic Families in America*, ed. C. Mindel, R. Habenstein and R. Wesley. 2d ed. New York: Elsevier North Holland.

Foner, N. 1994. *The Caregiving Dilemma*. Berkeley and Los Angeles: University of California Press.

Foster, B., J. Susman, K. Mueller, A. Bowman, and K. Lunt. 1994. "Delivering Services to the Rural Elderly: A Study of Policy Implementation." *Journal of Case Management* 3: 13–20.

Franklin, D. L. 1997. *Ensuring Inequality: The Structural Transformation of the African American Family*. New York: Oxford University Press.

Frazier, E. F. 1939. *The Negro Family in the United States*. Chicago: University of Chicago Press.

Fredman, L., M. P. Daly, and A. M. Lazur. 1995. "Burden among White and Black Caregivers to Elderly Adults." *Journal of Gerontology: Social Sciences* 50: 110–18.

Freudenberger Jett, K. M., R. T. Coward, N. E. Schoenberg, R. P. Duncan, and J. Dwyer. "The Influence of Community Context on the Decision to Enter a Nursing Home." *Journal of Aging Studies* 10: 237–54.

Friend, R. 1991. "Older Lesbian and Gay People: A Theory of Successful Aging." *Journal of Homosexuality* 20, no. 3/4: 99–118.

Fugita, S., K. L. Ito, J. Abe, and D. T. Takeuchi. 1991. "Japanese Americans." Pp. 61–96 in *Handbook of Social Services for Asian and Pacific Islanders,* ed. N. Mokuau. New York: Greenwood.

Fuji, Sharon M. 1976. "Elderly Asian Americans and Use of Public Services." *Social Casework* 57, no. 3: 202–7.

Fung, Ling-Wai. 1994. "Implementing the Patient Self-Determination Act (PSDA): How to Effectively Engage Chinese-American Elderly Persons in the Decision of Advance Directives." *Journal of Gerontological Social Work* 22, nos. 1–2: 161–91.

Fyans, J. Thomas. 1979. "Priesthood Administration of Welfare Services." *Ensign* 9 (November): 86–88.

Gallup, G. 1996. *Religion in America.* Princeton, N.J.: Princeton Religion Research Center.

Gallup, G., and J. Castelli. 1989. *The People's Religion: American Faith in the Nineties.* New York: Macmillan.

Gambino, R. 1974. *Blood of My Blood.* New York: Doubleday.

Ganguli, M., A. Fox, J. Gilby, and S. Belle. 1996. "Characteristics of Rural Homebound Older Adults: A Community-Based Study." *Journal of the American Geriatrics Society* 44, no. 4: 363–70.

Ganguli, M., B. Mulsant, S. Richards, G. Stoehr, and A. Mendelsohn. 1997. "Antidepressant Use over Time in a Rural Older Adult Population: The MOVIES Project." *Journal of the American Geriatrics Society* 45: 1501–3.

Gannon, L. G. 1999. *Women and Aging: Transcending the Myths.* New York: Routledge.

Gans, H. 1962. *Urban Villagers: Group and Class in the Life of Italian Americans.* New York: Free Press.

Garcia, A. 1990. "Social and Economic Well-Being of Elderly Minorities." In *Diversity in an Aging America: Challenges for the 1990s,* ed. S. Schoenrock, J. Roberts, and J. Hyde. San Diego, Calif.: National Resource Center on Minority Aging Populations.

Gardner, John W., and Joseph L. Lyon, "Cancer in Utah Mormon Men by Lay Priesthood Level." *American Journal of Epidemiology* 116: 1161–88.

Garnets, L., and A. D'Augelli. 1994. "Empowering Lesbian and Gay Communities: A Call for Collaboration with Community Psychology." *American Journal of Community Psychology* 22, no. 4: 447–70.

Gelfand, D. E. 1982. *Aging: The Ethnic Factor.* Boston: Little, Brown.

Gelfand, D. E., and C. M. Barresi. 1987a. "Current Perspectives in Ethnicity and Aging." In *Ethnic Dimensions of Aging,* ed. D. E. Gelfand and C. M. Barresi. New York: Springer.

———, eds. 1987b. *Ethnic Dimensions of Aging.* New York: Springer.

Gelfand, D. E., and Jody Olsen. 1979. "Aging in the Jewish Family and the Mormon Family." In *Ethnicity and Aging: Theory, Research, and Policy,* ed. D. E. Gelfand and A. J. Kutzik. New York: Springer.

Gelfand, D. E., and A. J. Kutzik, eds. 1979. *Ethnicity and Aging: Theory, Research, and Policy.* New York: Springer.

Gentry, S. 1992. "Caring for Lesbians in a Homophobic Society." *Health Care for Women International* 13: 173–80.

George, L. K., and L. P. Gwyther. 1986. "Caregiver Well-Being: A Multidimensional Examination of Family Caregivers of Demented Adults." *Gerontologist* 26: 253–59.

Gerbert, B., B. Maguire, and T. Bleecker. 1991. "Primary Care Physicians and AIDS." *JAMA* 226: 2837–42.

Glazer, N., and D. Moynihan. 1963. *Beyond the Melting Pot.* Cambridge: M.I.T. Press.

Glenn, Evelyn Nakano. 1983. "Split Household, Small Producer, and Dual Wage Earner: An Analysis of Chinese-American Family Strategies." *Journal of Marriage and the Family* 45: 35–46.

———. 1992. "From Servitude to Service Work: Historical Continuities in the Racial Division of Paid Reproductive Work." *Journal of Women in Culture and Society* 18, no. 1: 1–43.

Glicksman, A., and T. Cox. 1994. "Jewish Aged in the United States: Socio-Demographic and Socioeconomic Characteristics." Pp. 23–46 in *Jewish Aged in the United States and Israel: Diversity, Programs, and Services,* ed. Z. Harel, D. Biegel, and D. Guttmann. New York: Springer.

Goldscheider, C. 1986. *The American Jewish Community: Social Science Research and Policy Implications.* Atlanta: Scholars Press.

Goode, William J. 1963. *World Revolution and Family Patterns.* Glencoe, Ill.: Free Press.

Goodwin, J. S., S. A. Black, and S. Satish. 1999. "Aging versus Disease: The Opinions of Older Black, Hispanic, and Non-Hispanic White Americans about the Causes and Treatment of Common Medical Conditions." *Journal of the American Geriatrics Society* 47, no. 8 (August): 973–79.

Gordon, A. K. 1995. "Deterrents to Access and Service for Blacks and Hispanics: The Medicare Hospice Benefit, Health Care Utilization, and Cultural Barriers." *Hospice Journal* 10, no. 2: 65–83.

Gordon, Michael, Richard Vaughan, and Brendan Whelan. 1981. "The Irish Elderly Who Live Alone: Patterns of Contact and Aid." *Journal of Comparative Family Studies* 12, no. 4 (Autumn): 493–508.

Gould, J. 1999. *Dutiful Daughters: Caring for Our Parents As They Grow Old.* Seattle, Wash.: Seal Press.

Gould, K. 1988. "Asian and Pacific Islanders: Myth and Reality." *Social Work* 33: 142–47.

Granovetter, M. S. 1973. "The Strength of Weak Ties." *American Journal of Sociology* 78: 1360–80.

Grant, Heber J. 1936. "Conference Reports." *Ensign* (October): 3.

Graves, A. B., R. Lakshminarayan, J. D. Bowen, W. C. McCormick, W.C., S. M. McCurry, and E. B. Larson. 1999. "Cognitive Decline and Japanese Culture in a Cohort of Older Japanese Americans in King County, Washington: The Kame Project." *Journal of Gerontology: Social Sciences* 54: 154–61.

Greek Orthodox Archdiocese of America. 1999. *1999 Yearbook,* New York.

Greeley, Andrew M. 1972. *That Most Distressful Nation: The Taming of the American Irish.* Chicago: Quadrangle Books.

———. 1974. *Ethnicity in the United States.* New York: John Wiley & Sons.

———. 1981. *The Irish Americans.* New York: Harper & Row.

Greene, V. L., and D. J. Monahan. 1984. "Comparative Utilization of Community-Based Long-Term Care Services by Hispanic and Anglo Elderly in a Case Management System." *Journal of Gerontology: Social Sciences* 39, no. 6 (November): 730–35.

Gross, L. 1999. "Contested Closets: The Politics and Ethics of Outing." Pp. 421–28 in *On Lesbians and Gay Men in Media, Society, and Politics,* ed. L. Gross and J. Woods. New York: Columbia University Press.

Grube, J. 1991. "Natives and Settlers: An Ethnographic Note on Early Interactions of

Older Homosexual Men with Younger Gay Liberationists." Pp. 119–35 in *Gay Mid-Life and Maturity,* ed. J. A. Lee. New York: Haworth Press.

Guttmann, D. 1979. "Use of Informal and Formal Supports by White Ethnic Aged." Pp. 246–62 in *Ethnicity and Aging: Theory, Research, and Policy,* ed. D. E. Gelfand and A. J. Kutzik. New York: Springer.

Hamman, R. F., J. A. Marshall, J. Baxter, L. B. Kahn, E. J. Mayer, M. Orleans, J. R. Murphy, and D. C. Lezotte. 1989. "Methods and Prevalence of Non-Insulin-Dependent Diabetes in a Biethnic Colorado Population: The San Luis Valley Diabetes Study." *American Journal of Epidemiology* 129, no. 2: 295–311.

Hamman, R. F., C. L. Mulgrew, J. Baxter, S. M. Shetterly, C. Swenson, and N. E. Morgenstern. 1999. "Methods and Prevalence of ADL Limitations in Hispanic and Non-Hispanic White Subjects in Rural Colorado: The San Luis Valley Health and Aging Study." *Annals of Epidemiology* 9, no. 4 (May): 225–35.

Hammond, J. 1985. "Analysis of County-Level Data Concerning the Use of Medicare Home Health Benefits." *Public Health Reports* 100: 48–55.

Handlin, Oscar. 1979. *Boston's Immigrants: A Study in Acculturation.* Cambridge: Harvard University Press.

Hanson, B. 1996. "The Violence We Face as Lesbians and Gay Men: The Landscape Both outside and inside Our Communities." *Journal of Gay and Lesbian Social Services* 4, no. 2: 95–113.

Harel, Z. 1986. "Ethnicity and Aging: Implications for Service Organizations." In *European American Elderly: A Guide to Practice,* ed. C. Hays, R. Kalish, and D. Guttmann. New York: Springer.

———. 1990. "Ethnicity and Aging: Implications for the Jewish Community." *Contemporary Jewry* 11, no. 2: 77–91.

Harel, Z., and L. Noelker. 1995. "Severe Vulnerability and Long-Term Care." Pp. 5–24 in *Matching People and Services in Long-Term Care,* ed. Z. Harel and R. Dunkle. New York: Springer.

Harel, Z., L. Noelker, and B. F. Blake. 1985. "Comprehensive Services for the Aged: Theoretical and Empirical Perspectives." *Gerontologist* 25, no. 6: 644–49.

Harel, Z., E. A. McKinney, and M. Williams. 1987. "Aging, Ethnicity, and Services." In *Ethnic Dimensions of Aging,* ed. D. E. Gelfand and C. M. Barresi. New York: Springer.

———. 1990. *Black Aged: Understanding Diversity and Service Needs.* Newbury Park, Calif.: Sage.

Haremski, R. L. 1940. "The Unattached, Aged Immigrant: A Descriptive Analysis of the Problems Experienced in Old Age by Three Groups of Poles Living Apart from Their Families in Baltimore." Ph.D. diss., Catholic University of America.

Harlan, Heather. 1998. "Elderly Battle NYC Chinatown Condo Board." *Asian Week* 20, no. 1 (September 2): 11.

Harrington, C. 1996. "Nursing Facility Quality, Staffing, and Economic Issues." Pp. 453–94 in *Nursing Staff in Hospitals and Nursing Homes: Is It Adequate?* ed. G. Wunderlich, F. Sloan, and C. Davis. Institute of Medicine. Washington, D.C.: National Academy Press.

Harris, Ruth-Ann. 1989. Introduction to *The Search for Missing Friends: Irish Immigrant Advertisements Placed in the Boston Pilot.* Vol. 1, *1831–1850,* ed. Ruth-Ann Harris and Donald M. Jacobs. Boston: New England Genealogical Society.

Harris, Ruth-Ann, and Donald M. Jacobs, eds. 1989. *The Search for Missing Friends: Irish*

Immigrant Advertisements Placed in the Boston Pilot. Vol. 1, *1831–1850.* Boston: New England Genealogical Society.

Harrison, A. 1996. "Primary Care of Lesbian and Gay Patients: Educating Ourselves and Our Students." *Family Medicine* 28, no. 1: 10–23.

Hatch, J. W., and C. Jackson. 1981. "North Carolina Baptist Church Program." *Urban Health,* (May): 70–71.

Hayward, R., and J. Weissfeld. 1993. "Coming to Terms with the Era of AIDS: Attitudes of Physicians in US Residency Programs." *Journal of General Internal Medicine* 3, no. 8: 10–18.

Hazuda, H. P., S. M. Haffner, and M. P. Stern. 1988. "Acculturation and Assimilation among Mexican Americans: Scales and Population-Based Data." *Social Science Quarterly* 69: 687–705.

Hazuda, H. P., S. M. Haffner, M. P. Stern, and C. W. Eifler. 1988. "Effects of Acculturation and Socioeconomic Status on Obesity and Diabetes in Mexican Americans." *American Journal of Epidemiology* 128: 1289–1301.

Heer, David M. 1961. "The Marital Status of Second-Generation Americans." *American Sociological Review* 26, no. 2: 233–41.

Hendy, H., G. Nelson, and M. Greco. 1998. "Social Cognitive Predictors of Nutritional Risk in Rural Elderly Adults." *International Journal of Aging and Human Development* 47: 299–327.

Herek, G. 1984. "Beyond Homophobia: A Social Psychological Perspective on Attitudes towards Lesbians and Gay Men." *Journal of Homosexuality* 10: 1–21.

———. 1986. "The Social Psychology of Homophobia: Toward a Practical Theory," *Review of Law and Social Change* 14, no. 4: 923–34. .

Hessler, Richard M., M. F. Nolan, B. Ogbru, and Peter K. M. New. 1975. "Intraethnic Diversity and Health Care of Chinese Americans." *Human Organization* 34, no. 3: 253–362.

Hill, R. 1970. *Family Development in Three Generations.* Cambridge, Mass.: Schenkman.

Himes, C. L., D. P. Hogan, and D. J. Eggebeen. 1996. "Living Arrangements of Minority Elders." *Journal of Gerontology: Social Sciences* 51: 542–48.

Ho, Man Keung. 1976. "Social Work with Asian Americans." *Social Casework* (March): 195–201.

Holstein, M., and T. Cole. 1996. "The Evolution of Long-Term Care in America." Pp. 19–47 in *The Future of Long-Term Care: Social and Policy Issues,* ed. R. H. Binstock, L. E. Cluff, and O. von Mering. Baltimore, Md.: Johns Hopkins University Press.

Hong, G. K., and M. D. C. Ham. 1992. "Impact of Immigration on the Family Life Cycle: Clinical Implications for Chinese Americans." *Journal of Family Psychotherapy* 3, no. 3: 27–39.

Hong, Lawrence K. 1976. "Recent Immigrants in the Chinese-American Community: Issues of Adaptations and Impacts." *International Migration Review* 10: 509–14.

Hooyman, N. R. 1992. "Social Policy and Gender Inequities in Caregiving." Pp. 181–201 in *Gender, Families, and Eldercare,* ed. J. Dwyer and R. T. Coward. Newbury Park, Calif.: Sage.

———. 1997. "Is Aging More Problematic for Women than Men? Yes." Pp. 125–31 in *Controversial Issues in Aging,* ed. A. Scharlach and L. Kaye. Needham Heights, Mass.: Allyn & Bacon.

————. 1999. "Research on Older Women: Where Is Feminism?" *Gerontologist* 39: 115–18.

Hooyman, N. R., and J. Gonyea. 1995. *Feminist Perspectives on Family Care: Policies for Gender Justice.* Thousand Oaks, Calif.: Sage.

Hoppe, S. K., and P. L. Heller. 1975. "Alienation, Familism, and the Utilization of Health Services by Mexican Americans." *Journal of Health and Social Behavior* 16: 304–14.

Horgan, Ellen Somers. 1998. "The Irish-American Family." Pp. 39–67 in *Ethnic Families in America: Patterns and Variations,* ed. Charles H. Mindel, Robert W. Habenstein, and Roosevelt Wright Jr. 4th ed. Upper Saddle River, N.J.: Prentice Hall.

Hostetler, John A., ed. 1992. *Amish Roots: A Treasury of History, Wisdom, and Lore.* 3d ed. Baltimore: Johns Hopkins University Press.

Hostetler, John A., and Gertrude Enders Huntington. 1992. *Amish Children: Education in the Family, School, and Community.* 2d ed. Fort Worth, Texas: Harcourt Brace Jovanovich College Publishers.

Hsu, Francis L. K. 1970. *Americans and Chinese.* Garden City, N.Y.: Doubleday Natural History Press.

————. 1971a. *The Challenge of the American Dream: The Chinese in the United States.* Belmont, Calif.: Wadsworth.

————. 1971b. "Filial Piety in Japan and China." *Journal of Comparative Study* 2: 67–74.

Huang, K. 1991. "Chinese Americans." Pp. 79–96 in *Handbook of Social Services for Asian and Pacific Islanders,* ed. N. Mokuau. New York: Greenwood.

Huberman, S. 1984. "Growing Old in Jewish America: A Study of Jewish Aged in Los Angeles." *Journal of Jewish Communal Service* 60, no. 4: 314–23.

————. 1986. "Jews in Economic Distress." *Journal of Jewish Communal Service* 62, no. 3: 197–208.

Humphreys, Alexander. 1966. *The New Dubliners.* New York: Fordham University Press.

Ikels, Charlotte. 1983a. *Aging and Adaptation: Chinese in Hong Kong and the United States.* Hamden, Conn.: Archor Books.

————. 1983b. "The Process of Caretaker Selection." *Research on Aging* 5, no. 4 (December): 491–509.

————. 1988. "Delayed Reciprocity and the Support Networks of the Childless Elderly." *Journal of Comparative Family Studies* 19, no. 1 (Spring): 99–112.

Indian Health Service. 1997. *Trends in Indian Health, 1997. Statistical Review of Native North Americans.* Washington, D.C.: U.S. Department of Health and Human Services, Indian Health Service, Office of Planning, Evaluation, and Legislation, Division of Program Statistics.

Institute for the Future. 2000. *Health and Health Care 2010: The Forecast, the Challenge.* San Francisco: Jossey-Bass.

Ishii-Kuntz, M. 1997. "Intergenerational Relationships among Chinese, Japanese, and Korean Americans." *Family Relations* 46: 23–32.

Jackson, J. J. 1980. *Minorities and Aging.* Belmont, Calif.: Wadsworth.

Jacobson, Matthew Frye. 1995. *Song of Sorrows: The Diasporic Imagination of Irish, Polish, and Jewish Immigrants in the United States.* Cambridge: Harvard University Press.

Jacobson, R., and Wright, J. 1992. "Financial Planning: Making the Best Use of Your Money." Pp. 183–94 in *Positively Gay: New Approaches to Gay and Lesbian Life,* ed. B. Berson. Berkeley, Calif.: Celestial Arts.

Jacobson, S., and A. H. Grossman. 1996. "Older Lesbians and Gay Men: Old Myths,

New Images, and Future Directions." Pp. 345–73 in *The Lives of Lesbians, Gays, and Bisexuals: Children to Adults,* ed. R. C. Savin-Williams and K. M. Cohen. Philadelphia: Harcourt Brace.

Janowska, Halina. 1975. "An Introductory Outline of the Mass Polish Emigrations, Their Directions and Problems." Pp. 121–45 in *Employment Seeking Emigrations of the Poles World-Wide, Nineteenth and Twentieth Century,* ed. Celina Bobinska and Andrzej Pilch. Krakow: Jagiellonian University.

Jarrett, R. L., and L. M. Burton. 1999. "Dynamic Dimensions of Family Structure in Low-Income African American Families: Emergent Themes in Qualitative Research." *Journal of Comparative Family Studies* 30: 177–87.

Jay, K. A., and A. Young, eds. 1992. *Out of the Closets.* New York: New York University Press.

Johnson, A., and A. Taylor. 1991. *Prevalence of Chronic Diseases: A Summary of Data from the Survey of American Indian and Alaska Natives, National Medical Expenditure Survey Data, Summary 3.* Rockville, Md.: Public Health Service, Agency for Health Care and Policy Research.

Johnson, C. L. 1982. "Sibling Solidarity: Its Origin and Functioning in Italian American Families." *Journal of Marriage and the Family* 44: 155–68.

———. 1985. *Growing Up and Growing Old in Italian American Families.* New Brunswick, N.J.: Rutgers University Press.

Johnson, D., and R. Campbell. 1981. *Black Migration in America: A Social Demographic History.* Durham, N.C.: Duke University Press.

Johnson, F. A. 1993. *Dependency and Japanese Socialization: Psychoanalytic and Anthropological Investigations into Amae.* New York: New York University Press.

Johnson, F. A., and A. J. Marsella. 1978. "Differential Attitudes toward Verbal Behavior in Students of Japanese and European Ancestry." *Genetic Psychology Monographs* 97: 43–76.

Johnson, J. 1995. "Rural Elders and the Decision to Stop Driving." *Journal of Community Health Nursing* 12: 131–38.

Johnson, Sonia. 1981. *From Housewife to Heretic.* Garden City, N.Y.: Doubleday.

Jones, J. 1985. *Labor of Love, Labor of Sorrow: Black Women, Work, and the Family from Slavery to the Present.* New York: Basic Books.

Kahana, B., Z. Harel, Z., and E. Kahana. 1988. "Predictors of Psychological Well-Being among Survivors of the Holocaust." In *Human Adaptation to Extreme Stress: From the Holocaust to Vietnam,* ed. J. Wilson, Z. Harel, and B. Kahana. New York: Plenum.

Kahana, E., et al. 1993. "Adaptation to Institutional Life among Polish, Jewish, and Western European Elderly." Pp. 144–58 in *Ethnic Elderly in Long-Term Care,* ed. C. M. Barresi and D. E. Stul. New York: Springer.

Kahana, E., and B. Kahana. 1984. "Jews." In *Handbook of the Aged in the United States,* ed. E. B. Pallmore. Westport, Conn.: Greenwood.

Kalish, Richard A., and Sharon Moriwaki. 1973. "The World of the Elderly Asian American." *Journal of Social Issues* 29, no. 2: 187–209.

Kalish, Richard A., and Sam Yuen. 1971. "Americans of East Asian Ancestry: Aging and the Aged." *Gerontologist* 11, no. 1: 36–47.

Kamikawa, L. M. 1981. "The Elderly: A Pacific/Asian Perspective." *Aging,* no. 319/320: 2–9.

Kamo, Yoshimori, and Zhou Min. 1994. "Living Arrangements of Elderly Chinese and Japanese in the United States." *Journal of Marriage and the Family* 56: 544–58.

Kane, Eileen. 1968. "Man and Kin in Donegal: A Study of Kinship Functions in a Rural Irish and an Irish-American Community." *Ethnology* 7, no. 3 (July): 245–58.

Kane, R., and R. Kane. 1981. *Assessing the Elderly: A Practical Guide to Measurement.* Los Angeles: Rand.

Kane, R. A., and J. Penrod. 1995. "Toward a Caregiving Policy for the Aging Family." In *Family Caregiving in an Aging Society,* ed. R. A. Kane and J. Penrod. Thousand Oaks, Calif.: Sage.

Kane, R. A., R. L. Kane, and R. Ladd. 1998. *The Heart of Long-Term Care.* New York: Oxford University Press.

Kane, R. L. 1993. "Lessons in Long-Term Care: The Benefits of a Northern Exposure." Pp. 91–110 in *North American Health Care Policy in the 1990s,* ed. A. King, T. Hyclak, R. Thorton, and S. Mc Mahon. New York: John Wiley & Sons.

———. 1994. "Long-Term Care in the U.S.: Problems and Promise." In *Economic Security and Intergenerational Justice,* ed. T. R. Marmor, T. Smeeding, and V. L. Greene. Washington, D.C.: Urban Institute Press.

Kang, T. S., and G. E. Kang. 1981. "Adjustment Problems of Recently Immigrated Korean-American Elderly: Case Studies in New York City." Paper presented at the thirty-fourth annual meeting of the American Gerontological Society, Toronto.

Kantowicz, Edward. 1977. "Polish Chicago: Survival through Solidarity." Pp. 180–209 in *The Ethnic Frontier,* ed. Melvin Holli and Peter Jones. Grand Rapids, Mich.: Eerdmans.

Kauh, Tac-ock. 1997. "Intergenerational Relations: Older Korean-Americans' Experience." *Journal of Cross-Cultural Gerontology* 12: 245–71.

Kehoe, M. 1986. "Lesbians over Sixty-five: A Triple Invisible Minority." *Journal of Homosexuality* 12, no. 3/4: 139–52.

Keigher, S. 1995. "Compensation of Family Care for the Elderly." In *Family Caregiving in an Aging Society,* ed. R. Kane and J. Penrod. Thousand Oaks, Calif.: Sage.

Keith, J. 1982. *Old People as People: Social and Cultural Influences on Aging and Old Age.* Boston: Little, Brown.

Kelley, J., J. Lawrence, H. Hood, S. Smith, and D. Cook. 1988. "Nurses' Attitudes towards AIDS." *Journal of Continuing Education for Nurses* 19: 78–83.

Kelley, M. L., and M. J. MacLean. 1997. "I Want to Live Here for the Rest of My Life: The Challenge of Case Management for Rural Seniors." *Journal of Case Management* 6: 174–82.

Kemp, B. J., F. Staples, and W. Lopez-Aqueres. 1987. "Epidemiology of Depression and Dysphoria in Our Elderly Hispanic Population: Prevalence and Correlates." *Journal of the American Geriatrics Society* 35: 920–26.

Kennedy, Robert F., Jr. 1973. *The Irish: Emigration, Marriage, and Fertility.* Berkeley and Los Angeles: University of California Press, 1973.

Kenney, G. M. 1991. "Access to Home Health Services: Is It a Problem for the Rural Elderly?" Working paper 3971-05, Urban Institute, Washington D.C.

Kenney, G. M., and L. C. Dubay. 1992. "Explaining Area Variation in the Use of Medicare Home Health Services." *Medical Care* 30: 43–57.

Ketzer, J. K., R. T. Coward, C. W. Peek, J. C. Henretta, R. P. Duncan, and M. C. Dougherty. 1997. "Race and Residence Differences in the Use of Formal Services by Older Adults." *Research on Aging* 19: 300–332.

Kiefer, C. 1974. "Lessons from the Issei." Pp. 167–97 in *Late Life Communities and Environmental Policy,* ed. J. Gubrium. Springfield, Ill.: Charles C. Thomas.

Kim, Cheong-Seok, and Ka-Oak Rhee. 1997. "Variations in Preferred Living Arrangements among Korean Elderly Parents." *Journal of Cross-Cultural Gerontology* 12: 189–202.

Kim, Kwang Chung, and Won Moo Hurh. 1991. "The Extended Conjugal Family: Family-Kinship System of Korean Immigrants in the United States." Pp. 115–33 in *The Korean-American Community Present and Future,* ed. T. H. Kwak and S. H. Lee. Seoul: Kyungnam University Press.

Kim, Kwang Chung, Won Moo Hurh, and Shin Kim. 1993. "Generation Differences in Korean Immigrants' Life Conditions in the USA." *Sociological Perspectives* 36: 257–70.

Kim, Kwang Chung, Shin Kim, and Won Moo Hurh. 1991. "Filial Piety and Intergenerational Relationship in Korean Immigrant Families." *International Journal of Aging and Human Development* 33: 233–45.

Kim, Seung-Kyung. 2000. "Pennies Do Count: Korean American Elderly Women and Poverty." Paper presented at the tenth annual meeting of the International Council on Korean Studies, Washington, D.C., June 2–4.

Kimmel, D. C. 1992. "The Families of Older Gay Men and Lesbians." *Generations* 16, no 3: 37–38.

Kingson, Eric. 1996. "Population Aging and the Risk of Disability." In *From Nursing Homes to Home Care,* ed. Marie E. Cowart and Jill S. Quadagno. New York: Haworth.

Kington, R. S., and J. P. Smith. 1997. "Socioeconomic Status and Racial and Ethnic Differences in Functional Status Associated with Chronic Diseases." *American Journal of Public Health* 87, no. 5 (May): 805–10.

Kinoshita, Y., and C. W. Kiefer. 1992. *Refuge of the Honored: Social Organization in a Japanese Retirement Community.* Berkeley and Los Angeles: University of California Press.

Kitano, H. H. L. 1976. *Japanese Americans: The Evolution of a Subculture.* 2d ed. Englewood Cliffs, N.J.: Prentice Hall.

———. 1988. "The Japanese American Family." In *Ethnic Families in America: Patterns and Validations,* ed. C. H. Mindel, R. W. Habenstein, and R. Wesley. 3d ed. Englewood Cliffs, N.J.: Prentice Hall.

Kitano, H. H. L., and R. Daniels. 1988. *Asian Americans: Emerging Minorities.* Englewood Cliffs, N.J.: Prentice Hall.

Kitano, H. H. L., J. E. Lubben, E. Berkanovic, E. Chi, and N. Harada. 1995. *Study of Japanese American Elderly in Los Angeles.* Berkeley and Los Angeles: University of California Press.

Kitano, H. H. L., T. Shibusawa, and K. J. Kitano. 1997. "Asian American Elderly Mental Health." Pp. 295–324 in *Minorities, Aging, and Health,* ed. K. S. Markides and M. Miranda. Thousand Oaks, Calif.: Sage.

Klassen, Peter James. 1963. *Mutual Aid among the Anabaptists: Doctrine and Practice.* Bluffton, Ohio: Association of Mennonite Aid Society.

Koh, James Y., and William C. Bell. 1987. "Korean Elderly in the United States: Intergenerational Relations and Living Arrangements." *Gerontologist* 27: 66–71.

Kourvetaris, G. A. 1988. "The Greek American Family." Pp. 76–107 in *Ethnic Families in America: Patterns and Variations,* ed. C. H. Mindel, R. W. Habenstein, and R. Wright Jr. 3d ed. Englewood Cliffs, N.J.: Prentice Hall.

Kozaitis, K. A. 1987. "Being Old and Greek in America." In *Ethnic Dimensions of Aging,* ed. D. E. Gelfand and C. M. Barresi. New York: Springer.

Kramer, Josea B., Donna Polisar, and Jeffrey C. Hyde. 1990. *The Study of Urban American Indian Aging.* City of Industry, Calif.: Public Health Foundation of Los Angeles County.

Krause, N., and L. M. Goldenhar. 1992. "Acculturation and Psychological Distress in Three Groups of Elderly Hispanics." *Journal of Gerontology: Social Sciences* 47: 279–288.

Kraut, A. M. 1990. "Healers and Strangers: Immigrant Attitudes toward the Physician in America." *JAMA* 263, no. 13: 1807–11.

Kraybill, Donald. 1989. *The Riddle of Amish Culture.* Baltimore, Md.: Johns Hopkins University Press.

Krippner, S. 1995. "A Cross-Cultural Comparison of Four Healing Models." *Alternative Therapies* 1, no. 3: 21.

Kroeber, T., and R. F. Helzer. 1968. *Almost Ancestors: The First Californians.* Edited by F. D. Hales. San Francisco: Sierra Club.

Krout, J. A. 1997. "Barriers to Providing Case Management to Older Rural Persons." *Journal of Case Management* 6: 142–50.

Kung, S. W. 1962. *Chinese in American Life: Some Aspects of Their History, Status, Problems, and Contributions.* Seattle: University of Washington Press.

Kuo, Chien-Lin, and Kathryn Hopkins Kavanagh. 1994. "Chinese Perspectives on Culture and Mental Health." *Issues in Mental Health Nursing* 15: 551–67.

Kurashige, S. 2000. "The Problem of Biculturalism: Japanese American Identity and Festivals before World War II." *Journal of American History* 86: 1632–54.

Kutzik, A. J. 1979. "American Social Provision for the Aged: An Historical Perspective." Pp. 32–65 in *Ethnicity and Aging: Theory, Research, and Policy,* ed. D. E. Gelfand and A. J. Kutzik. New York: Springer.

Laczko, F. 1994. *Older People in Eastern and Central Europe: The Price of Transition to a Market Economy.* London: HelpAge International.

Ladner, J. A. 1971. *Tomorrow's Tomorrow: The Black Woman.* New York: Anchor Books.

Laguerre, M. S. 1984. *American Odyssey.* Ithaca, N.Y.: Cornell University Press.

———. 1998. *Diasporic Citizenship.* London: Macmillan.

———. 2000. *The Global Ethnopolis: Chinatown, Japantown, and Manilatown in American Society.* Basingstoke, England: Macmillan.

Lam, Lawrence. 1994. "Self-Assessment of Health Status of Aged Chinese-Canadians." *JAAS* 29: 77–90.

Larragy, Joe. 1993. "Views and Perceptions of Older Irish People." *Social Policy and Administration* 27, no. 3: 235–47.

Lauria, A. 1972. "Respeto, Relajo, and Interpersonal Relations in Puerto Rico." In *The Puerto Rican Community and Its Children on the Mainland.* Metuchen, N.J.: Scarecrow.

Le, Trung Vu, ed. 1992. *Le hoi co truyen* (Traditional Fold festivals). Hanoi: Nha Xuat Ban Khoa Hoc Xa Hoi.

Lee, G. R., J. K. Netzer, and T. C. Raymond. 1994. "Filial Responsibility Expectations and

Patterns of Intergenerational Assistance." *Journal of Marriage and the Family* 56, no. 3: 559–65.

Lee, Jik-Joen. 1986. "Asian American Elderly: A Neglected Minority Group." *Journal of Gerontological Social Work* 9: 103–16.

Lee, Rose Hum. 1956. "The Recent Immigrant Chinese Families of the San Francisco–Oakland Area." *Marriage and Family Living* 18: 14–24.

Lee, S. M. 1998. "Asian Americans: Diverse and Growing." *Population Bulletin* 53: 2–40.

Lee, S. M., and K. Yamanaka. 1990. "Patterns of Asian American Intermarriage and Marital Assimilation." *Journal of Comparative Family Studies* 21: 287–305.

Leung, P. 1990. "Asian Americans and Psychology: Unresolved Issues." *Journal of Training and Practice in Professional Psychology* 4, no. 1: 3–13.

Levkoff, Sue. 1997. Study on the impact on the care family members provide to elderly relatives who have Alzheimer's disease or related dementia. Available at www.hms.harvard.edu/news/releases/0997dement.html. Accessed February 1999.

Leyes de Puerto Rico. 1986. *Leyes anotadas de Puerto Rico.* Ley 121 del 12 de julio (8): 341–47.

Li, W. L. 1977. "Occupational Achievement and Kinship Assistance among Chinese Immigrants in Chicago." *Sociological Quarterly* 18: 478–89.

Liebig, P. 1998. "Housing and Supportive Services for the Elderly: Intergenerational Perspectives and Options." Pp. 51–71 in *New Directions in Old-Age Policies,* ed. J. Steckenrider and T. Parrott. Albany: State University of New York Press.

Lincoln, C. L., and L. H. Mamiya. 1991. *The Black Church in the American Experience.* Durham, N.C.: Duke University Press.

Linsk, Nathan, and S. Keigher. 1995. "Compensation of Family Care for the Elderly." In *Family Caregiving in an Aging Society,* ed. R. Kane and J. Penrod. Thousand Oaks, Calif.: Sage.

Lipman, A. 1986. "Homosexuals." Pp. 323–37 in *Handbook of the Aged in the United States,* ed. E. B. Palmore. Westport, Conn.: Greenwood.

Lipton, James A., and Joseph J. Marbach. 1984. "Ethnicity and the Pain Experience." *Social Science and Medicine* 19, no. 12: 1279–98.

Liu, William T. 1986. "Health Services for Asian Elderly." *Research on Aging* 8, no. 1: 156–75.

Liu, William T., and Elena S. H. Yu. 1985. "Asian/Pacific American Elderly: Mortality Differentials, Health Status, and Use of Health Services." *Journal of Applied Gerontology* 4: 35–64.

Lockery, S. A. 1992. "Caregiving among Racial and Ethnic Minority Elders: Family and Social Supports." Pp. 113–22 in *Diversity: New Approaches to Ethnic Minority Aging,* ed. E. P. Stanford and F. M. Torres-Gil. Amityville, N.Y.: Baywood.

Logan, J. R., and G. Spitze. 1994. "Informal Support and the Use of Formal Services by Older Americans." *Journal of Gerontology: Social Sciences* 49: 25–34.

Lopata, Helena. 1976. *Polish Americans: Status Competition in an Ethnic Community.* Englewood Cliffs, N.J.: Prentice Hall.

———. 1977. "Widowhood in Polonia." *Polish American Studies* 34: 7–25.

———. 1978. "Contributions of the Extended Families to the Social Support Systems of Metropolitan Area Widows: Limitations of the Modified Kin Network." *Journal of Marriage and the Family* 40: 358–64.

———. 1981. "The Polish American Family." Pp. 15–40 in *Ethnic Families in America,* ed. C. H. Mindel, R. W. Habenstein and R. Wesley. 2d ed. New York: Elsevier North Holland.

———. 1994. *Polish Americans*. 2d ed. New Brunswick, N.J.: Transaction Publishers.

Lopreato, J. 1970. *Italian Americans*. New York: Random House.

Lorenz, F., R. Conger, R. Montague, and K. Wickrama. 1993. "Economic Conditions, Spouse Support, and Psychological Distress of Rural Husbands and Wives." *Rural Sociology* 58: 247–68.

Loughman, Celeste. 1985. "'Old Now, and Good to Her': J. T. Farrell's Last Novels." *Eire Ireland* 20, no. 3 (Fall): 43–55.

Lubben, J. E., and A. Lee. 2000. "Social Support Networks among Older Chinese Americans in Los Angeles." In *Elderly Chinese in Pacific Rim Countries*, ed. I. Chi, N. L. Chappell, and J. Lubben.Hong Kong: Hong Kong University Press.

Lum, D. 1983. "Asian Americans and Their Aged." Pp. 85–95 in *Aging in Minority Groups*, ed. R. L. McNeely and J. L. Colen. Beverly Hills, Calif.: Sage.

Lum, D., Lucia Yim-San Cheung, Eric Ray Cho, Tze-Yee Tang, and How Boa Yau. 1980. "The Psychosocial Needs of the Chinese Elderly." *Social Casework* 61, no. 2: 100–106.

Lund, Dale A., Michael S. Caserta, and Margaret Diamond. 1998. "A Comparison of Bereavement Adjustments between Mormon and Non-Mormon Older Adults." *Journal of Religion and Aging* 5: 75–92.

Lyman, Stanford. 1974. *Chinese Americans*. New York: Random House.

Lyon, Joseph, M. R. Lauber, John Gardner, et al. "Cancer Incidence in Mormons and Non-Mormons in Utah, 1966–1970." *New England Journal of Medicine* 294: 129–33.

MacKinnon, Marian E., Lan Gien, and Douglas Durst. 1996. "Chinese Elders Speak Out: Implicatons for Caregivers." *Clinical Nursing Research* 5, no. 3: 326–42.

Macklin, E. 1987. "No Traditional Family Forms."Pp. 317–53 in *Handbook of Marriage and Family*, ed. M. S. Sussman and S. K. Steinmetz. New York: Plenum.

MacMaster, R. K. 1985. *Land, Piety, and Peoplehood: The Establishment of Mennonite Communities in America, 1683–1790*. Scottdale, Pa.: Herald Press.

Maly Rocznik Statystyczny. 1997. Warsaw: Glowny Urzad Statystyczny.

Mann, W. 1999. "Gray Gays: Aging Gay Men and Lesbians Face Unique Challenges." Available at www.bostonphoenix.com/archive/. Accessed April 1999.

Manson, Spero M. 1989. "Provider Assumptions about Long-Term Care in American Indian Communities." *Gerontologist* 29, no. 3: 355–64.

Manton, K. G., B. H. Singer, R. M. Suzman, eds. 1993. *Forecasting the Health of Elderly Populations*. New York: Springer-Verlag.

Marin, G., and B. V. Marin. 1991. *Research with Hispanic Populations*. Applied Social Research Methods 23. Newbury Park, Calif.: Sage.

Markides, K. S., and C. H. Mindel. 1987. *Aging and Ethnicity*. Newbury Park, Calif.: Sage.

Markides, K. S., and D. J. Lee. 1991. "Predictors of Health Status in Middle-Aged and Older Mexican Americans." *Journal of Gerontology: Social Sciences* 46, no. 5 (September): 243–49.

Martin, L. J. 1990. "The Status of South Asia's Growing Elderly Population." *Journal of Cross Cultural Gerontology* 5: 93–117.

Markides, K. S., C. A. Stroup-Benham, J. S. Goodwin, L. C. Perkowski, M. Lichtenstein, and L. A. Ray. 1996. "The Effect of Medical Conditions on the Functional Limitations of Mexican-American Elderly." *Annals of Epidemiology* 6, no. 5 (September): 386–91.

Mass, A. 1991. "Psychological Effects of the Camps on the Japanese Americans." Pp.

159–62 in *Japanese Americans: From Relocation to Redress,* ed. R. Daniels, S. C. Taylor, and H. H. L. Kitano. Seattle: University of Washington Press.

Massey, D. S. 1990. "American Apartheid: Segregation and the Making of the Underclass." *American Journal of Sociology* 96: 329–58.

Massey, D. S., R. Alarcon, J. Durand, and H. Gonzalez. 1987. *Return to Aztlan: The Social Process of International Migration from Western Mexico.* Berkeley and Los Angeles: University of California Press.

Matsui, W. T. 1996. "Japanese Families." Pp. 268–80 in *Ethnicity and Family Therapy,* ed. M. McGoldrick, J. K. Pearce, and J. Giordano. 2d ed. New York: Guilford.

Matsuoka, A. 1999. "Preferred Care in Later Life among Japanese Canadians." *Journal of Multicultural Social Work* 7: 127–48.

Matthes, W., M. Booth, J. Turner, and T. Kessner. 1986. "Physicians' Attitudes toward Homosexuality: A Survey of a California Medical Society." *Western Journal of Medicine* 144: 106–10.

McCaffrey, Lawrence J. 1997. *The Irish Catholic Diaspora in America.* Washington, D.C.: Catholic University of America Press.

McCormick, W. C., J. Uomoto, H. Young, A. B. Graves, P. Vitaliano, J. A. Mortimer, S. D. Edland, and E. B. Larson. 1996. "Attitudes toward the Use of Nusing Homes and Home Care in Older Japanese Americans." *Journal of the American Geriatrics Society* 44: 769–77.

McGivern, Elaine P. 1979. "Ethnic Identity and Its Relation to Group Norms: Irish Americans in Metropolitan Pittsburgh." Ph.D. diss., University of Pittsburgh.

McGoldrick, Monica. 1996. "Irish Families." Pp. 544–66 in *Ethnicity and Family Therapy,* ed. M. McGoldrick, J. Giordano, and J. K. Pearce. 2d ed. New York: Guilford.

McLaughlin, D., and L. Jensen. 1998. "The Rural Elderly: A Demographic Portrait." Pp. 15–43 *Aging in Rural Settings: Life Circumstances and Distinctive Features,* ed. R. T. Coward and J. A. Krout. New York: Springer.

McLaughlin, V. 1971. "Patterns of Work and Family Organization: Buffalo Italians." *Journal of Interdisciplinary History* 2: 229–314.

McNeely, R. L., and J. L. Colen, eds. 1983. *Aging in Minority Groups.* Beverly Hills, Calif.: Sage.

Mercer, S., P. Heacock, and C. Beck. 1994. "Nurse's Aides in Nursing Homes: A Study of Caregivers." *Journal of Women and Aging* 6: 107–20.

Metress, Seamus P. 1985. "The History of Irish-American Care of the Aged." *Social Science Review* 59, no. 1 (March): 18–31.

Miah, Mizanur Rahman, and Dean R. Kahler. 1997. "Asian-American Elderly: A Review of the Quality of Life and Social Service Needs." *Journal of Sociology and Social Welfare* 24, no. 1: 79–89.

Mick, Cynthia. 1983. *A Summary of Recent Long-Term Care Initiatives in the Fifty States.* Tucson: Arizona's Long-Term Care Gerontology Center.

Midre, Georges, and Brunon Synak. 1989. "Between Family and State: Ageing in Poland and Norway." *Ageing and Society* 9: 241–59.

Miller, B., and S. McFall. 1991. "The Effect of Caregiver's Burden on Change in Frail Older Persons' Use of Formal Helpers." *Journal of Health and Social Behavior* 32: 165–79.

Miller, Kerby A. 1985. *Emigrants and Exiles: Ireland and the Irish Exodus to North America.* New York: Oxford University Press.

Miller, Mark. 2000. "To Be Gay—and Mormon." *Newsweek* 135, no. 19 (May 8): 38–39.

Miller, Paul D. 1950. "Amish Acculturation." Master's thesis, University of Nebraska.

Min, Pyong Gap. 1998. *Changes and Conflicts: Korean Immigrant Families in New York.* Boston: Allyn & Bacon.

Misener, T., R. Sowell, T. Phillips, and C. Harris. 1997. "Sexual orientation: A Cultural Diversity Issue for Nursing." *Nursing Outlook* 45, no. 4: 178–81.

Mitchell, B. D., M. P. Stern, S. M. Haffner, H. P. Hazuda, and J. K. Patterson. 1990. "Risk Factors for Cardiovascular Mortality in Mexican Americans and Non-Hispanic Whites: The San Antonio Heart Study." *American Journal of Epidemiology* 131: 423–33.

Miyamoto, F. 1986–1987. "Problems of Interpersonal Style among the Nisei." *Amerasia Journal* 13: 29–45.

Mobily, P. R., K. A. Herr, M. K. Clark, and R. B. Wallace. 1994. "An Epidemiologic Analysis of Pain in the Elderly: The Iowa 65+ Rural Health Study." *Journal of Aging and Health* 6 (May): 139–54.

Molina, C. W., R. E. Zambrana, and M. Aguirre-Molina. 1994. *Latino Health in the U.S.: A Growing Challenge.* Washington D.C.: American Public Health Association.

Monk, A., and B. Warach. 1994. "Factors Shaping Policies and Programs for the Jewish Aged in the United States." Pp. 123–40 in *Jewish Aged in the United States and Israel: Diversity, Programs, and Services,* ed. Z. Harel, D. Biegel, and D. Guttmann. New York: Springer.

Monson, Thomas S. 1981. "The Long Line of the Lonely." *Ensign* 11 (May): 47–48.

Montgomery, R. 1995. "Examining Respite Care: Promises and Limitations." In *Family Caregiving in an Aging Society,* ed. R. Kane and J. Penrod. Thousand Oaks, Calif.: Sage.

Moody, Harry R. 1998. "Cross-Cultural Geriatric Ethics: Negotiating Our Differences." *Generations* 22, no. 3: 32–39.

Morawska, Ewa. 1985. *For Bread with Butter: The Life Worlds of East Central Europeans in Johnstown, Pennsylvania, 1890–1940.* Cambridge: Cambridge University Press.

———. 1991. "Aging under State Socialism: The Case of Poland." Pp. 175–205 in *State, Labor Markets, and the Future of Old-Age Policy,* ed. John Myles and Jill S. Quadagno. Philadelphia: Temple University Press.

Morrissey, M. 1996. "Attitudes of Practitioners to Lesbian, Gay and Bisexual Clients." *British Journal of Nursing* 5, no. 18: 980–82.

Morrisey, M., R. Ohsfeldt, V. Johnson, and R. Treat. 1995. "Rural Emergency Medical Services: Patients, Destinations, Times, Services." *Journal of Rural Health* 11: 286–94.

Morton, D. J., S. A. Schoenrock, E. P. Stanford, K. M. Peddecord, and C. A. Molgaard. 1989. "Use of the CES-D among a Community Sample of Older Mexican Americans." *Journal of Cross-Cultural Gerontology* 64: 289–306.

Moskos, C. 1989. *Greek Americans: Struggle and Success.* 2d ed. New Brunswick, N.J.: Transaction Publishers.

Moss, L., and W. Thompson. 1959. "The Southern Italian Family: Literature and Observations." *Human Organization* 18: 354–64.

Mostwin, Danuta. 1971. "The Transplanted Family: A Study of Social Adjustment of the Polish Immigrant Family to the United States after the Second World War." Ph.D. diss., Columbia University.

———. 1979. "Emotional Needs of Elderly Americans of Central and Eastern European

Background." Pp. 263–76 in *Ethnicity and Aging: Theory, Research, and Policy,* ed. D. E. Gelfand and A. J. Kutzik. New York: Springer.

Mui, Ada C. 1996. "Depression among Elderly Chinese Immigrants: An Exploratory Study." *Social Work* 41, no. 6: 633–45.

————. 1998. "Living Alone and Depression among Older Chinese Immigrants." *Journal of Gerontological Social Work* 30, no. 3/4: 147–66.

Murphy, B. 1992. "Educating Mental Health Professionals about Gay and Lesbian Issues." *Journal of Homosexuality* 22, no. 3/4: 229–46.

Myerhoff, B. 1978. *Number Our Days.* New York: E. P. Dutton.

Nagasawa, R. 1980. *The Elderly Chinese: A Forgotten Minority.* Chicago: Pacific Asian American Mental Health Research Center.

Nagata, D. 1993. *Legacy of Silence: Exploring the Long-Term Effects of the Japanese American Internment.* New York: Plenum.

National Indian Council on Aging. 1981. *American Indian Elderly: A National Profile.* Albuquerque: NICOA.

Nelson, G. 1994. "In-Home Services for Rural Elders." Pp. 65–83 in *Health Services for Rural Elders,* ed. R. T. Coward, C. N. Bull, G. Kukulka, and J. M. Galliher. New York: Springer.

Newton, F. C. 1980. "Issues in Research and Service Delivery among Mexican American Elderly: A Concise Statement with Recommendations." *Gerontologist* 20, no. 2 (April): 208–13.

Nguyen, Giai The. 1993. *Luat hon nhan va gia dinh: Tra loi mot so cau hoi* (Marriage and family law: Questions and answers). Hanoi: Chinh Tri Quoc Gia.

Nguyen, Quang Ngoc. 1993. *Ve mot so lang buon o dong bang bac bo the ky 18–19* (Northern Vietnamese villages in the eighteenth and nineteenth centuries). Hanoi: Hoi Su Hoc Vietnam.

Nhat, Thanh. 1968. *Dat le que thoi: Phong tuc Vietnam* (Traditions and mores of Vietnam). Saigon: Dai Nam.

Nishi, S. M. 1995. "Japanese Americans." Pp. 95–133 in *Asian Americans: Contemporary Issues and Trends,* ed. P. G. Min. Thousand Oaks, Calif.: Sage.

Nolan, Janet A. 1989. *Ourselves Alone: Female Emigration from Ireland, 1885–1920.* Lexington: University Press of Kentucky.

Novak, M. 1972. *The Rise of the Unmeltable Ethnics.* New York: Macmillan.

Oaks, Dallin. 1991. "Honour Thy Father and Thy Mother."*Ensign* 21 (May).

Ober, Barbara. 1988. "Unobtrusive Measures of the Amish: Aging and Death—A Preliminary Report." Paper presented at the North Central Sociological Association Conference, Shippensburg University, Shippensburg, Pa.

O'Brien, D. J., and S. S. Fugita. 1991. *Japanese American Ethnicity: The Persistence of Community.* Seattle: University of Washington Press.

Ogawa, N., and R. D. Retherford. 1993. "Care of Elderly in Japan: Changing Norms and Expectations." *Journal of Marriage and the Family* 55: 585–97.

O'Hare, William P., and Judy C. Felt. 1991. *Asian-Americans: America's Fastest-Growing Minority Group.* Washington, D.C.: Population Reference Bureau.

Okada, T. 1988. "Teachings of Confucianism on Health and Old Age." *Journal of Religion and Aging* 4, no. 3/4: 101–7.

Older Americans Report (OAR), 1999. Vol. 23, no. 41 (October 22). Silver Spring, Md.: Business Publishers.

Omidian, P. A. 1996. *Aging and Family in an Afghan Refugee Community: Transitions and Transformations*. New York: Garland.

O'Neill, J., and P. Shalit. 1992. "Health Care of the Gay Male Patient." *Primary Care* 19, no. 1: 191–201.

Opler, Marvin K., and Jerome L. Singer. 1956. "Ethnic Differences in Behavior and Psychopathology: Italian and Irish." *International Journal of Social Psychiatry* 2: 11–23.

Orona, C., B. Koenig, and A. Davis. 1994. "Cultural Aspects of Nondisclosure." *Cambridge Quarterly of Healthcare Ethics* 3: 338–46.

Osako, M. 1979. "Aging and Family among Japanese Americans: The Role of Ethnic Tradition in the Adjustment to Old Age." *Gerontologist* 19: 448–55.

Osako, M., and W. Liu. 1986. "Intergenerational Relations and the Aged among Japanese Americans." *Research on Aging* 8: 128–55.

Otsuka, Yoshimi. 1999. "Kin ON Expands Services: Home Care Help Available." *International Examiner* 26, no. 4 (March 3): 6.

Oyer, John S., and Robert S. Kreider. 1990. *Mirror of the Martyrs*. Intercourse, Pa.: Good Books.

Padilla, A., M. Carlos, and S. Keefe. 1976. "Mental Health Service Utilization by Mexican Americans." In *Psychotherapy with Spanish-Speaking: Issues in Research and Service Delivery*, ed. Manuel R. Miranda. Los Angeles: Spanish Speaking Mental Health Research Center.

Padilla, E. 1958. *Up from Puerto Rico*. New York: Columbia University Press.

Parot, Joseph John. 1981. *Polish Catholics in Chicago, 1850–1920*. DeKalb: Northern Illinois University Press.

Parra, E. O., and D. V. Espino. 1992. "Barriers to Health Care Access Faced by Elderly Mexican Americans." Pp. 171–77 in *Hispanic Aged Mental Health*, ed. T. L. Brink. New York: Haworth.

Pattillo-McCoy, M. 1998. "Church Culture as a Strategy of Action in the Black Community." *American Sociological Review* 63: 767–84.

Pearlin, L. 1970. *Class, Context, and Famly Relations*. Boston: Little, Brown.

Peck, Eldon. 1992. "Number of LDS Young Men Choosing Missions Remains Constant." *Sunstone: Mormon Experience, Scholarship, Issues, and Art*, September, 60.

———. 1995. "Church Explains Welfare System to Senate." *Sunstone: Mormon Experience, Scholarship, Issues, and Art*, December, 90.

Perez-Stable, E. J., M. M. McMillen, M. I. Harris, R. Z. Jaurez, W. C. Knowler, M. P. Stern, and S. G. Haynes.1989. "Self-Reported Diabetes in Mexican Americans: HHANES 1982–84." *American Journal of Public Health* 79: 770–72.

Phan, Doan Dai. 1992. *Lang Viet Nam: Mot so van de kinh te xa hoi* (Vietnamese villages: Some economic and social issues). Vietnam: Nha Xuat Ban Khoa Hoc Xa Hoi.

Piercy, K. W. 1998. "Theorizing about Family Caregiving: The Role of Responsibility." *Journal of Marriage and the Family* 60, no. 1: 109–18.

Pilemer, K., and D. Moore. 1989. "Abuse of Patients in Nursing Homes: Findings from a Survey of Staff." *Gerontologist* 29, no. 3: 314–20.

Pinkowski, Edward. 1978. "The Great Influx of Polish Immigrants and the Industries They Entered." Pp. 303–70 in *Poles in America: Bicentennial Essays*, ed. Frank Mocha. Stevens Point, Wis.: Worzalla.

Pinnock, Hugh W. 1979. "We Will Go with Our Young and with Our Old." *Ensign* 11 (November): 74–76.

Piotrowski, J. 1973. *Miejsce czlowieka starego w rodzinie i spoleczenstwie* (Old people in family and society). Warsaw: Interpress.

Ploch, D., and D. Hastings. 1994. "Graphic Presentations of Church Attendance Using General Social Survey Data." *Journal for the Scientific Study of Religion* 33: 16–33.

Popenoe, D. 1993. "American Family Decline, 1960–1990: A Review and Appraisal." *Journal of Marriage and the Family* 55: 527–55.

Pousada, L. 1995. "Hispanic-American Elders: Implications for Health-Care Providers." *Clinics in Geriatric Medicine* 11, no. 1 (February): 39–52.

Pugh, J. A., M. P. Stern, S. M. Haffner, C. W. Eifler, and M. Zapata. 1988. "Excess Incidence of Treatment of End-Stage Renal Disease in Mexican Americans." *American Journal of Epidemiology* 127, no. 1: 135–43.

Pula, James. 1995. *Polish Americans: An Ethnic Community.* New York: Twayne.

Pyke, K. 1999. "The Micropolitics of Care in Relationships Between Aging Parents and Adult Children: Individualism, Collectivism, and Power." *Journal of Marriage and the Family* 61, no. 3: 661–72.

Pyke, K., and V. L. Bengtson. 1996. "Caring More or Less: Individualistic and Collectivistic Systems of Family Elder Care." *Journal of Marriage and the Family* 58, no. 2: 379–92.

Quam, J. 1993. "Gay and Lesbian Aging." *Siecus Report,* www.cyc.umn.edu/Diversity, Gay/gayaging.html. Accessed March 1999.

Quam J., and G. Whitford. 1992. "Adaptation and Age-Related Expectations of Older Gay and Lesbian Adults." *Gerontologist* 32, no. 3: 367–74.

Quandt, S. A., T. A. Arcury, and R. A. Bell. 1998. "Self-Management of Nutritional Risk among Older Adults: A Conceptual Model and Case Studies from Rural Communities." *Journal of Aging Studies* 12: 351–68.

Queralt, M. 1983. "The Elderly of Cuban Origin: Characteristics and Problems." In *Aging in Minority Groups,* ed. R. L. McNeely and J. L. Colen. Beverly Hills, Calif.: Sage.

Queseda, G. M., and P. L. Heller. 1977. "Sociocultural Barriers to Medical Care among Mexican Americans in Texas: A Summary Report of Research Conducted by the Southwest Medical Sociology Ad Hoc Committee." *Medical Care* 15 (May supp.): 93–101.

Rabiner, D. 1995. "Patterns and Predictors of Noninstitutional Health Care Utilization by Older Adults in Rural and Urban America." *Journal of Rural Health* 11: 259–73.

Raichilson, S. 1994. "The Jewish Home for the Aged in the United States." Pp. 219–39 in *Jewish Aged: Ethnicity, Diversity, and Services,* ed. Z. Harel, D. Biegel, and D. Guttmann. New York: Springer.

Rainbow Gardens. 1999. Available at www.rainbow-gardens.com/prognf.htm. Accessed March 1999.

Rankow, E. J. 1995. "Lesbian Health Issues for the Primary Care Provider." *Journal of Family Practice* 40, no. 5: 486–93.

Ray, R. 1996. "A Postmodern Perspective on Feminist Gerontology." *Gerontologist* 36: 674–80.

Rayned, Marybeth, and Erin Parsons. 1983. "Single Cursedness: An Overview of LDS Authorities' Statements about Unmarried People." *Dialogue: A Journal of Mormon Thought* 16, no. 3: 35–45.

Reed, D., D. McGee, K. Yano, M. Feinleib. 1983. "Social Networks and Coronary Heart Disease among Japanese Men in Hawaii." *American Journal of Epidemiology* 117: 384–96.

Reid, Ira de A. 1939. *The Negro Immigrant*. New York: Columbia University Press.

Reid, J. 1995. "Development in Late Life: Older Lesbian and Gay Lives." Pp. 215–40 in *Lesbian, Gay, and Bisexual Identities over the Lifespan*, ed. A. D'Augelli and C. Patterson. New York: Oxford University Press.

Richards, Marty, Colette V. Browne, and Alice Broderick. 1994. "Strategies for Teaching Clinical Social Work Practice with Asian and Pacific Island Elders." *Gerontology and Geriatrics Education* 14, no. 3: 49–63.

Robb, N. 1996. "Medical Schools Seek to Overcome 'Invisibility' of Gay Patients, Gay Issues in Curriculum." *Canadian Medical Association Journal* 155, no. 6: 765–70.

Roberts, S., and L. Sorensen. 1995. "Lesbian Health Care: A Review and Recommendations for Health Promotion in Primary Care Settings." *Nurse Practitioner* 20, no. 6: 42–47.

Robertson, P., and J. Schachter. 1981. "Failure to Identify Venereal Disease in a Lesbian Population." *Sexually Transmitted Diseases* 9, no. 2: 75–76.

Rodríguez, J. 1999. *Impacto poblacional de adultos mayores ante el umbral del nuevo milenio*. Conferencia del Gobernador Hacia una Vejez Exitosa, San Juan, Puerto Rico, May 18.

Rokke, P., and D. Klenow. 1998. "Prevalence of Depressive Symptoms among Rural Elderly: Examining the Need for Mental Health Services." *Psychotherapy* 35: 545–58.

Root, M. P. P. 1996. "The Multiracial Experience: Racial Borders as a Significant Frontier in Race Relations." In *The Multiracial Experience: Racial Borders as the New Frontier*, ed. M. P. P. Root. Thousand Oaks, Calif.: Sage.

Rosenberg, S. 1970. *The Worker Grows Old*. San Francisco: Jossey Bass.

Rosenblatt R. 1990. "Survey: Abuse of Elderly Increasing. " *Santa Rosa (Calif.) Press Democrat*, May 1, A3.

Rosenthal, D. J. 1986. "Family Supports in Later Life: Does Ethnicity Make a Difference?" *Gerontologist* 26: 19–24.

Ross, G. W., R. D. Abbott, H. Petrovitch, K. H. Masaki, C. Murdaugh, C. Trockman, J. D. Curb, L. R. White. 1997. "Frequency and Characteristics of Silent Dementia among Elderly Japanese American Men: The Honolulu–Asia Aging Study." *JAMA* 227: 800–805.

Ruiz, P. 1993. "Access to Health Care for Uninsured Hispanics: Policy Recommendations." *Hospital and Community Psychiatry* 44, no.10 (October): 958–62.

Ryff, C. D., and M. J. Essex. 1991 "Psychological Well-Being in Adulthood and Old Age." *Annual Review of Gerontology and Geriatrics* 11: 144–71.

Safilios-Rothschild, C., and J. Georgiopoulos. 1970. "A Comparative Study of Parental and Filial Role Definitions." *Journal of Marriage and the Family* 32: 381–90.

Saghri, E. 2000. "Certified Nursing Assistants and Care Settings in San Diego County." Master's thesis, San Diego State University.

Sakayue, K. M. 1989. "Ethnic Variations in Family Support of the Frail Elderly." Pp. 65–106 in *Family Involvement in Treatment of the Frail Elderly*, ed. M. Z. Goldstein. Washington, D.C.: American Psychiatric Association Press.

Salcido, Ramon M., Carol Nakano, and Sally Jue. 1980. "The Use of Formal and Informal Health and Welfare Services of the Asian-American Elderly: An Exploratory Study." *California Sociologist* 3, no. 2: 213–29.

Saloutos, T. 1964. *The Greeks in the United States*. Cambridge: Harvard University Press.

Sánchez, C. D. 1987. "Self-Help: Model for Strengthening the Informal Support System of the Hispanic Elderly." *Journal of Gerontological Social Work* 9, no. 4: 117–31.

———. 1989. "Informal Support Systems of Widows over Sixty in Puerto Rico." Pp. 265–77 in *Mid-Life and Older Women in Latin America and the Caribbean*, ed. Pan American Health Organization and American Association of Retired Persons. Washington, D.C.: PAHO and AARP.

———. 1992. "Mental Health Issues: The Elderly Hispanic." *Journal of Geriatric Psychiatry* 25, no. 1: 25–30.

———. 1999. *Gerontología social*. San Juan: Ediciones Puertorriqueñas.

Sánchez-Ayendez, M. 1986. "Puerto Rican Elderly Women: Shared Meaning and Informal Supportive Networks." In *All American Women: Lines That Divide and Ties That Bind*. New York: Free Press.

———. 1998. "Middle-Aged Puerto Rican Women as Primary Caregivers to the Elderly: A Qualitative Analysis of Everyday Dynamics." *Journal of Gerontological Social Work* 30, no. 1/2: 75–97.

Sanchez-Jankowski, M. 1999. "The Concentration of African American Poverty and the Dispersal of the Working Class: An Ethnographic Study of Three Inner-City Areas." *International Journal of Urban and Regional Research* 23: 619–37.

Sandmeyer, Elmer Clarence. 1973. *The Anti-Chinese Movement in California*. Urbana: University of Illinois Press.

Sarason, B. R., I. G. Sarason, and G. R. Pierce. 1990. "Traditional Views of Social Support and Their Impact on Assessment." Pp. 9–25 in *Social Support: An Interactional View*, ed. B. R. Sarason, I. G. Sarason, and G. R. Pierce. New York: John Wiley & Sons.

Sarbaugh, T. J. 1991. "Irish America at the Crossroads." *Migration World* 19, no. 3: 5–8.

Saxton, Alexander. 1971. *The Indispensable Enemy: Labor and the Anti-Chinese Movement in California*. Berkeley and Los Angeles: University of California Press.

Schatz, B., and K. O'Hanlan. 1994. *Anti-Gay Discrimination in Medicine: Results of a National Survey of Lesbian, Gay, and Bisexual Physicians*. San Francisco: American Association of Physicians for Human Rights.

Schick, F., and R. Schick, eds. 1994. *Statistical Handbook on Aging Americans*. Phoenix: Oryx.

Schneider, D., and R. Smith. 1973. *Class Differences and Sex Roles: American Kinship and Family Situations*. Englewood Cliffs, N.J.: Prentice Hall.

Schoenberg, N. E., and R. T. Coward. 1997. "Attitudes about Entering a Nursing Home: Comparisons of Older Rural and Urban African-American Women." *Journal of Aging Studies* 11: 27–47.

Schorr, A. 1960. *Filial Responsibility in the Modern American Family*. Washington, D.C.: U.S. Department of Health, Education and Welfare, Social Security Administration, Division of Program Research.

Schrier, Arnold. 1958. *Ireland and the American Emigration, 1850–1900*. Minneapolis: University of Minnesota Press.

Schur, C. L., and L. A. Albers. 1996. "Language, Sociodemographics, and Health Care of Hispanic Adults." *Journal of Health Care for the Poor and Underserved* 7, no. 2 (May): 140–58.

Schwanberg, S. 1990. "Attitudes towards Homosexuality in American Health Care Literature." *Journal of Homosexuality* 19, no. 3: 117–36.

Scott, J. P., and K. A. Roberto. 1987. "Informal Supports of Older Adults: A Rural–Urban Comparison." *Family Relations* 36 (October): 444–49.

————. 1985. "Use of Informal and Formal Support Networks by Rural Elderly Poor." *Gerontologist* 25: 624–30.

Scourby, A. 1984. *The Greek Americans.* Boston: Twayne.

Shannon, William V. 1963. *The American Irish.* New York: Macmillan.

Shaughnessy, P. W. 1994 "Changing Institutional Long-Term Care to Improve Rural Health Care." In *Health Services for Rural Elders,* ed. R. T. Coward, C. N. Bull, G. Kukulka, and J. M. Galliher: 144–81. New York: Springer.

Shibusawa, T., H. Ishikawa, A. C. Mui. 1999. "Help-Seeking Attitudes among Japanese American Older Adults." Paper presented at the fifty-second annual scientific program of the Gerontological Society of America, November, San Francisco.

Simpson, George, and Milton Yinger. 1965. *Racial and Cultural Minorities: An Analysis of Prejudice and Discrimination.* New York: Harper & Row.

Singer, Jerome L., and Marvin K. Opler. 1956. "Contrasting Patterns of Fantasy and Motility in Irish and Italian Schizophrenics." *Journal of Abnormal Social Psychology* 53: 42–47.

Skerrett, Ellen, ed. 1997. *At the Crossroads: Old Saint Patrick's and the Chicago Irish.* Chicago: Loyola University Press.

Skolnick, A. 1991. *Embattled Paradise: The American Family in an Age of Uncertainty.* New York: Basic Books.

Slusher, M., C. Mayer, and R. Dunkle. 1996. "Gays and Lesbians Older and Wiser (GLOW): A Support Group for Older Gay People." *Gerontologist* 36, no. 1: 118–23.

Smith, E., S. Johnson, and S. Guenther. 1985. "Health Care Attitudes and Experiences during Gynecological Care among Lesbians and Bisexuals." *American Journal of Public Health* 75: 1085–87.

Smith, Barbara. 1987. "In the Time of Old Age." *Ensign* 8 (May): 85–87.

Sokolovsky, Jay. 1997. "Bringing Culture Back Home: Aging, Ethnicity, and Family Support." Pp. 263–75 in *The Cultural Context of Aging: Worldwide Perspectives,* ed. Jay Sokolovsky. Wesport, Conn.: Bergin & Garvey.

Solis, J. M., G. Marks, M. Garcia, and D. Shelton. 1990. "Acculturation, Access to Care, and Use of Preventive Services by Hispanics: Findings from HHANES 1982–84." *American Journal of Public Health* 80 supp. (December): 11–19.

Sotomayor, M., and S. Randolph. 1988. "A Preliminary Review of Caregiving Issues among Hispanic Elderly." Pp. 137–61 in *Hispanic Elderly: A Cultural Signature,* ed. M. Sotomayor and H. Curiel. Edinburg, Texas: Pan American University Press.

Spalter-Roth, R., and H. Hartman. 1988. *Unnecessary Losses: Costs to Americans of the Lack of Family and Medical Leave. Executive Summary.* Washington, D.C.: Institute for Women's Policy Research.

Spiegel, J. 1971. "Cultural Strain, Family Role Patterns, and Intrapsychic Conflict." In *Theory and Practice of Family Psychiatry,* ed. J. G. Howells. New York: Brunner/Mazel.

Squier, D. A., and Quadagno, J. S. 1988 (3d ed.), 1998 (4th ed.). "The Italian American Family." In *Ethnic Families in America,* ed. C. H. Mindel, R. W. Habenstein, and R. Wesley. 3d ed.; ed. C. H. Mindel, R. W. Habenstein, and R. Wright Jr. 4th ed. Englewood Cliffs, N.J.: Prentice Hall.

Steckenrider, J. 1998. "Aging as a Female Phenomenon: The Plight of Older Women." Pp. 235–60 in *New Directions in Old-Age Policies,* ed. J. Steckenrider and T. Parrott. Albany: State University of New York Press.

Stein, T. 1993. "Overview of New Developments in Understanding Homosexuality." Pp.

9–40 in *Review of Psychiatry,* ed. J. Olham, M. Riba, and A. Tasman. Washington, D.C.: American Psychiatric Association.

Stern, M. P., M. Rosenthal, S. M. Haffner, H. P. Hazuda, and L. J. Franco. 1984. "Sex Differences in the Effects of Sociocultural Status on Diabetes and Cardiovascular Factors in Mexican Amercians: The San Antonio Heart Study." *International Journal of Epidemiology* 120: 834–51.

Stevens, P., and J. Hall. 1988. "Stigma, Health Beliefs, and Experiences with Health Care in Lesbian Women." *Images* 20, no. 2: 69–73.

Stuart, P., and E. Rathbone-McCuan. 1988. "Indian Elderly in the United States." In *North American Elders,* ed. E. Rathbone-McCuan and B. Havens. Westport, Conn.: Greenwood.

Stuck, A. E., C. Minder, I. Peter-Woecz, G. Gillma, C. Egli, A. Kesserling, R. E. Liu, and J. Beck. 2000. "A Randomized Trial of In-Home Visits for Disability Prevention in Community Dwelling Older People at Low and High Risk for Nursing Home Admissions." *Archives of Internal Medicine* 160, no. 8: 977–85.

Suarez, L., and A. G. Ramirez. 1998. "Hispanic/Latino Health and Disease." Pp. 115–37 in *Promoting Health in Multicultural Populations: A Handbook for Practitioners,* ed. R. M. Huff and M. V. Kline. Thousand Oaks, Calif.: Sage.

Suchman, Edward A. 1964. "Sociomedical Variations among Ethnic Groups." *American Journal of Sociology* 70: 319–31.

Sue, Derald, and Stanley Sue. 1977. "Barriers to Effective Cross-Cultural Counseling." *Journal of Counseling Psychology* 24: 420–29.

Suleiman, Michael W., ed. 1999. *Arabs in America: Building a New Future.* Philadelphia: Temple University Press.

Sung, Betty Lee. 1971. *The Story of the Chinese in America.* New York: Collier.

———. 1977. "Changing Chinese." *Society* 14, no. 6: 44–99.

Suzuki, P. T. 1978. "Social Work, Culture-Specific Mediators, and Delivering Services to Aged Turks in Germany and Aged Chinese in San Francisco." *International Social Work* 21, no. 3: 13–19.

Synak, Brunon. 1987. "The Elderly in Poland: An Overview of Selected Problems and Changes." *Ageing and Society* 7: 19–35.

———. 1989. "Formal Care for Elderly People in Poland." *Journal of Cross-Cultural Gerontology* 4: 107–27.

Tabachnik, S. 1985. "Jewish Identity Development in Young Adulthood." Ph.D. diss., Wright Institute, Berkeley, Calif.

Takamura, J. C. 1991. "Asian and Pacific Islander Elderly." Pp. 185–202 in *Handbook of Social Services for Asian and Pacific Islanders,* ed. N. Mokuau. New York: Greenwood.

Tanjasiri, S. P., S. P. Wallace, and K. Shibata. 1995. "Picture Imperfect: Hidden Problems among Asian Pacific Islander Elderly." *Gerontologist* 35: 753–60.

Tavuchis, N. 1972. *Family and Mobility among Greek Americans.* Athens: National Center for Social Research.

Taylor, L., and A. Robertson. 1994. "The Health Needs of Gay Men." *Journal of Advanced Nursing* 20, no. 3: 560–66.

Taylor, R. J. 1986. "Receipt of Support from Family among Black Americans: Demographic and Familial Differences." *Journal of Marriage and the Family* 48: 67–77.

Taylor, R. J., C. G. Ellison, L. M. Chatters, J. S. Levin, and K. D. Lincoln. 2000. "Mental

Health Services in Faith Communities: The Role of Clergy in Black Churches." *Social Work* 45, no. 1: 73–87.

Tellis-Nayek, V., and M. Tellis-Nayek. 1989. "Quality of Care and the Burden of Two Cultures: When the World of the Nurse's Aide Enters the World of Nursing Homes." *Gerontologist* 29, no. 3: 307–13.

Thomas, William, and Florian Znaniecki. 1958 [1918]. *The Polish Peasant in Europe and America.* Chicago: University of Chicago Press.

Tingy, Earl C. 2000. "Widows of Zion." *Ensign* 30 (May): 62–63.

Toan, Anh. 1965. *Nep cu: Con nguoi Viet Nam* (Old ways: The people of Vietnam). Saigon: Dai Nam.

Tobin, S. S. 1994. "Jewish Aged in the United States: Policies and Programs." Pp. 161–80 in *Jewish Aged in the United States and Israel: Diversity, Programs, and Services,* ed. Z. Harel, D. Biegel, and D. Guttmann. New York: Springer.

Tolnay, S. E. 1997. "The Great Migration and Changes in the Northern Black Family, 1940 to 1990." *Social Forces* 75: 1213–39.

Tomita, S. K. 1998. "The Consequences of Belonging: Conflict Management Techniques among Japanese Americans." *Journal of Elder Abuse and Neglect* 9: 41–68.

Torres-Gil, Fernando. 1987. "Aging in an Ethnic Society: Policy Issues for Aging among Minority Groups." Pp. 239–57 in *Ethnic Dimensions of Aging,* ed. D. E. Gelfand and C. M. Barresi. New York: Springer.

Tran, T. V., and L. F. Williams. 1998. "Poverty and Impairment in Activities of Living among Elderly Hispanics." *Social Work in Health Care* 26, no. 4: 59–78.

Trippet, S., and J. Bain. "Preliminary Study of Lesbian Health Concerns." *Health Values* 14, no. 6 (November): 30.

———. 1993. "Physical Health Problems and Concerns of Lesbians." *Women and Health* 20, no. 2: 59–70.

Tsai, Debra Tzuling, and Rebecca A. Lopez. 1997. "The Use of Social Supports by Elderly Chinese Immigrants." *Journal of Gerontological Social Work* 29, no. 1: 77–94.

Ujimoto, K. V., H. K. Nishio, P. T. P. Wong, and L. Lam. 1993. "Cultural Factors Affecting Self-Assessment of Health Satisfaction of Asian Canadian Elderly." Pp. 229–41 in *Health and Cultures: Exploring Relationship,* ed. R. Masi, L. Mensah, and K. A. McLeod. Oakville, Ontario: Mosaic.

Urv-Wong, K., and D. McDowell. 1994. "Case Management in a Rural Setting." Pp. 65–89 in *Providing Community-Based Services to the Rural Elderly,* ed. J. Krout. Thousand Oaks, Calif.: Sage.

U.S. Bureau of the Census. 1988. *1980 Census of Population.* Vol. 2, *Subject Reports: Asian and Pacific Islander Population in the United States, 1980.* PC80-2-1E. Washington, D.C.: U.S. Government Printing Office.

———. 1990a. *Censo de población y vivienda de Puerto Rico.* Washington, D.C.: U.S. Government Printing Office.

———. 1990b. *Social and economic characteristics.* Washington, D.C.: U.S. Government Printing Office.

———. 1992a. *Census of Population and Housing, 1990.* Public use microdata sample U.S. technical documentation. Washington, D.C.: U.S. Government Printing Office.

———. 1992b. *U.S. Census of the Population, 1990. Detailed Ancestry Groups for States.* Washington, D.C.: U.S. Government Printing Office.

———. 1993a. *1990 Census of the Population. Social and Economic Characteristics of the Asian American Population.* CP-2-1. Washington, D.C.: U.S. Government Printing Office.

———. 1993b. *1990 Census of the Population. United States Summary. Asian and Pacific Islanders.* Washington, D.C.: U.S. Government Printing Office.

———. 1993c. *U.S. Census of the Population, 1990. Detailed Ancestry Groups for States.* Washington, D.C.: U.S. Government Printing Office.

———. 1993d. *We the American Asians.* Washington, D.C.: U.S. Government Printing Office.

———. 1995. *The Middle Series Projections.* Available at www.census.gov/socdemo/www. Accessed March 1999.

———. 1996a. *Population Projections of the United States by Age, Race, and Hispanic Origin: 1995 to 2050.* Current Population Reports, P25-1130. Washington, D.C.: U.S. Government Printing Office.

———. 1996b. *U.S. Population Estimates by Race, 65+ in the United States.* Washington, D.C.: U.S. Government Printing Office.

———. 1997. *Statistical Abstracts of the United States, 1997.* Washington, D.C.: U.S. Government Printing Office.

———. 1998. *Poverty in the U.S.,* Current Population Reports. Washington, D.C.: U.S. Government Printing Office.

———. 1999a. *American Housing Survey for the United States in 1997.* Current Housing Reports. Washington, D.C.: U.S. Government Printing Office.

———. 1999b. *Poverty Status of Families by Type of Family, Presence of Related Children, and Hispanic Origin: 1959–1998.* Washington, D.C.: U.S. Government Printing Office.

U.S. Department of Justice. 1977–1999 (annual). *Statistical Yearbook of the Immigration and Naturalization Service..* Washington, D.C.: U.S. Government Printing Office.

U.S. General Accounting Office (GAO). 1987. *Medicare and Medicaid: Stronger Enforcement of Nursing Home Requirements Needed.* Washington, D.C.: U.S. Government Printing Office.

———. 1998. *California Nursing Homes: Care Problems Persist Despite Federal and State Oversight.* July. Washington, D.C.: U.S. Government Printing Office.

———. 1999. *Nursing Homes: Additional Steps Needed to Strengthen Enforcement of Federal Quality Standards.* Washington, D.C.: U.S. Government Printing Office.

U.S. Office of Technology Assessment (OTA). 1986. *Indian Health Care.* OTA-H-290. Washington, D.C.: U.S. Government Printing Office.

U.S. Senate, Special Committee on Aging. 1987. *The Continuum of Health Care for Indian Elders.* Washington, D.C.: U.S. Government Printing Office.

———. 1989. *Aging America: Trends and Projections.* Washington, D.C.: U.S. Government Printing Office.

———. 1995. *Medicaid Reform: Quality of Care in Nursing Homes at Risk.* October 26. 104th Cong., 1st sess. Washington, D.C.: U.S. Government Printing Office.

———. 1997. *The Risk of Malnutrition in Nursing Homes.* October 22. 105th Cong., 1st sess., Washington, D.C.: U.S. Government Printing Office.

———. 1998a. *California Nursing Homes: Care Problems Persist Despite Federal and State Oversight.* July 28, 105th Cong., 2nd sess. Washington, D.C.: U.S. Government Printing Office.

———. 1998b. *The Cash Crunch: The Financial Challenge of Long-Term Care for the*

Baby Boom Generation. March 9, 105th Cong. 2nd sess., Washington, D.C.: U.S. Government Printing Office.

———. 1998c. *The Many Faces of Long-Term Care: Today's Bitter Pill or Tomorrow's Cure.* January 12, 105th Cong., 1st sess., Washington, D.C.: U.S. Government Printing Office.

———. 1999. *Nursing Homes: Stronger Complaint and Enforcement Practices Needed to Better Ensure Adequate Care.* March 22, 106th Cong., 1st sess. Washington, D.C.: U.S. Government Printing Office.

Valle, R. 1998. *Caregiving across Cultures: Working with Dementing Illness and Ethnically Diverse Populations.* Washington, D.C.: Taylor & Francis.

Valle, R., and L. Mendoza. 1978. *The Latino Elder.* San Diego: Campanile Press.

Van Biema, David. 1997. "Kingdom Come." *Time* 155, (August 4): 50–58.

Van Braguth, Thieleman J. 1984. *The Bloody Theater, or Martyrs Mirror of the Defenseless Christians.* Trans. Joseph F. Sohm. Scottdale, Pa: Mennonite Publishing House.

Villa, M. L., J. Cuellar, N. Gamel, and G. Yeo. 1993. "Aging and Health: Hispanic American Elders." Stanford Geriatric Education Center Working Paper 5, Ethnographic Reviews: 1–46.

Villa, Valentine. 1998. "Aging Policy and the Experience of Older Minorities." Pp. 211–33 in *New Directions in Old-Age Policies,* ed. J. S. Steckenrider and T. M. Parrott. Albany: State University of New York Press.

Vissing, Y. M., J. C. Salloway, and D. L. Siress. 1994. "Training for Expertise versus Training for Trust: Issues in Rural Gerontology." *Educational Gerontology* 20: 797–808.

Vosburgh, Miriam G., and Richard N. Juliani. 1990. "Contrasts in Ethnic Family Patterns: The Irish and the Italians." *Journal of Comparative Family Studies* 21, no. 2: 269–86.

Wagner, Norma. 1997. "Utah Slips in Health Rankings." *Salt Lake Tribune.* October 9, A1, A7.

Wailing, L., M. Seltzer, and J. S. Greenberg. 1997. "Social Support and Depressive Symptoms: Differential Patterns in Wife and Daughter Caregivers." *Journal of Gerontology: Social Sciences* 52: 200–211.

Wake, S. B., and M. J. Sporakowski. 1972. "An Intergenerational Comparison of Attitudes toward Supporting Aged Parents." *Journal of Marriage and the Family* 34: 42–48.

Walker, A. J., C. C. Pratt, and L. Eddy. 1995. "Informal Caregiving to Family Members: A Critical Review." *Family Relations* 44: 402–11.

Wallace, S. P., and C. Y. Lew-Ting. 1992. "Getting By at Home: Community-Based Long-Term Care of Latinos." *Western Journal of Medicine* 157, no. 3 (September): 337–44.

Wallace, S. P., K. Campbell, and C. Y. Lew-Ting. 1994. "Structural Barriers to the Use of Formal In-Home Services by Elderly Latinos." *Journal of Gerontology: Social Sciences* 49, no. 5 (September): 253–63.

Wallace, S. P., L. Levy-Storms, and L. R. Ferguson. 1995. "Access to Paid In-Home Assistance among Disabled Elderly People: Do Latinos Differ from Non-Latino Whites?" *American Journal of Public Health* 85, no. 7 (July): 970–75.

Wallick, M., K. Cambre, and M. Townsend. 1992. "How the Topic of Homosexuality Is Taught at US Medical Schools." *Academy of Medicine* 67, no. 9: 601–3.

Walls, C. T., and S. Zarit. 1991. "Informal Support from Black Churches and the Well-Being of Elderly Blacks." *Gerontologist* 31: 490–95.

Weeks, J. 1981. "The Problems of Older Homosexuals." Pp. 177–84 in *The Theory and*

Practice of Homosexuality, ed. J. Hart and D. Richardson. London: Routledge & Kegan Paul.

Weeks, J., and J. Cuellar. 1981. "The Role of Family Members in the Helping Networks of Older People." *Gerontologist* 21, no. 4: 388–94.

———. 1983. "The Influence of Immigration and Length of Residence on the Isolation of Older Persons." *Research on Aging* 5: 369–88.

Weibel-Orlando, J., and J. Kramer. 1994. "Indians: Ethnicity as a Resource and Aging—You Can Go Home Again." *Journal of Cross-Cultural Gerontology* 9: 18–32.

Weismehl, R. 1994. "Social Services for the Jewish Aged in the United States." Pp. 201–18 in *Jewish Aged in the United States and Israel: Diversity, Programs, and Services,* ed. Z. Harel, D. Biegel and D. Guttmann. New York: Springer.

Westefeld, J., and J. Winkelpeck. 1983. "University Counseling Service Groups for Gay Students." *Small Group Behavior* 14: 121–28.

Weston, K. 1991. *Families We Choose.* New York: Columbia University Press.

"Where You Live Determines How You Will Die." 1997. *Salt Lake Tribune,* October 15.

White, T. 1979. "Attitudes of Psychiatric Nurses toward Same-Sex Orientation." *Nursing Research* 28: 276–81.

White-Means, S. I., M. C. Thornton, and J. S. Yeo.1989. "Sociodemographic and Health Factors Influencing Black and Hispanic Use of the Hospital Emergency Room." *JAMA* 82, no. 1: 72–80.

Wiener, Joshua M., and David G. Stevenson. 1998. *Long-Term Care for the Elderly: Profiles of Thirteen States.* Occasional Paper 12. Washington, D.C.: Urban Institute.

Williams, J., and S. Rogers. 1993. "The Multicultural Workplace: Preparing Preceptors." *Journal of Continuing Education in Nursing* 24, no. 3 (May–June): 101–4.

Williams, M. P. 1992. *Blacks and Alzheimer's Disease: A Caregiver's Information Project.* Final Report to the Administration on Aging. Morehouse School of Medicine, Atlanta.

Williams, T. F. 1991. "The Health Needs of Older Hispanics." Letter. *JAMA* 265: 2065.

Williams, T. F., and H. Temkin-Greener. 1996. "Older People, Dependency, and Trends in Supportive Care." In *The Future of Long-Term Care: Social and Policy Issues,* ed. R. H. Binstock, L. E. Cluff, and O. von Mering. Baltimore, Md.: Johns Hopkins University Press.

Wilson, W. J. 1987. *The Truly Disadvantaged: The Inner City, the Underclass, and Public Policy.* Chicago: University of Chicago Press,

———. 1996. *When Work Disappears: The World of the New Urban Poor.* New York: Alfred Knopf.

———. 1999. *The Bridge over the Racial Divide: Rising Inequality and Coalition Politics.* Berkeley and Los Angeles: University of California Press.

Wilson-Ford, V. 1992. "Health-Protective Behaviors of Rural Black Elderly Women." *Health and Social Work* 17: 28–36.

Witt, Judith LaBorde. 1994. "The Gendered Division of Labor in Parental Caretaking: Biology or Socialization?" *Journal of Women and Aging* 6, no. 1/2: 65–89.

Woehrer, C. E. 1978. "Cultural Pluralism in American Families: The Influence of Ethnicity on Social Aspects of Aging." *Family Coordinator* 27: 329–38.

Wojciechowski, C. 1998. "Issues in Caring for Older Lesbians." *Journal of Gerontological Nursing* 24, no. 7: 28–33.

Wong, B. P. 1979. *A Chinese American Community: Ethnicity and Survival Strategies.* Singapore: Chopmen Enterprises.

Wong, Morrison G. 1980. "Model Students? Teachers' Perceptions and Expectations of Their Asian and White Students." *Sociology of Education* 53: 236–46.

———. 1984a. "Asian Students as Model Students?" Pp. 283–98 in *Preparing for Reflective Teaching,* ed. Carl A. Grant. Boston: Allyn & Bacon.

———. 1984b. "Economic Survival: The Case of Asian-American Elderly." *Sociological Perspectives* 27: 197–217.

———. 1985. "Post-1965 Immigrants: Demographic and Socioeconomic Profile." Pp. 51–71 in *Urban Ethnicity: New Immigrants and Old Minorities,* ed. Lionel A. Maldonado and Joan W. Moore. Beverly Hills, Calif.: Sage.

———. 1986. "Post-1965 Asian Immigrants: Where Do They Come From, Where Are They Now, and Where Are They Going?" *Annals of the American Academy of Political and Social Science,* no. 487: 150–68.

———. "The Education of White, Chinese, Filipino, and Japanese Students: A Look at 'High School and Beyond.'" *Sociological Perspectives* 33: 355–74.

———. 1994. "Chinese Americans." Pp. 58–94 in *Asian Americans: An Overview of Ethnic Groups,* ed. P. G. Min. Newbury Park, Calif.: Sage.

———. 1998. "The Chinese American Family." Pp. 284–310 in *Ethnic Families in America,* ed. C. H. Mindel, R. W. Habenstein, and R. Wright Jr. 4th ed. Upper Saddle River, N.J.: Prentice Hall.

Wong, Morrison G., and Charles Hirschman. 1983. "The New Asian Immigrants." Pp. 381–403 in *Culture, Ethnicity, and Identity: Current Issues in Research,* ed. William McCready. New York: Academic.

Woodham-Smith, Cecelia. 1963. *The Great Hunger.* New York: Harper & Row.

Worach-Kardas, Halina. 1979. "Family and Neighborly Relations: Their Role for the Elderly." Pp. 39–47 in *Family Life in Old Age: Proceedings of the Meetings of the European Social Sciences Research Committee in Dubrovnik, Yugoslavia, October 19–23, 1976,* ed. G. Dooghe and J. Helandel. The Hague: M. Nijhoff.

———. 1987. "Retirement in Poland." Pp. 271–86 in *Retirement in Industrialized Societies,* ed. K. S. Markides and C. L. Cooper: New York: John Wiley & Sons.

Wright, Scott D. 1998. *Utah Sourcebook on Aging.* Salt Lake City: Empire Publishing.

Wu, Frances Y. T. 1975. "Mandarin-Speaking Chinese in the Los Angeles Area." *Gerontologist* 15, no. 3: 271–75.

Wunderlich, G., F. Sloan, and C. Davis, eds. 1996. *Nursing Staff in Hospitals and Nursing Homes: Is It Adequate?* Washington, D.C.: Institute of Medicine, National Academy Press.

Wylan, Louise, and Norbett L. Mintz. 1976. "Ethnic Differences in Family Attitudes towards Psychotic Manifestations, with Implications for Treatment Programs." *International Journal of Social Psychiatry* 2, no. 2: 86–95.

Yanagisako, S. J. 1985. *Transforming the Past: Tradition and Kinship among Japanese Americans.* Stanford, Calif.: Stanford University Press.

Yancey, W., E. Ericsen, and R. Juliani. 1976. "Emergent Ethnicity: A Review and Reformulation." *American Sociological Review* 41: 391–403.

Yano, K., R. D. Wasnich, J. M. Vogel, and L. K. Heilbrun. 1984. "Bone Mineral Measurements among Middle-Aged and Elderly Japanese Residents in Hawaii." *American Journal of Epidemiology* 119: 751–64.

Yee, Barbara W. K., and Gayle D. Weaver. 1994. "Ethnic Minorities and Health Promotion: Developing a 'Culturally Competent' Agenda." *Generations* 18, no. 1 (Spring): 39–44.

Yeo, Gwen. 1995. "Ethical Considerations in Asian and Pacific Elders." *Clinics Geriatric Medicine* 2: 139–52.

———. 1996–1997. "Ethnogeriatrics: Cross-Cultural Care of Older Adults." *Generations* 20: no. 4 (Winter): 72–77.

Ying, Yu Wen. 1988. "Depressive Symptomatology among Chinese-Americans as Measured by the CES-D." *Journal of Clinical Psychology* 44: 739–46.

Yoo, D. K. 2000. *Growing Up Nisei: Race, Generation, and Culture among Japanese Americans of California, 1924–49.* Urbana: University of Illinois Press.

Yoo, Seung Ho, and Kyu-Taik Sung. 1997. "Elderly Koreans' Tendency to Live Independently from Their Adult Children: Adaptation to Cultural Differences in America." *Journal of Cross-Cultural Gerontology* 12: 225–44.

Yu, Elena S. H. 1986. "Health of the Chinese Elderly in America." *Research on Aging* 8, no. 1: 84–109.

Zane, N., D. T. Takeuchi, and K. N. J. Young. 1994. *Confronting Critical Health Issues of Asian and Pacific Islander Americans.* Thousand Oaks, Calif.: Sage.

Zborowski, Mark. 1969. *People in Pain.* San Francisco: Jossey-Bass.

Zeidenstein, L. 1990. "Gynecological and Childbearing Needs of Lesbians." *Journal of Nurse Midwifery* 35, no. 1: 10–18.

Zhou, Min. 1999. "Coming of Age: The Current Situation of Asian American Children." *Americas Journal* 25: 1–27.

Zill, N., and C. C. Rogers. 1988. "Recent Trends in the Well-Being of Children in the United States and Their Implications for Public Health." Pp. 31–115 in *The Changing American Family and Public Policy,* ed. A. Cherlin. Washington, D.C.: Urban Institute.

Zola, Irving K. 1966. "Culture and Symptoms: An Analysis of Patients' Presenting Complaints." *American Sociological Review* 31, no. 5: 615–30.

———. 1973."Pathways to the Doctor: From Person to Patient." *Social Science and Medicine* 7, no. 9: 677–89.

Zubrzycki, Jerzy. 1953. "Emigration from Poland in the Nineteenth and Twentieth Centuries." *Population Studies* 6: 248–72.

Zych, Adam A., and Roland Bartel. 1988. *Zur Lebenssituation alternder Menschen in Polen und in der Bundesrepublik Deutschland: Eine komparative Survey-Studie.* (Living situation of older people in Poland and in the Federal Republic of Germany: A comparative survey). Giessen: Institut fuer Heil- und Sonderpaedagogik, Justus-Liebig-Universität.

———. 1990. *Sytucja zyciowa ludzi w podeszlym wieku w Polsce i w Republice Federalnej Niemiec: Studium metodyczno-porownawcze* (Living situation of older people in Poland and in the Federal Republic of Germany: A comparative survey). Kielce, Poland: Wyzsza Szkola Pedagogiczna im. Jana Kochanowskiego.

Index

AAAs (Area Agencies on Aging), 247–48
abuse of elders, 11, 69, 117, 228–29, 238–39
activities of daily living (ADL), 76–77
activity theory, 104
Administration on Aging, 116, 121
African Americans, 2, 3, 13; church and social support, 97, 100–102; cultural views of disease, 79; demographics, 4, 95–96, 101; family relations and support, 98–99; Great Migration, 96–98; policy implications, 102; socioeconomic status, 5, 97
AHEPA (American Hellenic Progressive Association), 215
AI/AN. See American Indians/Alaska Natives
AIDS, 13, 99, 217, 223
Alaska Natives. See American Indians/Alaska Natives
amae, 36
American Association of Physicians for Human Rights, 222–23
American Hellenic Educational Progressive Association, 7
American Hellenic Progressive Association (AHEPA), 215
American Indians/Alaska Natives, 3, 5; attitudes about aging, 9, 121–22; communication, 119–20; cultural aspects, 117–18; demographics, 113–15; dietary practices, 120; education, 115; families, 117; federal government and, 113–14; health and social services, 116; language barriers, 118; long-term

care, 120–21; policy implications, 122; socioeconomic status, 6; stressful experiences, 13; traditional healing and spirituality, 118–19, 122
Americanization, 2, 12, 15–16, 25–26
American Medical Association, 119, 225
American Psychiatric Association, 223
Amish, 5, 9; attitudes toward aging, elders, and care of elders, 136–39; attitudes toward government programs and welfare, 140–42; bishops, 136–37; childless elders, 142–43; gender roles, 137–38; *Grossdaadi Haus,* 134, 136, 138, 142; independence, 136; migration, 135–36; mutual aid, 134–35, 140, 141–44; *Ordnung,* 140; policy implications, 143–44; Social Security and, 135, 140–41, 144; view of death, 139–40; women, 137, 142
Amish Church Aid, 142
Amish Liability Aid, 141–42
Amish Roots, 140
Anabaptists, 134, 135, 140. *See also* Amish
Arab American and Chaldean Council, 9, 169
Arab Americans, 14, 160; attitudes and values, 9, 161, 164; community agencies and, 168–69; country of birth, 167; demographics, 165–66; education, 166–67; families, 161; historical context, 160–61; living arrangements, 162–69; occupation, 167–68; policy implications, 169–70; Quran, 9, 163–64; research methodology, 161;

About the Contributors

CELIA BERDES is associate director of the Buehler Center on Aging at Northwestern University and assistant professor of medicine at Northwestern University Medical School. She is coauthor of "Subjective Quality of Life of Polish, Polish Immigrant and Polish American Elderly," which appeared in the *International Journal of Aging and Human Development,* and the author of "Race Relations and Caregiving Relationships: A Qualitative Examination of Perspectives from Residents and Aides in Three Nursing Homes," in *Research on Aging.* She is presently working on a study on the sense of community in residential facilities for the aging.

BRUCE L. CAMPBELL is associate professor of administration and counseling at California State University, Los Angeles. His publications have focused on the Mormon family, including research on polygamy and early historical developments in Utah. He teaches life-span development, counseling theories, and parenting. He has served as the token liberal in several Mormon wards.

JACALYN A. CLAES is assistant professor of social work at the University of North Carolina at Greensboro. She has presented numerous papers at national conferences on issues affecting the family at all stages of the life cycle. She is coauthor of "Gender Issues and Elder Care," in *The Aging Family,* and "Issues Confronting Lesbians and Gay Elders: The Challenge for Health and Human Service Providers," in *The Politics and Policies of Caring in an Age of Retrenchment.* She draws for her research upon her ongoing clinical practice of twenty-five years.

CHRYSIE M. CONSTANTAKOS is professor emerita at Brooklyn College of the City University of New York. She has conducted research on Greek ethnicity and authored *The American Greek Subculture: Processes of Continuity* (1971). She has published numerous chapters and/or articles in scholarly books and journals, among them "Ethnic Language as a Variable in Subcultural Continuity," "The Greek American Subcommunity: Intergroup Conflict," "Greece in Modern Times," "Variations in Adaptation by Greek Home Region: Stories to Live By," and "The Role of Elder Adults in Transmitting Ethnic Heritage."

PEGGYE DILWORTH-ANDERSON is Elizabeth Rosenthal Excellence Professor in human development and family studies at the University of North Carolina at Greensboro. Her recent publications include "A Sociohistorical View of African American Women and Their Caregiving Roles"(2000), "Ethnic Minority Perspectives on Dementia, Family Caregiving, and Interventions" (1999), "The Contexts of Experiencing Emotional Distress among Family Caregivers to Elderly African Americans" (1999), "Family Caregiving to Elderly African Americans: Caregiver Types and Structures" (1999), and "Full Color Aging: Facts, Goals, and Recommendations for America's Diverse Population" (1999).

BARBARA C. DU BOIS is director of research and a faculty member at the University Center on Aging at San Diego State University. She is the associate director of the National Resource Center on Aging and Injury. Currently she is co-principal investigator of a community-based intervention project examining the role of community health advocates representing at-risk older people participating in a managed health care plan. Her interests are in Medicare managed care systems; access issues related to utilization of long-term care and health services; and community-based health promotion programs. In collaboration with the Union of Pan Asian Communities, she received the C. Everett Koop National Health Service Award for cost effectively improving the health status and exercise behaviors of a Pacific Islander community.

MARY PATRICE ERDMANS is a visiting associate professor of sociology at College of the Holy Cross. Her areas of interest include ethnicity and immigration, with a special focus on Poles in the United States. Her most recent book is *Opposite Poles: Immigrants and Ethnics in Polish Chicago, 1976–1990* (1998). She is currently studying white working-class women through oral histories of fourth-generation Polish American women.

HANI FAKHOURI is professor emeritus of anthropology at the University of Michigan, Flint. His research and writing focus on the impact of industrialization and the new urban trends in Egypt; the Arab American elderly population; multiculturalism and ethnic diversity; and the Middle East as a culture area study. He has authored two books and has published numerous articles in professional journals.

PATRICIA J. FANNING is assistant professor of sociology and anthropology at Bridgewater State College. Her essays on Irish Americans have appeared in *New Hibernia Review,* the *Historical Journal of Massachusetts,* and *New Perspectives on the Irish Diaspora.*

ZEV HAREL is professor of social work at Cleveland State University. He has written over sixty journal articles and book chapters on extreme stress and aging, ethnicity and aging, and vulnerable older populations. His recent edited books include *Human Adaptation to Extreme Stress: From the Holocaust to Vietnam* (1988); *The Black Aged: Understanding Diversity and Service Needs* (1990); *The Jewish Aged in the United States and Israel* (1994); *The Vulnerable Aged: People, Services, and Policies* (1990); *Matching People and Services in Long-Term Care* (1995); and *Quality of Long-Term Care and Its Impact on Quality of Life* (2001). He serves in leadership roles with local, state, and national organizations in aging.

COLLEEN L. JOHNSON is professor of anthropology, history, and social medicine at the University of California, San Francisco. In addition to her work with Italian Americans, she has conducted research on Japanese Americans and black Americans. She has published numerous articles on ethnicity, ethnic families, and the family in later life. She received a MERIT Award from the National Institute on Aging for a ten-year study on the oldest old, which is described in *Life Beyond Eighty-five Years: The Aura of Survivorship* (1997).

KWANG CHUNG KIM is professor of sociology at Western Illinois University. His areas of interest are sociology of family, race/ethnic relations, and life experiences of recent immigrants and their children. His numerous publications include *Korean Immigrants in America: Structural Analysis of Ethnic Confinement and Adhesive Adaptation* (1984), *Koreans in the Hood: Conflict with African Americans* (1999), and *Korean Americans and Their Religions: Pilgrims and Missionaries from a Different Shore* (2001).

SHIN KIM, formerly professor of economics at Chicago State University, is an adjunct professor of social work at the University of Chicago and McCormick Theological Seminary. Her interests are welfare and immigration policies, economics of gender and race/ethnic minorities, and sociology of religion of recent immigrants. Her publications include over twenty articles. She is coeditor of *The Emerging Generation of Korean Americans* (1993).

HARRY H. L. KITANO is professor emeritus of social welfare and sociology at the University of California, Los Angeles. He was the first person to hold the endowed chair of Japanese American studies. He is the author of numerous scholarly articles and books, including the much acclaimed *Achieving the Impossible Dream: How Japanese Americans Obtained Redress* (1999) and *Race Relations* (1998), now in its fifth edition. He spent his teenage years in the Topaz Concentration Camp in Utah. He continues to teach and conduct research on the Asian American experience.

MICHEL S. LAGUERRE is professor and director of the Berkeley Center for Globalization and Information Technology at the University of California at Berkeley.

He has written fourteen books, among them *American Odyssey: Haitians in New York City* (1984), *Urban Poverty in the Caribbean* (1990), *The Military and Society in Haiti* (1993), *Diasporic Citizenship* (1998), and *The Global Ethnopolis: Chinatown, Japantown, and Manilatown in American Society* (2000). He is completing *The Global Chronopolis: Globalization, Diasporic Temporalities, and Internet Time* (forthcoming).

JAMES LUBBEN is professor of social welfare and urban planning at the University of California, Los Angeles. He has developed an abbreviated social network scale for both research and clinical use among older populations. Much of his gerontological research involves cross-cultural and cross-national comparisons. Most often these consider Asian and Asian American populations. He has been a visiting scholar in Canada, Hong Kong, Japan, and Singapore.

WAYNE R. MOORE is assistant professor of social work at North Carolina A&T State University, Greensboro. He has presented numerous papers and workshops at national, state, and regional conferences on issues dealing with Alzheimer's disease and dementia, bereavement, and developing support groups for caregivers of people with cancer, dementia, and HIV/AIDS. He has worked in various health care settings, establishing and directing clinical social work departments.

DUNG NGO is a doctoral candidate in clinical psychology at St. Louis University. His dissertation focuses on mental health issues in the Vietnamese American community.

LAURA KATZ OLSON is professor of political science at Lehigh University, where she specializes in women's issues, aging, and public policy. Her publications include *The Political Economy of Aging: The State, Private Power and Social Welfare* (1982), *Aging and Public Policy: The Politics of Growing Old in American* (1983), *The Graying of the World: Who Will Take Care of the Frail Elderly* (1994), and *The Politics and Policies of Caring in an Age of Retrenchment* (2000). She has been a Gerontological Fellow, NASPAA faculty fellow, and a senior Fulbright-Hays scholar. She currently is lecturing in Pennsylvania on Social Security and Medicare policies through a grant funded by the Pennsylvania Humanities Council.

MONA POLACCA is a senior research specialist at the University of Arizona, where she currently is overseeing data collection for research on alcoholism prevalence and gene/environment interactions in American Indian tribes. Her publications include *Primary Care of Native American Patients: Diagnosis, Therapy, and Epidemiology* (1999) and *Rural Mental Health Training Project: Mental Health and the Aging Native American* (1996). She is Hopi and Havasupai and an enrolled member of the Colorado River Indian Tribes of Parker, Arizona.

CARMEN DELIA SÁNCHEZ is a professor at the graduate school of social work of the University of Puerto Rico. She has published three books on gerontology in Latin America and is the author of over fifty articles and book chapters on social work, the aged, support systems, and elder abuse. Her most recent publication is *Gerontologia Social* (1999). She has been a visiting professor in universities in Brazil, Colombia, Spain, and the Dominican Republic.

JEAN PEARSON SCOTT is professor of human development and family studies at Texas Tech University, Lubbock. Her recent publications focus on informal and formal support networks of older rural women, late-life sibling relationships, and family caregiving.

TAZUKO SHIBUSAWA is an assistant professor at the Columbia University School of Social Work. Her research areas include mental health among older immigrants and their families, help-seeking among ethnic elders, and clinical practice with Asian and Asian American families.

E. PERCIL STANFORD is professor and director of the University Center on Aging at San Diego State University. He also is director of the National Resource Center on Aging and Injury, and the National Institute on Minority Aging. He is widely recognized as a national expert on cultural diversity and aging. He has been the codirector of the National Resource Center on Long-Term Care and Diversity and director of the National Resource Center on Minority Aging Populations. He serves on several national committees, boards, and commissions focusing on issues affecting older adults. He has been appointed twice to the White House Conference on Aging and has served as a commissioner on the California Commission on Aging.

TRICIA H. SUNG is a doctoral student in cultural and developmental psychology at Boston College. Her research interests include acculturation; end-of-life and long-term care decision making among older Americans and their families; culture, self, and emotions over the life span; and culturally fair measurement and assessment among immigrant and minority older adults.

THANH VAN TRAN is professor of social work at the Boston College Graduate School of Social Work. He has published in the *Journal of Gerontology: Social Sciences, Psychology of Aging*, the *Gerontologist, Gerontological Social Work*, and other social welfare journals. His research projects have been funded by the National Institute of Mental Health and the Medical Foundation. His work focuses on the health and well-being of Indochinese Americans and more recently that of elderly Russian and Chinese Americans.

ISHAN CANTY WILLIAMS is a Ph.D. candidate in human development and family studies at the University of North Carolina at Greensboro. She currently is working on her dissertation, "The Caregiving Career among African American Caregivers: After Institutionalization and the Death of the Care Recipient." Her research interests include African American elderly, minority caregivers, caregiver relationships, family togetherness, institutional placement/long-term care, and end-of-life decisions.

SHARON WALLACE WILLIAMS currently is completing a postdoctoral fellowship in gerontology at the Wake Forest University School of Medicine. Her research focuses on individuals with chronic diseases and the ways in which family interventions can lead to improved outcomes. She also examines relationships between informal and formal support systems for the elderly.

MORRISON G. WONG is professor of sociology at Texas Christian University. He has published articles and chapters on the Asian experience in the United States, examining such aspects as immigration trends, socioeconomic status and achievement, model student stereotypes, hate crimes and Asian Americans, and the Chinese elderly, the Chinese family, and the Chinese experience in the United States.

CAROL H. YAVNO is an adjunct faculty member at the University Center on Aging at San Diego State University and is coordinator of the National Resource Center on Aging and Injury. Her research interests include community-based health promotion and risk perceptions of older adults. She also has participated in social science research for the U.S. Census Bureau; the National Institute on Drug Abuse; and the Survey Research Lab, University of Illinois at Urbana. She also has worked with professional training programs for older adults at the U.S. Department of Defense.

LEE J. ZOOK is professor of social work at Luther College. He is currently writing about the Amish migration to the Upper Midwest, an area where he has served as an expert witness in court cases for the Amish. He grew up in a Mennonite Amish community in central Pennsylvania.